INTERIOR PRAISE PAGE

"No field needs a new paradigm more than healthcare, which is exactly what Gunderson and Cochrane offer us in this timely volume. Here are carefully wrought ideas on which to build partnerships across the disciplines and specialities that now divide hospitals from community, so necessary to advance population health. Administrators, physicians, policy makers, and community leaders should welcome this as a way to move forward—together."

—Bob Waller, ex-CEO and president of the Mayo Clinic,
Board of Directors of the Institute for
Health Improvement, Cambridge, MA

"*Religion and the Health of the Public* is a remarkable book in its broad academic scope combined with a focused argument about public health and religious communities. To anyone interested in salutogenic conceptions of health, it is mandatory reading."

—Ola Sigurdson, professor and director of the Centre
for Culture and Health, University of Gothenburg

"Drawing on the moral commitments and empirical insights of religion and public health in Africa and the United States, this groundbreaking and inspiring book also engages the connection of religion and the health of the public."

—Abdullahi A. An-Na'im, Charles Howard
Candler Professor of Law, Emory University

RELIGION AND THE HEALTH OF THE PUBLIC

SHIFTING THE PARADIGM

Gary R. Gunderson and James R. Cochrane

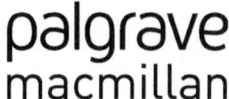

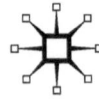
First published in 2012 by
PALGRAVE MACMILLAN®
in the United States—a division of St. Martin's Press LLC,
175 Fifth Avenue, New York, NY 10010.

Where this book is distributed in the UK, Europe and the rest of the world,
this is by Palgrave Macmillan, a division of Macmillan Publishers Limited,
registered in England, company number 785998, of Houndmills,
Basingstoke, Hampshire RG21 6XS.

Palgrave Macmillan is the global academic imprint of the above companies
and has companies and representatives throughout the world.

Palgrave® and Macmillan® are registered trademarks in the United States,
the United Kingdom, Europe and other countries.

ISBN: 978–0–230–34127–2 (HC)
ISBN: 978–0–230–34152–4 (PB)

Library of Congress Cataloging-in-Publication Data

Gunderson, Gary.
    Religion and the health of the public : shifting the paradigm / Gary
R. Gunderson and Jim R. Cochrane.
        p. cm.
    ISBN 978–0–230–34127–2 (hardback)—
    ISBN 978–0–230–34152–4 (Paperback)
    1. Medical care—Religious aspects. 2. Public health.
    I. Cochrane, Jim R., 1946– II. Title.

BL65.M4G86 2012
201'.7621—dc23   2011036151

A catalogue record of the book is available from the British Library.

Design by Newgen Imaging Systems (P) Ltd., Chennai, India.

First edition: March 2012

10 9 8 7 6 5 4 3 2 1

In memory of Steve and in gratitude to the many warm friends and colleagues with whom we have journeyed along the way from the Interfaith Health Program, the African Religious Health Religious Health Assets Programme and the Center of Excellence for Faith and Health

CONTENTS

FIGURES

Acronyms

ABCD	Asset based community development
AIDS	Acquired immune deficiency syndrome
ARHAP	African Religious Health Assets Programme
ART	Anti-retroviral treatment
CDC	Centers for Disease Control and Prevention
CHAM	Christian Health Association of Malawi
CHAZ	Christian Health Association of Zambia
CHEP	Copperbelt Health Education Project
CHN	Congregational Health Network
CI	Christian Institute of South Africa
CMC	Christian Medical Commission
CPE	Clinical pastoral education
CTS	Chicago Theological Seminary
DCPP	Disease Control Priorities Project
EIS	Epidemic Intelligence Service
EQUINET	Regional Network for Equity in Health in Southern Africa
ER	Emergency room
FBOs	Faith-based organizations
FES	Focused ethnographic studies
FFEs	Faith-forming entities
HIV	Human immunodeficiency virus
IHI	Institute for Healthcare Improvement
IHP	Interfaith Health Program
ILO	International Labor Organization
IMF	International Monetary Fund
IOM	Institute of Medicine
IY	Imizamo Yethu
KAP	Knowledge, Attitudes and Practices surveys
LCL	Leading Causes of Life
MLH	Methodist Le Bonheur Healthcare
NGOs	Nongovernmental organizations
PHC	Primary health care
PIRHANA	Participatory Inquiry into Religious Health Assets, Networks and Agency

PLHIV	People living with HIV
PRSPs	Poverty Reduction Strategy Papers
RHAs	Religious health assets
SAPs	Structural Adjustment Programs
SLF	Sustainable livelihoods framework
SOC	Sense of coherence
STEEEP	Safe, timely, effective, efficient, equitable, and patient-centered
STIs	Sexually transmitted infections
TB	Tuberculosis
UNESCO	United Nations Educational Scientific and Cultural Organization
UNICEF	United Nations International Children's Emergency Fund
WCC	World Council of Churches
WHO	World Health Organization
World Bank	International Bank for Reconstruction and Development

Acknowledgments

The book that you have before you has had the benefit of all sorts of contributions to our thinking and writing over a considerable period of time, as well as some vital assistance in getting things right or adequately expressed. Much has been achieved through these several collaborative efforts, particularly with the Interfaith Health Program (IHP), now at the Rollins School of Public Health at Emory University; the African Religious Health Assets Programme (ARHAP), previously directed from the Department of Religious Studies and now located in the School of Public Health and Family Medicine at the University of Cape Town; and the recently established Center of Excellence in Faith and Health at Methodist Le Bonheur Healthcare, Memphis, Tennessee.

We are deeply grateful for the collegial and friendship relationships that have produced significant contributions to understanding religion in the context of public health well beyond the ideas captured in this particular volume. Throughout our text, we reference many other works that our colleagues or we have produced as we have together traveled the terrain that makes up that complex interface, and in that way show our debt to them. At the same time, a number of people have made particular contributions to helping us get this book in place and in the good shape it is in, its weaknesses being entirely our own.

Above all, we must acknowledge Teresa Cutts, who has read draft after draft with a penetrating eye that never misses the errors, the gaps, the critical additions that are necessary, and the well-worked (or badly written) phrases and sentences. Her intellectual sharpness and rich experience have been an invaluable addition to our efforts. Equally, her willingness to sort through what we wanted and needed to say, has been hugely generous, besides debts of substance (you will notice her input in several endnotes, and she provided much needed additional detail on the Congregational Health Network, on sickle cell anemia, and on stories of diabetes, among other things). To her, we give special thanks.

Among others who have read bits of chapters or drafts we would particularly like to mention Barbara Schmid at the University of Cape Town, Deb McFarland at the Rollins School of Public Health at Emory University, Chip Clay and Liz Dover of Methodist Le Bonheur Healthcare, and Dr. Reinward Bastian and Beate Jakob of the German Institute for Medical Mission (Difäm) in Tübingen. The three anonymous reviewers of our manuscript were also particularly helpful in pulling the final product into much better shape, and presuming they know who they are, we give them special thanks too. Patrick Denning and Stephanie Harrison have our deep thanks for their meticulous final technical review of the for-publication-draft using fresher eyes. Special thanks, too, to Kathryn Gunderson, who did a wonderful job of providing us with the cover picture, an illustration of the multiple channels of how a river flows through time.

Our own intellectual journey would not have been possible without those whom we accompanied in exploring the interface of religion and public health, especially our friends and colleagues (pretty much the same thing) of the ARHAP international collaborative, and even before that, of the IHP at Emory University. These are the people with whom we have journeyed closely, in research projects, seminars, workshops, conferences, and gatherings of fun and celebration, as we explored the world of religion and public health. They particularly include Mimi Kiser, Fred Smith, Debbie Jones, and Bob Sprinkle; Barbara Schmid, Jill Olivier, Steve de Gruchy, and Paul Germond; Sinatra Matimelo, Liz Thomas, Sepetla Molapo, Mary Mwiche, Tessa Dooms, Mary Baich, Frank Dimmock, and Stephanie Doan; Beate Jakob, John Blevins, and Tor Haugstad; and many more at one point or another.

At Methodist Le Bonheur Healthcare in Memphis, Tennessee, we owe particular gratitude to Gary Shorb for both creative room and intellectual participation in the Memphis field of practice, Bobby Baker for blending his practical intelligence with our theoretical bent, the Covenant Committee of Congregational Health Network and the Methodist Le Bonheur Healthcare Board of Directors Committee on Faith and Health for such knowledgeable and supportive leadership, and partners at Memphis Theological Seminary, notably Dr. Barbara Holmes and Stan Wood.

Others that deserve special mention include: Canon Ted Karpf, for believing that religious health assets had something to give to the World Health Organization and all those upon whom it impacts; Fred Smith, Professor of Urban Ministry at Wesley Theological Seminary for nearly twenty years of intellectual cocreation in the field of faith and health; Dr. William Foege and President Jimmy Carter for providing the ground of experimental practice, the IHP, out of which came much of this thought; Dr. Jim Curran, Dean of Rollins School of Public Health, who gave the IHP space, and who has kindly provided the foreword for our book; Mary Baich of the Vesper Society, a particularly close and exemplary partner and a critical catalytic funder of much of the work of ARHAP; Jerry Paul, president of the Deaconess Foundation in St. Louis for early creative support of ARHAP and IHP; Wheat Ridge Ministries for early support of IHP and ARHAP and creative engagement with the stream of ideas of faith and health; Heather Wood Ion, for insights into the epidemic of health; Tom Peterson of Heifer Project International for intellectual generosity on how things move; Larry Pray for constantly emergent thought of life; Liz Dover, Niels French, and Chip Clay for incalculable bits of help; John Kilzer, for his insights into recovery and heatlhworlds; Doug McGaughey for talking to us about the reality of the possible; and Herman Waetjen for reminding us of John Fowles' reminder that the writer, though pretending to know all, does not in fact stand next to God.

Between us, we taught early versions of this book, either as a whole or in part, in several places, including the University of Cape Town, Memphis Theological Seminary, and Wesleyan Theological Seminary in Washington,

DC. Through many speaking engagements, we have also had opportunities to share one or another part of what has eventually appeared in the book, including at the Eberhard Karl's University of Tübingen, the Sawyer Seminar Series at the University of Cape Town, the Research in Progress seminar at Boston University, and the Indianapolis Consultation with Duke Divinity School and the Lilly Endowment. We thank our colleagues in these institutions for making this possible and, in this way, contributing to this work.

Funding for many aspects of the work that allowed us to complete this project came from Methodist Le Bonheur Healthcare's Center of Excellence in Faith and Health, the ARHAP, the University of Cape Town Research Committee, and the National Research Foundation of South Africa. Author James Cochrane also expresses his thanks for two periods of research leave from the University of Cape Town in 2009 and 2010 that were vital to being able to complete the product. In acknowledging our gratitude, we simultaneously absolve these institutions of any responsibility for the end product, which responsibility we of course hold.

One place should also be on our list of acknowledgments, for it enabled the necessary creative space to pursue ideas and sheltered a great deal of the hard task of finding a common style between us as we sought to craft the chapters of this book: so we give thanks for a rural cabin overlooking a national forest in northern Georgia, and a hot tub open to the skies. No wonder the Cherokee considered the land sacred.

Finally and vitally, our respective families were seasonally and variously interested or bored, supportive or wishing it was done, excited or living their own lives, impressed by our work or suspicious of our claims, among our best critics and partners or wondering when we would turn to something concrete and practical. This work is also for them: Karen and Renate for ground and grounding, Lauren, Thembisa, Thandeka, Kathryn, and Tebo. Who of them belongs to which of us is another question for those who do not know us—a playful reminder that linear relationships are not necessarily the way life works. Nevertheless, they are all very much part of our healthworld, our well-being, and our hope.

GARY R. GUNDERSON
Methodist Le Bonheur Healthcare
Memphis, Tennessee, USA

JAMES R. COCHRANE
University of Cape Town
Rondebosch, South Africa

FOREWORD

Advancing the health of the public has always relied on the gathering and interpretation of accurate information to clarify the pattern of threats that could be interrupted and prevented. This process is at the heart of epidemiology, a foundational science of public health. The most famous example of modern epidemiology is attributed to the physician John Snow who went against the expertise of the day to find the pattern of cholera deaths in London in 1854; this led to the closing of the Broad Street pump, the source of the contaminated water causing the outbreak. This epidemiologic mapping and the successful intervention reversed what was common knowledge about how disease spread and became a giant step toward the large-scale implementation of science to prevent not only cholera, but also many other contagions to follow.

It is often not recognized that Dr. Snow relied on the intelligence and rigorous neighborhood research of the local parish curate, the Reverend Henry Whitehead. Because Whitehead was deeply and intimately involved in the life of the people, he could talk to them (eventually 479 of the 896 residents) and understand the pattern of how they walked to get water, offering critical insights as to how the disease spread.

Since then, the field of public health has changed the prospects of billions of people who owe their extended life span to rational public choices and policies based on science that seem almost inevitable once the causal pathways and consequences are understood. From its earliest focus on sanitation and food inspection to more recent attempts to control tobacco and sexually transmitted diseases, science has made clear how much of the currently accepted patterns of disease and injury are unnecessary because they are preventable.

In each community, advancing public health begins with accurate information, but it also requires social and public policies that redefine what is unacceptable in terms of preventable illness and death. Conflicts are inevitable since this process demands change and requires a redefinition of the roles in necessary partnerships. For this reason, the notion that religion and religious leaders are unlikely, or even hostile, partners in the work of public health should be dismissed.

The early history of public health is replete with individual partnerships such as the one between Whitehead and Snow, and later ones such as the institutional collaboration between the young World Health Organization and World Council of Churches that promoted primary health care. Many more take place quite commonly around the world in communities where the social realities are woven through with religious structures and cultures of all faiths. In communities throughout the world, religious leaders recognize the need for a collaborative, science-based approach to protect the health of their constituents, and public health leaders recognize the importance of faith in peoples' lives and the need to harness the faith-based assets to improve health.

Nowhere has the relationship between public health and faith been filled with more friction and yet promise, than in the global confrontation with HIV/AIDS. Everything that is difficult in that relationship is visible in these three deadly decades with a disease that thrives in the silent spaces protected by religiously justified complicity, stigma, and denial. Moreover, much of what is hopeful is also found in the voices, practices, and patterns of care giving and truth telling now so common.

While examples of effective partnerships are very common, we have lacked a conceptual map to help public health and religious leaders understand their common values and shared intelligence that should so effectively serve their communities. This is the work that Gunderson and Cochrane offer in this important book. It is in a sense a kind of map that helps us see our communities and our work in a wholly new way. Each of the component chapters challenges the status quo: "leading causes of life," in a field that has long invested in understanding the leading causes of death; the idea of "religious health assets," in a field where many view religion as an impediment; linking how people act and behave to the idea of "healthworlds"; a new way of seeing the community systems that goes way beyond "public health systems." The authors offer an overarching paradigm in which a suite of challenging new ideas form an integrated map against which we all—religious and health leaders—may test our combined actions and ourselves.

It is not surprising that such a bold new intellectual map should emerge from scholars immersed in the long struggle with apartheid in South Africa, and racial and ethnic disparities in the United States. Both contexts point to fundamental determinants of health inequity. Both offer a sobering story of religious complicity as well as transformational hope. This work, arising within the Africa Religious Health Assets Programme, has served as an intellectual foil for dozens of scholars at Emory University and at the Universities of Cape Town, KwaZulu-Natal, and the Witwatersrand, among others, across the many distinctive disciplines so strong there. It was first envisioned at The Carter Center Interfaith Health Program (now the Interfaith Health Program at the Rollins School of Public Health), then expanded in Geneva, and finally rooted in field research in many African countries and in the United States. It has attracted hundreds of scholars, students, and practitioners, and it has gained the attention of many global public and philanthropic organizations. This stream of inquiry, research, and highly creative practice has captured the imagination of some of Emory's best students and faculty, just as it has in other institutions.

Gunderson and Cochrane provide an integrative model to see it all together as a field capable of effective large-scale practice. They would quickly acknowledge that their map would not be the last in this field. The best scholars in new fields offer themselves as a bridge to later work that may well eclipse theirs over time. That is the way that knowledge moves forward, especially knowledge developed for the urgent work of advancing the health of entire communities.

I am honored to be the dean of one of the anchoring institutions that have helped build and support this field. The health and well-being of individuals living in communities throughout the world depend upon strengthening these partnerships between religion and public health.

JAMES W. CURRAN, MD, MPH
Dean of Public Health
Rollins School of Public Health
Emory University
Atlanta, Georgia

1

SEEING DIFFERENTLY: CHANGING THE PARADIGM OF THE HEALTH OF THE PUBLIC

The scissors kick was a wonderful way to do the high jump. Until a guy said, "What the heck, I think I'll go over back first." He did. The rest is history.

Larry Pray[1]

At one level, this book is about the relationship between public health and religion. It is a relationship with deep historical roots that remain much closer to our time than what current intellectual formation and disciplinary training in either public health or religious leadership fully grasps. Reconnecting the two is more important than one might think. One of our major undertakings here, then, is to argue for that reconnection—for the sake of public health and for the best in religious traditions.

We do not need to defend the importance of public health. We are aware, however, that in the world of public health and of professional biomedicine, things "religious" or "faith-directed" are not easily grasped, absorbed, or even welcomed. Conversely, religious or faith leaders are often equally as misdirected or forgetful about the pertinence of their own traditions for public health, though religious faiths include strong transformative currents oriented toward greater well-being for all. Religion in its deepest foundations and public health in its genesis are not just about specific intellectual disciplines or fields of practice but, ultimately, about the health of the whole and health for all, the well-being of people and populations. The emphasis of this book is on why, and how, we can and should take religion and faith more seriously in the common task of contributing to healthy citizens in a whole world.

Paying attention to religion and public health also means, by definition, confronting the shape of the public in our time. This, too, is no small issue in the face of the erosion of public sphere proper through the seemingly inexorable penetration of the triumphant instrumental rationality of money and power, of markets and bureaucracies, which hold dominion over vast regions of our lives, not least, our health and well-being. This is so important, that we speak not only about religion and public health, but also about religion and the health of the public.

We write about these issues because we have an empirically grounded commitment to the necessary intellectual task of rethinking the relationship between religion and public health, honed through a combined twenty plus years of work in the field. In Gunderson's case, this work began with the establishment of the Interfaith Health Program (IHP) in 1991 at The Carter Center in Atlanta, US, after he had spent many years of work on poverty, hunger, and economic development in Africa. This informed his leadership as director of IHP at The Carter Center and after, when it moved to the Rollins School of Public Health at Emory University. Since then, he has carried the ideas and knowledge gained through multiple experiences, studies, and associations with others to Memphis and the large Methodist Le Bonheur Healthcare system located there. Here he has put into practice much of this learning in helping rethink and reshape the hospital in the light of a larger journey of health that includes congregations, communities, and other partners at every level. Cochrane was drawn into this work by Gunderson at a Carter Center meeting in 2002, though their relationship was predated by a series of events on religion and public life organized by Cochrane from the University of Cape Town in the late 1990s in which Gunderson participated. A focus on faith or religion and public life has shaped much of Cochrane's personal and academic life, beginning with his involvement from the late 1960s in well-known anti-Apartheid Christian movements in South Africa (particularly the Christian Institute, and the Institute for Contextual Theology), informing his teaching and research at the universities of KwaZulu-Natal and Cape Town as well as several international institutions, and continuing through to this work in religion and public health.

Both of us have been shaped by histories and contexts that are dominantly Christian. This introduces certain limitations into what we write and how we write it, though it also enables us to link phenomenological with analytical, internal with external understandings, and critiques of religious or faith traditions by paying attention to what we know in this regard, while providing some necessary concreteness to the general concepts we are introducing. Still, we have also engaged widely throughout the years of work reflected in this book with people of other religious traditions or none, well beyond any particular Christian narrative, and with many people trained in public health and allied disciplines. We think, therefore, that the theoretical framework introduced in this book is indeed generalizable, and that it readily opens up space for accounts from other religious or nonreligious perspectives. At least we hope so.

The book addresses public health and religious thinkers, leaders and practitioners. Its broad intention is to pose the possibility of another way of engaging with each other than the one that ignores what each brings to the other in working for the greater health of the public. More than an intellectual enterprise, the book also serves, against the instrumentalization of life, as a call for a recovery of the deep vocations of both public health and the vast majority of religious faiths. In this sense, it is a manifesto, advocating for a different way of seeing religion and public health that we believe, supported by concrete examples that are now emerging in practice, implies a different way of acting, one more hopeful than what we currently experience.

GLOBALIZING RELIGION AND PUBLIC HEALTH

The intellectual disciplines and fields of practice of religious and public health leaders differ, with their respective scientific guilds and faith communities seldom in sync. In reality, it nonetheless remains true that religion and health are intimately bound up with each other, within individuals, and in the lifeworlds of communities everywhere. The artifice that separates individual persons from their social relations is thus ultimately unsustainable. In our time, the social is not just local but also global, which affects both religion and public health. Let us begin there.

A Graveyard, the Pink Palace, and the Blues

Ironically, this particular graveyard is called no-man's-land, though it could be everyone's. In 1878, a few yards from where the busy US I55 Interstate highway runs through Memphis today, in a new cemetery on the edge of town, one and a half thousand unnamed people were buried in haste and fear, too quickly to be identified. Thousands were also buried elsewhere. Borne by mosquitoes, the cause was yellow fever, the "American Plague."[2]

Faced with this plague, Memphis was for those who came to care for the ill what physicists call a strange attractor; it wove together then odd patterns of faith and health that still echo a century and a third later. Almost anyone who could flee the pestilence did, barring some astonishing martyrs, mostly held there by their faith to care for those dying. Some came *moved* by their faith, converging from around the nation on Memphis' streets of sorrow, priests working alongside prostitutes and former slaves beyond logic and planning, though many fell within days of their arrival. Such patterns defy simplistic models of health intervention, particularly a purely medical approach, an instrumental politics of health, or a functionalist view of "faith-based" organizations as mere service providers.

The decimation of its population was Memphis' first documented health disparity. It was a flip of today's racial coin: about 80 percent of the dead were Euro-Americans who had less resilience to this tropical disease than what their African American peers had. Perhaps socially transmitted diseases are harder to overcome than those borne by insects, but then the link to faith and culture is probably even more profound. Elmwood Cemetery now holds seventy-five thousand, including Confederate veterans, governors, mayors, and princes of the globally connected cotton, hardwood, and medical industries that rebuilt Memphis after the American Plague. The ground tells stories, fanciful and tragic, of death and, through that dark mirror, of the life of a city that eventually found its way from the high bluffs over the Mississippi River across the world, connecting the surrounding region to global markets and purposes. The ways and means of cotton—how it was planted, tended, gathered, sold, shipped, and used—infuse the story of Memphis in the 1870s as much as the postcolonial dynamics of Africa affect AIDS today. In Memphis' surrounding county the quiet total of AIDS deaths will soon, if it has not already, pass the number of yellow fever victims buried long ago, many dying in destitution and finding their way into the soil only a hundred yards away from where their plague-struck cousins rest.

To take a history and a physical checkup of Memphis' health is to account for the global social and economic determinants that create a particular story of public health. This includes the rise of medical and educational institutions, with all their ironic entanglements in race or ethnicity, that produce the incongruity of elite institutions situated a few hundred yards from people who experience egregious disparities in health that persist decade after decade. In the inner city, the medical school turns some of the brightest people from other countries and of many faiths into front-line medical staff, using the Methodist system as their teaching hospital. Why is a *religious* institution the place where this happens? In part because other profit-seeking health care institutions, uninformed by any profound religious vision, have moved out to the city rim, to where the more affluent, insured clients live, leaving downtown Memphis—and its poor—to the university and the Methodists.

In 1908, Memphis gave birth to one of the great pharmaceutical firms—Sterling Plough—when twenty-one-year-old Abe Plough produced a highly questionable "antiseptic healing tonic" from a copper mixing vat. Now swarms of medical device manufacturers are found near the airport, the world's busiest cargo dispatching center and home of FedEx, which jets these devices around the world daily. The ER (Emergency Room) staff of the hospital joke darkly that the same aircraft bring diseases directly back to Memphis, so that if avian flu breaks out anywhere, it may well arrive in the Methodist Hospital system, the second largest employer in Tennessee after FedEx, the next morning. Since most of its thousands of staff attend one of the city's community churches or other places of worship, the flu could be at a place of worship the Sunday following. Disease is as global as trade.

Memphis has also long been home to a special kind of entrepreneur with eyes for new cutting-edge opportunities. Clarence Saunders invented the first modern grocery store here, where customers could browse the shelves themselves instead of asking a clerk for every item. With access to cheap and easy capital, Saunders's "Piggly Wiggly" store model spread across the nation, though he lost a Wall Street struggle for control of the highly leveraged stock—a fate experienced by others in the lightly regulated stock markets of the time—and went bankrupt before he was able to occupy his vast, newly built "Pink Palace" on the outskirts of Memphis, now a nice city museum. The first motels were conceived here as Holiday Inns, serving the newly mobile millions who had wheels, time, and government-funded highways to use. The confluence of wheels and highways also makes possible Memphis' three hundred trucking companies part of a global pattern of shipping that links China through Canada to the heartland of everconsuming America. Unsurprisingly, those factors feed the predictable patterns of diseases such as HIV that thrive on transience and mobility.

A superabundance of pastors, prostitutes, and entrepreneurs continues to define Memphis today, still a magnet for the adult industries that public health authorities recognize as vectors for all sorts of deadly infectious diseases. Memphis is an outlier in the wrong direction for AIDS, every sort of sexually transmitted disease, and the gendered social pathologies of extraordinary numbers of low birth-weight babies born out of wedlock, all in the context of one of the highest concentrations of religious structures in the United States, including more than two thousand congregations within an hour of Elmwood's no-man's-land.

Yellow fever was a mosquito-borne disease that thrived in the casual sewage and water supply of a city too busy with managing the global demand for cotton to bother with taking out the trash. Nobody understood that link until decades later, much as today we casually dismiss knowledge we find economically inconvenient. Once the science of the late 1800s had turned on the appropriate lights, engineers drained the mosquito infested swamps, found the deep aquifers of clean crystal water, built the sidewalks, invented food inspection, inaugurated public health departments, and established the massive tunnels that now lie under Memphis to guide the used waters to the river, providing protection that its 1 million citizens seldom realize they depend on for their very lives.

Making public health a story of scientists and engineers, however, leaves some of the most interesting parts in the shadow, for it fails to account for the relationship between human perception, knowledge, and action on a social scale. How *one* human seeks health is complicated enough. Hundreds of congregations in Memphis linked to the Methodist system now collaborate to help individuals navigate the treacherous and intimidating journey toward and through medical institutions, and back home again. How a *public* seeks health is more important, as the history of Memphis itself shows. What helps the public navigate its way, and how do faiths or religions make the course plain and possible or hidden and difficult?

Just as the affluent inherit historical privileges that enhance their health, others close by inherit historical traumas that do not. They present themselves at the hospital's trauma centers for treatment of violence and injury or the longer-term effects of grossly disparate patterns of housing, food, education, and employment that are often, woefully, regarded as matters merely of medical care. Eighty percent of those without insurance entering the ERs have at least one chronic disease condition, whatever else brings them there that day. Put this against another high statistic: 70 percent of them also say they have attended a place of worship within thirty days of attending the ER.

What then is the connection between those two doorways in the minds of citizens who experience life both as members and as patients? What connection, if any, is made in the minds of health planners and administrators, public, private, and faith based? Or in the minds of those leading the congregations who are praying, holding rituals of healing and hope—and who are, sometimes, complicit in failing the health of their community?

Not many miles south of Elmwood Cemetery lies another site of pilgrimage, Graceland, the home of Elvis Presley, whose presence still resonates decades after his death, partly because of his Mississippi hill country mélange of sexual grind and good church sweetness. Others are barely less known, like the great B. B. King, or platinum album artist Al Green, who now pastors one of the thousands of churches on this complex soil. Like other cities that are magnets for suffering, Memphis' music is a rich tapestry woven of blues and bombast, faith and failure.

Americans will say that the church is separate from the state. Music tells a more sophisticated story. Music in Memphis is the Blues—not really Elvis' sequins, though, shaped by Blues, he epitomizes the paradox of the good church boy who is also a demon hip-shaking rock and roller. Paradox, the ineluctable tension between hope and hurt, is the point. The Blues, born in the cotton fields along Route 61 deep in the Mississippi Delta above which Memphis sits, is the quintessential coping mechanism: sing the pain away, communicate in code, keep moving through the suffering, sorrow, and loss—hang in there as long as you can. Thus the most intriguing story at the intersection of faith and health is how communities of people near the dirt tease resilience out of oppression and nothingness, and live to sing about it.

Zambian Cotton, Copper, and Christianity: Same Beat, Different Blues

Memphis was founded as a minor cog of much larger global economic gears, and it only exists because of this continued mesh. The region's lowland hardwoods have long been cut and shipped elsewhere, its medical institutions long surpassed by others in Boston and Atlanta, not to mention Cape Town, or Vellore in India. Bales of cotton no longer fill the streets of Memphis in the fall, but the world's largest cotton trading firm is still there, a block south of a notorious strip club and within two blocks of six churches. Its third-generation leader, Bill Dunavant, manages not only the trading, but also the growing of cotton in nations precariously struggling on the edges of development. This includes an affiliate in Zambia: the largest employer there, it organizes more than a hundred thousand small farmers who each plant, tend, harvest, and sell small amounts of cotton that the Dunavants trade globally.

Zambia, despite good-health promotion campaigns and a relatively well-educated population, is notable for one of the highest global rates of HIV infection. The Dunavant company has won awards for a pitifully relevant innovation: including condoms and educational materials about HIV and AIDS, along with the seeds and fertilizer, in each starter kit for their local farmers. Zambia, now officially defining itself as Christian, is also remarkable for its exceptionally high rates of religious participation. Even more faith-soaked than Memphis, if that is possible; hardly any place where two dirt roads cross is devoid of a church of some sort.

Ndola and Kitwe in Zambia's famed Copperbelt, unmistakable signs of past British colonial presence on every street and façade, are crossroads of global economic significance, resting on vast reserves of copper and bordering Democratic Republic of the Congo, where wars for control over even larger mineral resources have long burned. This is Zambia's economic hub, with manufacturing, large-scale power production, mining and more mining, as well as churches, including rapidly growing Pentecostal congregations that serve thousands throughout rural and urban communities.

A collapse of the copper industry and the introduction of Structural Adjustment Programs (SAPs) in the 1990s, now superseded, radically changed the health profile of the Copperbelt. Virtually malaria free then thanks to a remarkably successful eradication program, malaria is once again endemic, while weakened health systems and broken public infrastructure now face HIV, a disease that also exposes religious complicity with gendered oppression and cultural norms of denial. How do faith leaders find their voice when facing complex global economic forces manipulated from afar and a disease carried by behaviors they can hardly bring themselves to speak about? How do public health leaders begin to engage the largest organized social assets in their nation—the churches—when the very subject creates a divided table before the conversation begins?

In Zambia, there is a level of active, considered collaboration between faith and public entities at multiple levels. The Christian Health Association of Zambia (CHAZ) thus manages funds from the Global Fund for AIDS, Tuberculosis (TB), and Malaria for the state Ministry of Health. However, there is much more too. The African Religious Health Assets Programme (ARHAP), mapping the scope, scale, and diversity of religious work in health in the area, discovered sixfold as many religious health programs on the ground than anyone in government or the World Health Organization (WHO) knew existed.[3] Many religious actors channel resources and expertise far beyond the reach of government programs, sometimes with the help of trusted intermediaries such as the Copperbelt Health Education Project (CHEP), which assists close on a hundred local community-based organizations at any one time, most faith linked, to strengthen and manage their activities, gain access to finance, and find the connections that enable them to thrive.[4]

Such intermediary bodies represent critical models for the practical alignment of resources, intelligence, and compassion capable of crossing many boundaries.[5] The many religious health assets on the ground—way beyond official records of health facilities and unaligned with formal health system structures, but providing a great deal to people who otherwise would be stranded or unsupported—are also a critical part of the picture. Understanding the implications of such realities is one purpose of this book.

PASSIONATE SCHOLARSHIP, COMMITTED ENGAGEMENT, AND TRANSFORMATIVE PRACTICE

We could call the interweaving of faith and health fractal. The patterns of complexity and multilevel interdependencies that appear repeatedly on the interface between religion and health weave through individual persons to global polity and back again. Tearing faith and health apart simply damages our ability to grasp their connection, often with significant negative practical consequences. Scholars necessarily draw conceptual boundaries around a particular phenomenon and domains of interest, but that is a functional strategy, no substitute for the complexity of reality.

The intersection between faith and health is properly understood not only as a reflection of the current condition of any one person, but also of their longer journey of health, where others are always present. It thus goes beyond individuals to include the journey of communities and of the bodies in which people congregate, as well as the social narrative that describes them in time and space. Even attempting to recount this complexity using the clumsy conjunction "and" misses how tight the relationship between these levels is, how conceptually interwoven the links are, and how easily their ecology fragments through the disentanglement that scholars perform with such automatic rigor.

In lived human experience, the relationship is better understood. In the mountain villages of Lesotho there are no words that distinguish between faith and health. Here it is impossible to speak of one without meaning the other, and the only relevant word, *bophelo*, representing the full ecology of faith/health, holds the whole intact and closer to life as actually lived.[6] Our mostly fragmented scholarship is not sophisticated enough to grasp the whole, but any scholar properly humbled by even a glimpse of that reality knows enough to pause in awe and wonder before setting out to describe and analyze it.

Scholarship should not only serve the arts of wonder, but also the arts of change. One of the great physicians of the body politic, Dr. Martin Luther King, Jr., observed that only maladjusted people changed anything. We assume he meant, by maladjustment, an inability to accept things as they are, a critical urge to move from the sapping inertia of what is to the generative innovations that signal how it might be. As part of our own thinking about shifting paradigms, we call this "boundary leadership."[7]

One great moral scandal of our times is how much suffering can be not only ameliorated but also prevented. Already from the late 1870s onwards, we began to notice enough about the patterns of disease to realize the enormous opportunities for interrupting the pathological pathways thought to be the normal and precarious way of human life: tuberculosis, cancer, cholera, yellow fever, and smallpox—a whole gamut of deadly companions taken simply as given. The genius of epidemiological attentiveness helps us see that these and other socially determined ills, including car wrecks and domestic violence, can be actively engaged sufficiently to prevent or at least seriously dent their destructive effects. The scandal is how little of what can be prevented is prevented; how much we still mimic the early Memphians' casual approach to drainage, water, and sanitation. A simple accounting of the economic asymmetries of health, in particular societies or globally, makes the point starkly clear. We know enough to inform our humility and more than enough for well-informed shame, even enough to inform systematic action to bend the curve of our communities' and societies' journeys toward well-being.

What scholarship can help us move toward that action? We think a part of the answer is thoughtful analysis of the intersection between two things imagined as distant that we understand to be intrinsically one—faith and health. We know, personally, in each of our own nations as well as intellectually, about the pathological possibilities of religion or faith. It takes little new scholarship to add to that sad tale. However, we have a different starting point.

We wonder about the obvious possibilities this intersection holds for our communities' well-being. Ideas do matter, and bad ones do result in bad structures, produce bad plans, and result in bad outcomes, even from otherwise intelligent people. Think, in our time, of the trillions of dollars lost because of patently bad economic ideas that religious leaders and philosophers, even economists, had warned about, a policy of deregulation that amounted to an agreement to let the greedy regulate themselves. As Alan Greenspan himself admitted, it was based not only on a fundamental "flaw" that missed the destructive power of deregulated mortgage lending and overestimated the ability of the free market to self-correct but, he ruefully admitted, "the whole intellectual edifice" had collapsed.[8] A large admission in its own context, something similar could be said about another context—the reduction of health to the idea of individual "consumers" or "patients" served by a small cadre of well-paid professionals.

What, then, is the thinking around which we should organize? One part is certainly that health is social, and that social assets include—have always included in every culture—some kind of religion or faith. Obviously not every norm, value, and practice of any particular religion or faith is an asset for health; we are not that naïve. Nonetheless, we ask, which are? How might religious assets helpfully overcome barriers to health or help us wisely harness new health technologies in service of human well-being? To answer such questions we need better ideas than those that mostly govern the minds of leaders of public, private, and religious bodies. Moreover, we need better-connected ideas, a coherent framing paradigm that holds together and makes actionable a comprehensive way of seeing the parts as a whole.

Thus, the ideas of this book, the reader will find, weave into and across each other; they are meant to be read together rather than singly. Covering a wide spectrum of themes, theories, and studies across several disciplines, we cannot always pursue all in depth, but we have provided a rich array of references that the reader may pursue.

The vast bulk of academic literature on religion and health focuses on microphenomena, individual existence, or personal experience. We, however, are interested in population health, in religion tested against hopes on a social scale. We seek to ground the connections of religion and health at the level of communities, societies, or the public in relation to their well-being, to root action in better choices about how one works with religion or faith in dealing with the inevitable complexity and ambiguity of the profound contemporary challenges posited by a vision of health for all in a healthy public realm.

These are not realities, scandals, and hopes in which we do not participate. We write therefore as passionate scholars, interested in the well-being of all, proposing a way of seeing religion in relation to health that we have become increasingly convinced is a necessary part of meeting that passion and vision—and a requirement for scholarship fitting not only to the demands of good science, but also to the realities of the world in which we live.

CRISIS IN THE HEALTH OF GLOBALIZED PUBLICS

Our interest in religious health assets, therefore, is not about some desire to rehabilitate "religion" or "faith" for its sake, or to enter into special pleading for religious bodies of one kind or another within the existing systems. That is simply not the point. We are motivated by a reasonable conviction that human beings everywhere—including ourselves and our families and friends—confront a crisis in public health and in the health of the public that is deep and likely to grow, just when new possibilities for doing something to address those crises are also present, including a much more productive alignment of religious health assets with those of public health and health care generally, and a stronger shared vision about a more hopeful future around which to mobilize.

Researchers of the Institute for Health and Social Justice and Partners in Health, articulating the depth of the current crisis in global public health, show "how specific growth-oriented policies have not only failed to improve living standards and health outcomes among the poor, but also have inflicted additional suffering on disenfranchised and vulnerable populations."[9] Human health is a particularly compelling lens on the nature and the health of society, best understood in relation to the commonweal, the *salus rei publicae*, the health of the public per se.[10] It cuts across all divisions and conflicts to reveal where society itself is diseased. If, in modern societies, well-being is heavily impacted by the system imperatives of markets (money) and bureaucracies (power) seen in the effects on the lifeworlds of people,[11] then the extent to which lifeworlds are respected and fittingly drawn into (or not) any social arrangement is a key indicator of good or bad policy. That implies a strong emphasis on the language of citizenship and of the commonweal, and a clear acknowledgment of the existing asymmetric distribution of power and money. Systems, governed by control over power and money, however, think mostly in instrumental, functionalist terms.

Similarly, the classic analytical tool of public health, epidemiology, rests upon generalizable, aggregate, population-scale measurements of disease and on the outcomes of particular interventions. Specific indicators (infant mortality rates, immunization levels, relative drug costs, number of hospital beds, etc.) act as proxies for the health of populations. A powerful and sophisticated range of tools and methods, buoyed by some spectacular successes (smallpox eradication, effective methods for dealing with cholera), has thus propelled into the foreground the mathematizable constructs of public health as the key drivers of policy and resource allocation. However, they have not solved the problems of public health.

Public health, in its modern origins, worked with an intrinsically social understanding of health.[12] Its principals saw the link between human suffering and key social determinants of health.[13] Moreover, if social, political, and economic life was integral to understanding population health, then, conversely, population health status also exposed the nature of such systems.[14]

At the time, a vision of the commonweal, with its associated notion of the common good, inspired public health. However, that vision was already under threat. The common good requires that individual interests find meaning amid generalized interests, but along with the industrial revolution came the idea of the sovereign, autonomous individual, rationally choosing according to self-interest. Here the public is simply the aggregate of individuals, whose competing interests must be refereed through contractual arrangements.

The early founders of modern public health were deeply discomforted by this perspective and, as Garrett notes: "At the dawn of the twentieth century the Western world fused the ideas of civic duty and public health. Conquering disease was viewed as a collective enterprise for the common good."[15] One problem is that science does not apply itself; groups of people have to decide to do so. However, how are those many faceted decisions made? How can we seek the health of the public when there is no public to be healthy?

WAYS OF SEEING: RELIGION IN HEALTH

Toward a New Paradigm: What This Book Is About

Religion and health are social realities, not just personal ones, implicated in each other both historically and practically. We seek to ground an understanding of their interface through multiple, congruent ideas that pattern a way of seeing and not just a disciplinary perspective. The ideas are fractal, their patterns repeating themselves in fresh ways at every level of practice. As such, they aim at grasping complexity rather than producing simplifications that are likely to repeat existing failures and prevent innovations.

Underlying these ideas is a broad conception of health that, not unlike the WHO definition, we call "comprehensive well-being."[16] The idea of well-being in relation to public health, though in widespread use, has been questioned as overly general and imprecise. Perhaps it is for some purposes, yet it can be defended. Cameron et al., reviewing recent debates, conclude that a tighter conceptual tie between well-being and public health requires that one pay attention to a disciplined inquiry into (1) the necessity and nature of engagement with and "partnerships" between different stakeholders, (2) the complexities of differing conceptions of health, (3) the widening of its evidence base to more fully include and value qualitative data, and (4) the boundaries and roles within health sectors and between health and other sectors.[17] Our ideas about religion and health fit well with this approach, though we also include other dimensions such as the social determinants of health.

At least seven interlocking ideas make up the pattern or paradigm we describe in this book. They are meant to be read neither separately nor sequentially but as linked pathways into the same whole. Though each may be pursued in its own right, to lose their connections is to strip any one idea of crucial dimensions.

First, in chapter 2, we unpack aspects of the embodied religious mind that critically contribute to insights necessary for a sustainable, enduring, and just health of the public. Three iconic narratives, much celebrated landmarks in the history of public health but largely repressing the role of religious mind in standard accounts, serve our purpose: Dr. John Snow's seminal contribution to the science of epidemiology in relation to the problem of cholera in industrializing England; the WHO's establishment of primary health care as its definitive mandate in the Alma-Ata Declaration; and Dr. William Foege's contribution to the global eradication of smallpox. If apathy or enmity toward religious experience and worldviews is common, we hope to dislodge it; it is simply silly, on empirical and strategic grounds if nothing else, to ignore their positive potentials and energies.

In chapter 3, we introduce the idea of religious health assets. A critical shift in thinking is to cultivate an active curiosity about the assets for health, tangible and intangible, that are already held and utilized by those seeking their health for whom public health interventions are intended, and how one can leverage such assets for greater health. Before diagnosing what is *not* there in a person, family, local community, or society that should be—a "needs-based" approach— an asset-based approach asserts that it is important to understand what *is* there of crucial significance for the health of the public. A needs-based approach insinuates, ipso facto, a deficit still to be overcome by those who have the need, inherently implying that external intervention by an outside agent is necessary. An intrinsic dependency relationship is then almost unavoidable. An assets-based approach reverses the priority, generating in the process several innovative and productive approaches to understanding religion and health, as we discuss in this chapter.

By now one might ask just what we mean by religion, for which we often use the term "faith" interchangeably. As any scholar of religion knows, all definitions of religion finally prove to be inadequate to the complex, rich stew of phenomena commonly, colloquially called "religion." We adopt a largely pragmatic definition, encompassing how people in local contexts define themselves, the historical traditions usually described as "religions," and the concrete manifestations of these traditions in specific people, groups, organizations, or movements. Our primary interest, however, is in its social embodiment, rather than its presence in the internal lives of individuals. Though the personal and the social, the private and the public dimensions of religion are finally never separate, often intimately bound up with each other, it is the social and the public that is at the center of our gaze.

A new paradigm of religion and health will be informed by a preferential option for life against death. As odd as that sounds, it simply means asking, first, "what generates health?" before being thoroughly absorbed by what causes ill-health, disease, or death. We need no scholarship to note that we all die at some point. However, it requires fresh thought to account for the dynamic, often surprising processes through which people do *not* run down, wear out, give up, catch some disease, and expire. While understanding and dealing with pathologies is undoubtedly vital, we require a fundamental shift in curiosity, somewhat analogous to the change in paradigm that helped physicists look beyond the idea of entropy (everything running down) to the regenerating logic of creative possibility. Life dissipates energy to be sure, but it also adapts and transforms in unpredictable patterns that are remarkable, if not beautiful, in their emergence. Things do run down, and it would be foolish not to notice that people get sick and societies fail to provide well-being. However, vitality, as a subject of curiosity, is more useful than death, if leaders want to know what might contribute to well-being.

In chapter 4, therefore, we ask what might be the leading causes of life. We do not understand the causes of life with anything near the precision with which we can analyze death and its causes, in individuals or societies. Physicians are trained to focus centuries of scientific knowledge of disease into the compact intellectual container of a fifteen-minute visit with one patient at a time. To a remarkable degree, those fifteen minutes do manage to produce a high level of relevant information about what is trying to kill a patient. However, any physician knows that half of their patients present with little that is medically wrong, making most of their sophisticated knowledge of disease an irrelevance. Public health practitioners are equally troubled by the relative irrelevance of their tools to the challenges of ill-health at social scale. Scholarship has done only part of its job, ignoring life, vitality, and flourishing as fit subjects for rigorous analysis. Theology too has been complicit in this process when it pathologically hammers on sin rather than announcing grace, forgiveness, love, hope, or justice. An adequate paradigm of religion also rests on the foundation of life.

In chapter 5, curious about how people find their way to health, survive, and even flourish, we ask how religion impacts upon their health-seeking behavior. Any particular health intervention is never a one-way street between the provider and the health seeker. The behavior of the latter can, and often does, make a huge difference in how successful or sustainable an intervention is. That behavior is mostly rooted in norms, values, and beliefs, often religious in character, that are critical to understand for achieving public health outcomes. While medical anthropologists and sociologists, psychologists and others, have drawn increasing attention to these issues, we seek to add here further insights into the role of religion in this context, and in the process, we introduce the concept of the healthworld.

Chapter 6 moves in another direction, exploring how religion creates the energy, hope, and imagination from which positive futures emerge. In almost every case we know, a community, not an individual, lies at the heart of the story. We are concerned here not about communities characterized by an exclusive, walled-off, primarily self-protective defense against perceived threats to their insularity, but with those that inspire inclusive, open, and generative life, not just for those who belong, but also for those who do not.

Neuroscientists suggest that we are wired for this kind of social generative intimacy, literally forming common bioelectric fields of influence, affection, and hope that allow for common action. Libraries of books describe how religion creates boundaries that defy common vision and action, that feed the worst and last bastions of fear and stigma. We would like at least a few scholarly works about the opposite. We therefore explore what we regard as the key strengths of people who congregate in the name of one religious tradition or another. These are strengths that can be identified and worked with, and they are significant for understanding how those who congregate can be part of a common vision relevant to the health of the public.

Particular persons, either in a defined role or by virtue of their personal influence and authority, usually lead groups of one kind or another. Leaders matter, not just by what they do or make happen, but in how they live their life in social transparency and through what they facilitate in the process. Social wholes, especially emergent ones, are marked by leading figures whose ways of living and influencing others help form the emergent possibilities of that whole. Here, it is the peculiar role of leaders to anticipate and consciously form the future into a chooseable, actionable pathway, and to help those choices be made. This is why we learn from such religious innovators as Dietrich Bonhoeffer, Mahatma Gandhi, and Dr. Martin Luther King, Jr.—one faced death in prison, the other two in the streets, but all died in expectation that their movements of life would survive them because they were held deeply in the vitality of living communities.

In chapter 7 we explore how that happens, and what leadership practices or characteristics make that more likely. This kind of leader, whom we call "boundary leader," is not set apart from the whole, as a catalyst might be, and certainly not above the whole in some privileged space removed from exposure to the path others are asked to tread. The life of such leaders is a journey in itself, of continued transformation in their own lives, and in the relationships they have with other leaders inside and across the boundaries of blood, discipline, geography, and resource capacities. How does religion shape, energize, and embolden the journey of such leaders in social spaces? Where does their courage and vision come from, or their caution, humility, grace, and patience? What enables them to reframe their imagination and reshape their actions, to see more clearly what can be done, and to act more intelligently in embodying how it is done?

Chapter 8 introduces another critical dimension, which has to do with the political and economic forces that shape so much of our world and daily lives, whether individually or socially. No discussion of religion or of health has any chance of grasping the complexity of life without taking into consideration these systemic dimensions of the social whole, and the social choices that shape the health of the public. In this regard, we focus specifically on the challenge of systems, particularly those mediated by money and power, that is, markets and bureaucracies. Such systems are driven by imperatives of their own that are inherently instrumental, aimed at achieving the purposes for which they exist, which are primarily about the economy and about governance. No one escapes this and many of us serve one or other system imperative. How do we live constructively, innovatively, toward life and the greater health of the public in this context? Here we turn to a consideration of how asymmetries of power (and by implication, money) generate pathologies, and what it means to be a "health citizen" in the face of such pathologies, with a view to imagining what it takes to produce a "healthy political economy."

One part of this equation has to do with the purposes of knowledge. Simply generating more and more basic and applied knowledge, however valuable, without considering for whom and why that knowledge is produced is wholly inadequate, if not dangerous. Knowledge sits within larger social norms and values, and how a society chooses to employ its resources and express its common will, or decides what kinds of science to apply in what kinds of ways to which parts of the society, is not just a matter of instrumental logic but also of communicative rationality. This, in turn, depends upon the capability that any one person or group in a society has to enter meaningfully into such choices or decisions, and these capabilities are directly related to economic and political dynamics and institutions. It is in this light that one must ask how social wholes might move forward toward well-being. And about what religion might have to do with the informed hopes, capacities for common imagination, and the will needed to implement the best social choices for all.

If one is to move all of this beyond theory into practice, it requires not just a conceptual framework of seven interrelated dimensions but also a commitment to the intentions that lie behind all of them and any others that may be congruent. A vision of the health of the public, accompanied by the transformative practices that would bring that vision more fully into being, calls forth some accountability to it, and to those for whom it is intended. Whether in faith institutions or among religious leadership, whether in public health agencies or the academy, this calls forth what we call "deep accountability." That is the theme of our final chapter.

In sum, the seven themes outlined above, taken together (we again emphasize), represent what we regard to be most basic starting points in crafting foundational concepts for transformative practice on the interface between religion and public health (see figure 1.1). They indicate the shape of the book and its chapters. Intimately interwoven with each other, our development of these points will indicate why there is a newly unfolding appreciation in public health

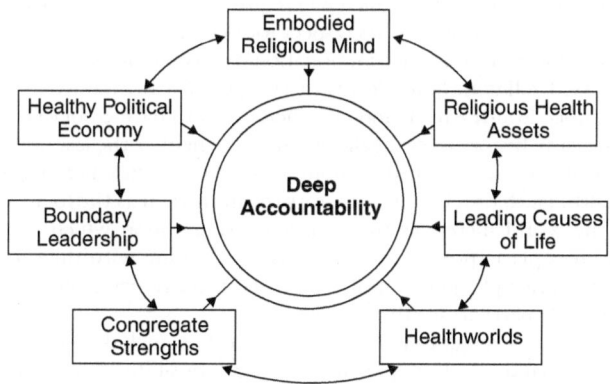

Figure 1.1   Religion and public health transformative ensemble.

circles of the role of religion. And why we believe them to be the basis of a necessary shift in the paradigm of religion in the health of the public.

Old Paradigm: What This Book Challenges

If a new paradigm is emerging, one may logically ask what it is about the existing, dominant paradigm that is failing. With no attempt at an exhaustive analysis, we underline four themes of particular relevance to understanding religion in relation to public health.

The first concerns religion. Under the aegis of the idea of secularism, an idea that has captivated social scientists for decades and that still holds wide sway despite its many critical deconstructions, religion was no longer regarded as a key variable in the development of modern societies. Theories of secularization argued that religion in "advanced" or "modernizing" societies would gradually shrivel away in the face of human autonomy and the authority of reason, or disappear from the public sphere to become a private matter of individuals. European societies offered some empirical content to this claim that soon acquired the status of scientific truth, of a law of evolving society under conditions of industrialization, urbanization, and democratization.

It is trite now to observe that this supposed law does not hold, with even ardent past theorists of secularization conceding their error in imagining that religion or communities of faith would fade from public life.[18] There is no law here—only a rapidly shifting, contextually determined, historically shaped pendulum that swings hither and thither in irregular arcs. The only sustainable aspect of the theory that remains is the tendency in modern states, because of increasing pluralism under globalizing conditions and the need to stabilize increasingly diverse societies, to separate the state from any established religion in order to serve all citizens or inhabitants without fear or favor. This obviously does not at all imply the absence of religion from the public sphere. It does imply that the public sphere is more likely to reflect a contestation between religious and nonreligious worldviews, which will require some respect for the other with whom one disagrees if one wishes respect for oneself.

More serious to us, is the accommodation of certain forms of faith to the idea of a privatized religion. Some forms of evangelical Christianity in the United States, Zambia, South Africa, and elsewhere seem to have embraced this idea—against the early history of evangelicals who were neither the last nor the least in pressing their energies and their passions into service of the emerging concerns of public health. Faith or religion that treats the individual as the focus of redemption, or the world merely as the temporary stage upon which the drama of salvation takes place, provides no impetus to engaging with the society or the world. Unsurprisingly, public health activists, practitioners, and policy makers find no sensible partners for their work there.

However, many religious people and institutions, including evangelicals, are engaged in social life and accept some public responsibility, including for public health. Zambia is full of such bodies, as is Africa generally, not to mention the United States. If the old paradigm is crudely expressed in the popular aphorism, "keep religion out of politics" (desired by some people of faith as much as secularists), then it no longer has purchase. In its place must come a search for a mutually responsible understanding of religion and health conjoined in a common passion and vision for the well-being of all.

Our second theme is related. If some treat faith and religion primarily as individual, others treat the significance of religion for health similarly. In Christian theological formation, in the United States originally but since exported worldwide, the classic paradigm for such a view can be found in what is known as "clinical pastoral education" (CPE). Originating with the groundbreaking work at Chicago Theological Seminary of Anton Boisen and influenced by the new psychoanalytic theories of Freud and Jung, the CPE model was first established as standard practice at Billings Hospital in Chicago. A powerful integration of medical and religious practice in a clinical setting, it has expanded the horizon of possibilities of all who have participated in it. However, it remains heavily focused on the individual and her or his family. Little of a public health perspective can be found. Certainly, individual CPE practitioners do by and by become aware of the social determinants of health that affect the people for whom they care, but the model itself gives them no way to conceive of those determinants in relation to its practice, for it is primarily organized around individual, at best family, health and spirituality.

Various medical practitioners and scientists, happily accompanied by religious scholars and social scientists, similarly place a heavy emphasis on the spirituality or religiosity of the individual health seeker as the most salient issue. Here the interest is on the impact upon health outcomes of religious practices such as prayer, liturgy, accompaniment, song, or touch: do they increase resilience, improve the immune system, or speed up recovery? The *Handbook of Religion and Health*, the most complete reference work to survey this field of interest, demonstrates the range and depth of interest in such topics.[19] However, rarely do these considerations extend to anything more than the health of the individual or the family. The paradigm within which these approaches operate is translated into the health of the public only with great difficulty, if at all, while an equivalent body of literature that might explore the role and effects of religion or faith in the health of the public barely exists.

A third theme, well represented in scientific and religious literature, bedeviling any attempt to find a meaningful interface between religion and public health, concerns two related metaphysical presumptions: one, an idealist predisposition, assumes a priority of spirit, mind, or cognition over the body; the other, a materialist bias, prioritizes physical reality over mind or spirit. The best thinkers usually avoid these dual prejudices, but the prejudices remain hardy and widespread. The default position largely remains that science and religion have to do with two unrelated, even incompatible realities.

The idea of disembodied spirit or thought is more deeply entrenched than we may suspect. One subtle example is the emphasis in scientific circles on measurement and measures, indicators and predictors, usually captured in sophisticated mathematical models. The language of mathematics, including statistics and biometrics, takes on an objective reality of its own, even though it is fundamentally an abstraction, a mental map and not an embodied territory with actual dirt. The models substitute for the reality itself, especially when—as in the very useful work done by epidemiologists on disease patterns—they prove useful enough to drive policy decisions.

The illusion or mystification lies not in the methods used or their utility but, as the challenges of HIV and AIDS have made abundantly clear, in the assumption that whole systems of health can be set up on the basis of utilitarian knowledge without simultaneously taking seriously the entirely communicative dimensions of human interaction that undo or reshape mathematics on a regular basis. Persons-are-bodies-are-minds-are-spirit. Any science or practice of health that reduces that complex reality to a single idea or a measure will succeed only to a certain point, and fail at other critical points. The current paradigm, unable yet to bridge the gaps that arise, cannot solve the inherent problems of complexity in ways that provide for long-term, sustainable, comprehensive health.

The other side of the picture, our fourth theme, concerns particular forms of religious thought and practice. This book has a clear bias: our focus is on what religion and religious people or groups do that promotes, sustains, or protects health on a communal or social scale. However, we know well, from personal experience too, of the many ways in which religion is dangerous for the health of persons or the body politic. Faced with patients forswearing the vital treatment offered to them for HIV, because a misinformed or alienated traditional healer has told them otherwise or a Pentecostal preacher has pronounced that faith alone heals, we know doctors who wish nothing more than to be rid of religion, and we sympathize.

Whether religious people here act from ignorance, fear of losing authority, a desire to hold together a community's belief, or an uncritical ideology, does not matter. What does matter is their implicit assertion of direct and unmediated access to divine or sacred knowledge that places them outside human limits. Self-critical questioning is thus, in principle, set aside, and it becomes impossible to enter with an inquiring mind into dialogue with scientific knowledge, whether it be the science of the ancients or of biomedicine.

Science works best when its wisdom is tested against new experience and knowledge in a continual cycle of deepened experience, expanded insight, enhanced judgment, and intelligent action. That is hard for many religious people to incorporate in their own claims, but it is essential. And it is not out of the question. We would argue that the best religious thinkers, whatever their tradition, embody just such an attitude in their ability to transcend the particularities of their time and place, and to introduce innovations into the midst of their own communities. That is what we must work with.

Why Does It Matter?

We are of course not alone in noticing the difficulties that plague the dominant health paradigm of the present, or in wondering about what may be emerging that embodies the shape of the future. If the situation of public health is much more critical than might have been anticipated, and the potential role of religion in the health of the public is insufficiently grasped by most health *and* religious leaders, then the question of shifting the paradigm to allow for aligning religion and public health is worth posing.

It may be that religions or systems of faith and belief inherently conserve the past, thus resisting any shift that appears to threaten their self-understanding and institutional foundations. Yet, the history of religions also demonstrates their astonishing capacities to innovate, invent, adjust, and even act as harbinger of the future: faith communities working against Apartheid in South Africa or racism in the United States being examples. The inherited crust of tradition and authority that marks much religion has had more than its share of critics. Our interest is in the innovative, life-giving, and life-sustaining capacities that people of faith or religious conviction bring to the table, especially those that contribute to the well-being of the widest community. Words such as the Sesotho bophelo, the Hebrew shalom, or the Arabic salaam evoke the underlying hope that what is possible to imagine might come to pass in the social spaces of our lives.

We know it is a long way from words to sustained communal action. We need a bridge of logic over the deep chasms separating the possible from the actual. That logic should be able to carry the weight of different kinds of component ideas, some more useful in medical environments, some in worshipping con- gregations, some in wild streets or rural villages, some in legislative hallways where policy is crafted, and yet others for scholars whose constant work is to notice, refine, and articulate questions that lead more deeply into the possibili- ties ahead. A conceptual framework matters if one wishes to go from where we are to where we might be, and words matter in service of better ideas to open up a different vision and better choices.

So we spend little, though some, time in this book detailing what is wrong with the current order that leaves stillborn the hopes of millions of people and thousands of communities. Not because we do not ache at the scandalous dis- tance between the obvious potentials of the twenty-first century and the equally dramatic pathologies that mock those potentials, but because our passion and commitment is to lend our minds to turning that situation around, to convert as many keystrokes and sentences as we can to energies going the other way. Thus, we pursue here another way of seeing the future, a shift in our cognitive mapping, that can align the assets relevant to health at community scale, some identified as religious and others as public. We argue for a conceptual frame- work that finds between them a deep commonality of purpose and possibility.

A conceptual framework may seem a rather indirect gift to offer in the face of urgent and overwhelming challenges. However, this is what scholars can do and must do if we are to give leaders more than a clutter of disconnected mus- ings and random projects that seem to work. We should spend less time on what keeps us apart and more on what keeps our mutual passions focused on what matters most. What we offer here is a paradigm of religion in the health of the public that helps us distinguish opportunities from distractions, that which is well for the whole from that which is good for only a part.

2

THE HEALTH OF THE PUBLIC AND THE RELIGIOUS MIND: CONNECTIONS AND DISCONNECTIONS

TERMS OF ENGAGEMENT

The history of religion can barely be separated from that of health. Most, if not all, religions are bound up with some comprehensive conception of health and well-being, whether cast in cyclical or linear patterns of redemption, salvation, or fullness of life. Health, here, means more than medicine.[1] However, even the term "medicine" has a deeper meaning than most realize, with surprising etymological origins in the pharaonic language of Egypt: the mediation (*medi*) of the healer (*sine*).[2]

However, neither the general history of health nor the specific conceptions of religious traditions are our focus here. Instead, we ask what in "the religious mind" enables a reconfiguration of paradigms of health, altering practice in the process. The metaphor of "the religious mind," as we mean it, includes discursive practices and human imagination as they are shaped by religion, how they shift language and conceptual frameworks through the capacity of the human mind to reflect on "what is" (actuality) and imagine "what is not yet" (possibility), and how this is embodied in action. The term "mind" is somewhat misleading, then, but it serves our purpose as long as one remembers that it does not refer to a disembodied, decontextualized Cartesian ego. Rather, it has to do with resources and strategies found in religious traditions for orienting one to, and negotiating one's way in the world.

Without making exclusive claims, two basic dynamics are hypothesized: (1) that religious discourses, often closely conformed to actual conditions in local communities, enable early identification of crises; and (2), that religious imagination, often deeply sensitive to the lure of new possibilities and their embodiment, enables existing ways of seeing and acting to be transcended.

We explore this through three archetypal historical case studies that, taken together, articulate the *longue durée* of the history of religion and the health of the public.[3] The term "the health of the public" indicates that we are dealing with something more than the field of public health and epidemiology, though the case studies include both. All three cases reflect a particular faith tradition, Christianity, which thus acts as our evidence base; all narrate a capacity to cross the boundaries of a particular hegemonic discourse of health, challenging an existing paradigm and establishing the elements of a new one; and each begins with a practical crisis in the existing paradigm, whose underlying metatheoretical assumptions about health no longer address the crisis adequately.

MAPPING THE BODY: CHRONICLES OF CHOLERA

If one narrative defines the spirit and the method of epidemiology, the core science of public health, it is the fearful 1854 cholera outbreak in Soho, London, the legendary case of the Broad Street pump. Its usual hero is Dr. John Snow, physician to Queen Victoria, inventor of modern anesthesia. This famous tale, however, should include Henry Whitehead, the local curate, without whom Snow's breakthrough insight into the nature of cholera would arguably not have seen the light of day.

A new disease, cholera came from the Ganges river in India, transported by the growing trade network of European colonizers, and arriving in England in 1831.[4] The great scourge of the time in Europe and North America, "no disease in history had been so widely heralded,"[5] and it caused panic wherever it struck. Cholera thrives in closely packed urban environments lacking decent sanitation systems. Mysterious and nasty, "the blue death"[6] kills people rapidly and terribly. It spreads when the *vibrio cholera* bacteria are transmitted from one infected small intestine into another; so the germ has to be swallowed for the disease to spread. In the 1850s this was not known, which made it difficult to prevent or ameliorate the spread of the disease.

Having confronted it earlier before moving to London, John Snow suspected that cholera was ingested rather than inhaled, and that contaminated water was its primary means of transmission. However, the data he gathered on water supplies in South London, where the disease occasionally appeared, was insufficient to prove his theory. Moreover, against him stood the reigning view on the cause of disease: foul air. This "miasma theory" of disease, the most compelling medical orthodoxy of its day, was assumed by all the leading health and public authorities of the time, not without reason. After all, "The defining feature of the heavily overstressed towns in the nineteenth century was their stench."[7] If air does transmit illnesses like colds, influenza, or tuberculosis, the theory was useless in dealing with cholera. In addition, germ theory, only then emerging, would not be accepted as standard for some decades to come.[8]

When Snow suggested that "animalculae" in water caused cholera, he was disregarded or ridiculed despite his fame, widespread respect for his methodological acuity and rigor, and his status as a royal physician. Not a year after the Broad Street outbreak, the *Lancet*'s editor mockingly wrote that Snow's "theory, of course, displaces all other theories .... *Therefore* [*sic*], says Dr. Snow, gases from vegetable and animal decomposition are innocuous! If this logic does not satisfy reason, it satisfies a theory; and we all know that theory is often more despotic than reason. . . . In riding his hobby very hard, he has fallen down through a gully-hole and has never since been able to get out again."[9]

The Broad Street cholera outbreak gave Snow the *experimentum crucis* he needed.[10] Sudden in its arrival, vicious in its attack, within five days of the first case some five hundred people had died, with the number soon rising to seven hundred.[11] The local population fled in panic and fear. Nothing similar had occurred before, and it had a lot to do with the crowded, dirty, and unhygienic conditions of the rising industrial city of London, already packed with over two million people.[12] Broad Street was among the most densely packed areas, with up to fifty people in a house (also living in Soho then, in two rooms with six others, was Karl Marx), and it was filthy. Human noses are able to pick up miniscule concentrations of odorous chemicals, and such areas in the heyday of industrial development literally stank. The connection between smell and disease seemed incontrovertible.

Hearing of the outbreak, Snow, living not ten minutes away in Piccadilly, began to work, visiting the houses of eighty-three victims in two days,[13] enquiring what water they had drunk. Quickly he established the Broad Street pump as the common source and persuaded the local Board of Governors to remove its handle, despite their belief in miasma theory.[14] The epidemic subsided, and Snow began to work on the map that was to make his name as an epidemiologist.

On Snow's first version of the map, using data from personal interviews and Farr's *Weekly Returns*, a black bar marked every death, creating a "dot map" graphically depicting the distribution of cases in the area, with victims clearly concentrated around Broad Street. Edmund Cooper, an engineer, had made a similar map for the Board of Health, but it was virtually useless in establishing any clear pattern; it marked too much, including sewers, gullies, pits, ventilation areas, burial grounds, and more.[15] Snow's map incorporated one decisive element: a theory behind it. Since he was interested in where water was acquired, the pattern was far clearer, but still inconclusive if one viewed Broad Street as an airborne source of the disease. Moreover, one confusing fact could derail Snow's arguments, with the city authorities, about drinking water: many people living near the well did not get sick.

The person to provide Snow with the data needed to clinch the case was the local curate, Reverend Henry Whitehead. Locals were not happy about the Board removing the handle of the Broad Street pump, for this was the source of their best water and they had no reason to doubt that odorous air carried the cholera blight. Whitehead, who knew the neighborhood as no other, and skeptical of Snow's waterborne theory, assured the Board that he would "carry out such an inquiry himself with the aim either of confirming or refuting the 'Snovian' hypothesis."[16] So began the long process of visiting everyone he could find, some repeatedly, taking copious notes about those afflicted, recording the circumstances and—crucially—who had drawn water from the Broad Street pump at any time.

Gradually he debunked some popular theories: that sanitary conditions were causal (some filthy homes were spared, some of the cleanest not); that fear or a weak constitution were responsible; or that class status was crucial (measured by whether one lived in the lower or upper floors of a house).[17] Whitehead himself held three objections to Snow's hypothesis: the generally recognized and confirmed quality of the Broad Street pump water; his own personal experience in his pastoral visitations that many survivors of the disease drank copious amounts of the water without succumbing; and, a Paving Board inspection that found no fissures in the pump well or connections either to drains or underground sewer lines.[18]

Snow had by now shared his first report with Whitehead, who had also written on the epidemic. It helped Whitehead set aside his first objection, for Snow did not question the quality of the pump water. Instead, he suggested that a special contamination must be involved. However, it could not address the survival of those who drank lots of this water. Later it became clear that dehydration was the most deadly feature of cholera, and rehydration an effective antidote, explaining why those who drank large amounts of the infected water during their illness (one girl drank seventeen quarts in one day!) nevertheless survived. Moreover, because the highest intensity of contamination was short-lived, the death rate would have tailed rapidly after the first days, before the pump handle had been removed, indicating a self-cleansing mechanism in the well itself.

However, what had caused the initial contamination? In epidemiology, this is the index case, a crucial piece of information in determining the nature and spread of a disease. Snow had none; Whitehead provided it.[19] Searching the records, he noticed a brief reference to a baby Lewis who had expired in 40 Broad Street, directly abutting the pump, just before the epidemic began. The attendant doctor had reported the baby's diarrhea, but did not think it was cholera. Whitehead dug deeper. He knew the family, attending them in their illness, and now visited Mrs. Lewis, the surviving widow and mother. He established that for four days she had washed infected diapers in buckets, throwing some water into the backyard—a common practice—and some into a cistern in the basement of the house. This cistern was about two feet from the well, and its bricks were decayed and seeping. The pump well itself was now reinvestigated, and sure enough, soaking earth between the cistern and the well was found. The case was as good as sealed.

Throughout, and for some time after the outbreak, Whitehead went on locating people who had been in the thick of things, tracking the whereabouts of those who had fled, eventually interviewing 479 of the 896 Broad Street residents. This prodigious effort is hard to grasp unless one takes into account the intimacy of the tragedies for him as the person, responsible for his parish, who accompanied many of those who suffered and died or were left behind. His relationship with those who lived there allowed for his special contribution, and this peculiar advantage over Snow, of which he was aware, is seen in his own report on his work:[20]

> Long before the Cholera came upon us I was well acquainted with the street and its inhabitants. It so happened that during the outburst I was more in this street than any other, visiting very many of the families which suffered.... The ordinary

course of my duties taking me almost daily into the street, I was under no necessity to be either hasty or intrusive, but asked the needful questions just when and where opportunity occurred, making a point of letting scarcely a day pass without acquiring some information, and not caring how often I had to verify it in quarters where I rely upon a willingness to converse upon the subject.

Herein lies the key to our tale—and to Snow's second version of his iconic map. The parish Vestry Committee had meanwhile invited both men onto their investigating committee (other investigations included one by the General Board of Health, which refused to cooperate with the Vestry Committee). Snow thus began to add the details of Whitehead's investigations to his own data, and with this enriched data, reworked his map using a principle later formalized by Georgy Voronoi that traces patterns of proximity to key points. Snow included all water pumps in the area, focusing on the Broad Street pump, and instead of assessing distances as the crow flies, traced the time taken on foot from any particular house to the nearest pump.

The pattern was dramatic in its clarity; almost every arm of the star-like Voronoi diagram, with the Broad Street pump at its center, encompassed the otherwise inexplicable distribution of cholera deaths. Miasma theory could not explain this pattern. The few exceptions to the pattern could be explained on investigation too: some people preferred to walk further to fetch the better water at Broad Street rather than use a pump closer to them, whose water they found distasteful. The Voronoi map depended upon street-level knowledge of the behavior of ordinary people. It was able to "show lives, not just death," to indicate "the way the neighborhood was actually traversed by its residents."[21] It was an elegant and deservedly famous piece of epidemiology. Snow had spent only a couple of days there early on, however, and much of the data reflecting those lives came from Whitehead's dogged pursuit of information.

As Johnson puts it, "If part of the significance of Snow's second map lay in the way it empowered the community to represent itself, Whitehead was the conduit that made that representation possible. Whitehead was not an expert, an official, an authority. He was a local. That was his great strength."[22] Without Whitehead's persistent tracking of the lives (and deaths) of his parishioners, then, it is fair to say that Snow's work would have had little impact for lack of sufficiently persuasive evidence. Lacking Whitehead's direct access to the homes and workplaces of these traumatized and frightened people, their trust in him as their parish priest (though he acknowledges that he did not know everyone and faced some distrust among a few), and his intimate knowledge of their behavior and living conditions, Snow would more than likely have continued to suffer unabated ridicule. Moreover, until some future investigator finally established the case, cholera would probably have done far more damage than it did. Likewise, Whitehead was as decisive as Snow in challenging the prevailing paradigm of miasma theory, though he is neither celebrated in the annals of public health—nor is he entirely forgotten.[23] Working together, Whitehead and Snow resolved not only a critical public health problem but also undid a paradigmatic yet problematic construction of knowledge, miasma theory, no small matter.

Whitehead was not only a religious man, but also an ordained minister whose social intelligence had been developed through the normal work of a parish clergyman participating in and caring for its human beings, families, and social enterprises. It was his job to engage. Blending his personal curiosity and intelligence with a ministry of presence, caring, pathos, lament, and prophetic truth telling, his is a story of a form of religious health asset at work in a particular social context. However, even crediting Whitehead as Snow's intellectual partner does not quite get the story right, for it also ignores the Vestry Committee that decided to investigate the cholera outbreak. Recruiting both men, though they were initially at loggerheads with each other, the committee gave them the authority they needed to pursue their investigations and to publish their report in direct conflict with the city authorities.

The secularized world has difficulty seeing religion functioning except at the individual level. However, here we see religious health assets that are social in form, nature, and function. The Broad Street pump story is thus not just about one or two heroic individuals who found a way to join their respective insights and intellects. It is about a particular kind of community that held together the work they did and the passion they shared, from which they gained public purchase. More broadly, it is about how religion and the health of the public might interact. Historically, it represents only one development in the genesis of modern public health in which the religious mind and community have played a role.

ON NOT SEEING BODIES: LIMITS OF THE HOSPITAL

If London in mid-1800 was a center of globalization, then Geneva in mid-1900 has some claim to that title. Numerous global multilateral bodies were headquartered there in the post–Second World War reconstruction of international relations, including the World Health Organization (WHO). Earlier, in 1936, here too a rising Christian ecumenical movement established the World Council of Churches (WCC). Initially a mechanism for greater coordination and cooperation between worldwide missionary societies, the WCC rapidly became an influential body in international affairs. Among its many concerns was health.

Under the auspices of the medical missions of the eighteenth- and nineteenth century, hundreds, if not thousands, of hospitals and clinics sprang up in Africa, Asia, and elsewhere. By the 1950s, with the reshaping of post–World War II polity and economy, many medical missionaries had become increasingly self-critical of the work they were doing—not about their presence in various parts of the world, but about the limits to that presence. What they meant is that their care, however high in quality, was reaching far too few people, a concern that would subsequently inspire a paradigmatic revolution in health.

In a longer historical frame, because it has implications for our later discussion, it is worth recalling the origins of the hospital. Duffy believes that "[t]he hospital—as a place to undergo surgical procedures or receive treatment for major illnesses—is essentially a twentieth-century development," but that it was originally designed "to care for the sick poor or ill and destitute strangers."[24] Rosen agrees, noting that Roman *valetudinaria* or infirmaries primarily served the military, while the idea of the hospital fully emerged only later under Christian influence with "motives of benevolence."[25] At the time of Hippocrates, Greek *medici* or *iatroi* (doctors/physicians) shared their knowledge through societies (*koinon*) usually linked to worship,[26] and some may have been specifically responsible for public service (*iatroidēmosieuontes*), while sanctuaries to Asklepios, the god of healing, also existed.[27] Indeed, the earliest forms of the hospital might even trace back to Sinhalese culture under Buddhist influence around the fourth century B.C.E.[28] However, the key shift, Porter thinks, came with the emergence of hostels for "institutionalized charity" under Byzantine bishop Leontius (344–358 C.E.), *xenodokeia*, meaning "places for strangers."[29] An even more precise origin of the hospital may lie in institutions established by the Cappadocian Father Basil of Caesarea in early 370 C.E. These were independent of the monastery, where care for the sick was already common, and they were specifically dedicated to health care for all. Including the poor as a specific social category, van Minnen sees this as a "revolution in the organization of medical care,"[30] one which meant that "the Christian xenodocheion packed an ideological punch out of all proportion to its size and distribution."[31] What Basil did was to harmonize two distinct elements for "the necessary union of rational medicine with the distinctly Christian value of charity" to all, namely, "the markedly medical intentions he had for the institution he founded," and a clear directive to include "all passers-by who need somebody's attention."[32]

Under the Christian influence from the fourth century C.E. onwards, public hospitals spread, emerging in numerous cities,[33] and from the eleventh century, perhaps because of widespread illness and disease among Christian crusaders, they were to be found throughout Europe. One was Bedlam, the first for the mentally ill, whose name gave the English language a new word.[34] Throughout, the link between medicine, health care, and charity remained, shaped by an inclusive ethic and an orientation to the poor. It can also be traced in the later self-understanding of eighteenth- and nineteenth-century medical missions in Europe's newly colonized territories.

In these missions, the link sometimes produced deep tensions, especially between missionaries who happened to be doctors or others who saw their primary task as healing the body, and mission boards concerned primarily with evangelization.[35] Moreover, medical missions were not unambiguous blessings, with many medical missionaries generally dismissive of, even hostile toward, existing indigenous health practices, knowledge, and systems. They often also evidenced a systematic blindness to the effects of colonization on the health of colonized populations, and frequently served primarily the health of settlers, colonial administrators, and their military, rather than those who had been subjugated.[36] Nevertheless, positive dimensions to medical missions remained, and one of them was an intrinsic idea of service much like Basil of Caesarea's faith-based injunctions about inclusive access for all. So, for example, the Salvation Army in Natal, South Africa, at the end of the eighteenth century instructed its missionaries in every respect to "become Zulus to the Zulus" (other than con-suming alcohol), in effect ignoring reigning ideals of Victorian "civilization."[37]

Over time, leaders and doctors in the hospitals and clinics of the medical missions realized that their institutions were not adequately addressing the health of populations they served. Hospitals were treating no more than a small percentage of those who needed care, especially in rural areas. The relatively high cost of centralized tertiary medical care was another growing concern. Energizing a rethink of the role of medical missions was the mood of recon-struction of the post–World War II ethos, and the decolonization processes it inaugurated.[38] New ideas were needed to realign health assets at population scale with new insights on how to extend health care.

The WCC and its affiliates around the world provided exactly the right forum for a rethink of medical missions in the postwar decades. From the resulting fer-ment, fueled by voices raising similar questions elsewhere,[39] emerged ideas that helped inaugurate long-term structural shifts in health care, and not only in the context of Christianity or religion in general.

"Labels Cure Nobody": Transcending Exclusive Bodies

In the mid-1960s Malawi's Blantyre airport was the scene of a fortuitous encounter with long-lasting consequences. A skilled surveyor had arrived, com-ing to examine church-related medical programs in Malawi after three similar surveys of Protestant institutions in Nigeria, Uganda, and Kenya. These surveys were occasioned by the new responsibility placed upon local denominational bodies, because of decolonization, for programs and institutions inherited from external missions, especially hospitals and clinics. Inspired by the ecumeni-cal movement (from the Greek *ecuméne*, the "world as one household"), they were part of a concerted attempt to assess Protestant medical mission activities interdenominationally, with a view to the joint cooperation that now seemed imperative, especially where resources for health in needy communities were unconnected or misaligned.

The general secretary of the Malawian National Council of Churches, a member of the ecumenical movement, welcomed the surveyor. However, on this day, the roads from the airport into the city were closed for the arrival of the Lion of Africa, the Emperor Haile Selassie, the Ras Tafari, visiting Malawi's life president Hastings Banda. Having to wait until the hullaballoo around Haile Selassie was over, a chance encounter took place with the Roman Catholic bishop of Mzuzu who had flown in from dioceses in the north. When he learned of the mission of the surveyor, he immediately requested that Roman Catholic medi-cal programs be surveyed as well, and so began a process of enduring import for new alignments between Christian institutions and state health institutions in Malawi.[40]

The Christian denominations in fact controlled some 40 percent of all health facilities in the country, hospitals, and clinics in the main. They were no small part of the functioning national health system. Yet they had no place whatsoever in the Malawian government's development plan for health services, in part, as President

Banda had remarked regarding the twenty-six church bodies operating these various facilities, because "they are all playing in their own back yards and they never look over the wall."[41] To plan a national health system with them was too difficult. Unsurprisingly, then, the first recommendation from the survey, once completed, was that Christians should "disregard the labels on their doors which never cured anybody."[42] The consequence was the establishment of a single national Christian Health Association of Malawi (CHAM)—formed to coordinate activities, cooperate on developing the highest level and best distribution of health care, develop appropriate health personnel training programs, facilitate cooperation with state health services, and enter into joint planning with government. The President's response was to offer accommodation within the Ministry of Health.

A review of CHAM's work ten years later showed that, with support from international church-based partners from Canada and Ireland, it had taken on a broad responsibility for public health activities and outreach programs in a context of low per capita income and inadequate national financial resources. Equally importantly, because churches had close links through their congregations to local people, the association had begun to emphasize community health, and fully integrated preventive services.[43] What happened in Malawi was repeated in many other African countries, and today these religious health associations remain a highly significant part of their health systems.[44] They also reflect a trend toward community health that had other, related roots, deep within the WCC, of even wider significance for public health.

"No-one Heals Alone": Tübingen, the WCC, and the WHO

During the 1950s, medical missions faced a growing crisis driven by rising costs, competition from national state health facilities, and a destabilization of their identity as missions with something unique to offer. In 1964, to address these concerns, the WCC and the Lutheran World Federation called key stakeholders to an extended consultation in Tübingen, hosted by the German Institute for Medical Mission (*Difäm*).[45]

Querying the church's mission and ministry in health, the meeting concluded that health, beyond curative interventions for individual conditions, had to be understood in social terms.[46] Mission hospitals, driven largely by the medical model and its increasingly specialized, technologically driven innovations, not only reached too small a proportion of the population but also absorbed more and more resources. Health for all thus seemed utopian within this paradigm, and an expanded public health perspective seemed essential. It also brought into question the basic religious purpose of health and healing.

The participants at the first Tübingen meeting knew that compassion, discipline, responsibility, and a willingness to sacrifice for others were not virtues characteristic of people of faith alone. What then was characteristic, if anything? Their simple but profound answer lay in recognizing that no one heals alone: healing, they determined, incorporates the whole community; it is a mutual enterprise and an enterprise of mutuality, and it aims not merely at an individual person but at the totality of life. Tübingen I, one stream in a much wider river of doubt about the world's health systems in the postwar environment, generated further consultations on "a healing church," first in India, then in Africa. It also motivated the surveys that took place in Africa, including the one in Malawi. For Christians, above all, it acutely raised the question of the relationship between health and salvation or redemption. That, in 1967, was to be the theme of Tübingen II.

Again hosted by Difäm, this seminal consultation considered the question of the wholeness of the human being in society in relation to health. Dr. Robert A. Lambourne, a physician who had already written a considerable amount on the link between faith and health, provided a key preparatory paper. Intriguingly titled "Hospital Salt, Theological Savour and True Humanism," it took as incontrovertible that medical treatment in a hospital was meant to be a truly humanizing instrument. What then, he asked, does Christian faith have to say to clinical medicine in the treatment of an individual patient? His answer was forthright and forceful.

The humanizing vision of medicine, he bemoaned, had been displaced by the complexity of specialization, the growth of inanimate technologies, and the power of metrics. The consequence was a hospital environment that was less a place for the care of persons, including their "soul," than a factory for repairs. Worse, the epistemological basis of medicine had been eroded, reduced to a "concept of health as the absence of disease—a concern for rooting out objectifiable defects in isolated individuals."[47] Medicine's most basic rationale and modus operandi was thus increasingly less about life ("salvation") and progressively more about death ("evil"). Yet avoiding death, he argued, "did little if anything to remove the causes of sickness or to promote and maintain health."[48]

To be clear, Tübingen II held no enmity toward modern medicine, nor could it have—given the many physicians in its midst. Rather, drawing on theological notions of redemption, it sought to establish a new framework for understanding health. Medicine, it was argued, had to be located within a wider, holistic paradigm of health, including its social dimensions, attentive to the quality of life of all, and governed by the principles of love (esteem for the other) and justice (acting in accordance with the dignity of all).

Inspired by the thinking of Tübingen I and II, and supplemented by knowledge gained from the surveys of religious health services in Africa, the WCC in 1968 founded the Christian Medical Commission (CMC).[49] Dr. John H. Bryant, at that time writing a seminal work on health and the developing world, was its first chair.[50] Not designed to run programs, the CMC was intended as an enabling agent for people and organizations around the world who found themselves dealing with the same questions for the same reasons. Its only product would be a magazine, *Contact*. One aim of the CMC was to promote more effective use of resources for medical work through joint planning and action across six continents, including other religious communities, voluntary agencies, and governments. Another aim was to further study the foundations for this work in the Christian tradition.[51] Finally, it would establish links with appropriate United Nations agencies, particularly the WHO.

This last intention was propitious. Of the twenty-five people appointed by the WCC to the original Commission, eighteen were health professionals, and two of these were senior officials of the WHO.

Primary Health Care and the Social Body: The Role of the CMC

Dr. James McGilvray, a practiced hospital administrator and its first director, set the tone for the CMC. Deeply concerned about the growing dominance of "the medical model," he defined this model as "the provision of services by a whole range of professionals...(usually for a reward)" to those who seek help for a real or imagined disease, but with "an emphasis on specific, individual etiology resulting in individual cures with a tendency to concentrate on the disease rather than the total person."[52] This model shaped medical mission facilities equally, with a similar impact on the delivery of health care: increasing professionalization, rising costs as scientific discoveries brought more advanced technologies, and a specific structural effect, decreasing access to care for those who had lesser means.

Robert Lambourne provided the content for the first issue of *Contact*. A general practitioner in a working-class area of Birmingham, UK, he had served as a medical officer to an infantry battalion, had acquired degrees in theology and psychiatry,[53] and was a participant in Tübingen II. Again, passionately pursuing the crisis in medicine that was leading many to wonder whether healing lay outside, rather than with, the medical profession, he called the failure to deliver health care to the many people who needed it "the final injustice, the ultimate injustice" noting, "There is nothing so ultimate and so immediate as acts around your body-person."[54] The excellent medical services and care in hospitals increasingly existed only for those who could access them, he noted, a point oft repeated in *Contact*, so that the overall health status of poor or disadvantaged populations changed little.

As an example, Lambourne noted how little effect a "famous pediatric hospital in Africa" had had in its district on a persistently high infant mortality rate (about 282 in a thousand), though it was led by devoted Christian medical professionals offering excellent care over many years.[55] The situation changed only when a new head pediatrician, seeing the figures and noting the treatable or curable diseases afflicting many children, decided to train fifteen girls from the mission school as village health workers. Within five years, the infant mortality rate had dropped remarkably, to seventy-eight per thousand. "Now what was killing all those children before?" asked Lambourne, and answered himself, "A sacred, stereotyped view of excellence! That is, a graven image of excellence, tempting us to idolatry."[56]

Dr. John H. Bryant, chair of the CMC for many of its crucial years, not only shared these views but was also able to spread them, being a staff member of the Rockefeller Foundation, professor of medicine in Bangkok, director of the School of Public Health at Columbia University, and author of the seminal work *Health and the Developing World*.[57] Reflecting in *Contact* on the structuring of health services, Dr. Bryant reiterated the point that, despite massive efforts, "vast numbers of people do not benefit from modern knowledge and technology in relation to health." Moreover, he noted that the poorest, all too often excluded at every level, "are lost from sight; difficult to find."[58] Similarly, David Jenkins, a theologian who with Dr. Bryant shaped much of the Commission's self-understanding, wrote that the poor are "those who are not cared for and to whose care no prestige is attached," they are those who are "the neglected, the ignored, the unimportant, the rejected, the outcasts and dropouts of society at all levels."[59] Perhaps Dr. Bryant put it most succinctly: the poor are "they who are not."[60]

In the CMC, then, "[o]ne theme that recurred again and again was that the focus of care must change from the individual to the community which includes all individuals."[61] This meant designing an integrated system of care within which formal health facilities were linked to community care. "The direction for change," the CMC thought, "points to the adoption of a central concept in health care which recognizes the total needs of man [sic] in community." On this basis, the CMC called on churches to turn towards "comprehensive health care of man [sic], his family and his community."[62] More radically, it argued, "In the new healing ministry the community is the patient," and called for individual treatment and care to be placed within a "community ecology."[63]

Seeking to concretize this vision, the CMC actively searched for, and supported where possible, experiments in health care that offered glimpses of new models in practice. They could be found, driven by people who had struggled with the same questions, and who exercised leadership across the disciplinary and practical boundaries that normally were locked in place. Some inspiration came from introduction of community-based health workers, the so-called barefoot doctors, in the People's Republic of China.[64] Other experiments were uncovered in Indonesia, South Korea, Nigeria, India, and Thailand, and all were documented in *Contact*.[65]

The WHO became interested. The membership of the CMC certainly helped to attract attention, for it included Dr. Morley from the Institute of Child Health at the University of London, pioneer in Africa of the successful Under Fives Clinics, Dr. Taylor who was chair of International Health at Johns Hopkins University, and Dr. Bryant, the then dean of the School of Public Health at Columbia University. Crucially, however, the Commission also included two officially seconded staff members of the WHO. They regularly fed the substance of the CMC's work back to the WHO, including its formative ideas of just and equitable health for all (especially the poorest), of community or village based care as primary, of a specific focus on those not reached by existing formal health facilities, and of health as something other than the absence of disease. The CMC reports on the growing number of cases from around the world also demonstrated the viability of alternative practices compatible with greater access to health care, more equitable distribution of resources, and stronger rooting in the neediest communities.

It is no surprise, then, that the deputy director general of the WHO would approach the CMC in 1973 to explore closer cooperation, and the next year the director general himself, Dr. Halfdan Mahler, called a full consultation with the CMC to establish a joint working committee.[66] As a result, the WHO expanded the work that the CMC had begun on alternative experiments, and all of it was published in the influential 1975 WHO publication, *Health by the People*.[67] The concepts thrashed out in Tübingen and at the CMC were now global property, reaching audiences far beyond the confines of Christian agencies and denominations. The key principles were gathered under a new nomenclature that of primary health care. Introduced to the Executive Board of the WHO in December 1974, it was adopted in 1975 by the World Health Assembly, and three years later enshrined in the famous Alma-Ata Declaration, its slogan being "Health for All by the Year 2000."[68]

THE SURPRISING STORY OF SMALLPOX AND THE RELIGIOUS MIND

The Alma-Ata Declaration and its grand view of the possibilities of human action in the field of health reflect the overriding ethos of the times. Notwithstanding the shattering of earlier optimisms by two major wars and the horrors of the Holocaust and the atomic bomb, the post–World War II ethos was marked by renewed hope for progress driven by reason and science.[69] The wars had interrupted a dramatic globalization of the world political economy in the nineteenth century resulting from the industrial revolution and the colonizing enterprises of its major metropoles.[70] The interruption was now over, and new multilateral institutions such as the United Nations offered the possibility of coordinated global action in fields such as basic education, the sharing of scientific knowledge—United Nations Educational Scientific and Cultural Organization (UNESCO); children rights—United Nations International Children's Emergency Fund (UNICEF); labor—International Labor Organization (ILO); development—International Bank for Reconstruction and Development (World Bank); and health (WHO).

With the WHO, the idea of "global health" was born, a far-reaching convergence of ideas, institutions, and technologies. Primary health care, itself a radicalization of the idea of global health, was one outcome. However, there were also several dramatic developments of widespread import in the health sciences and the technologies they produced, such as the jet vaccination gun (allowing for simple and effective vaccine administration), the bifurcated needle (providing a consistently uniform and correct dosage of vaccine), and freeze-dried vaccine (making possible mass-immunization campaigns away from the electrical grid).[71]

By the 1970s, it was possible to think of immunizing entire regions to confront historically intractable diseases such as smallpox. The development and deployment of the polio vaccine had already moved immunization from being an individual privilege to being part of the social contract, a moral obligation to the whole public,[72] but engaging smallpox in severely underdeveloped countries in Africa required another order of imagination. At the time, the WHO and the Centers for Disease Control and Prevention (CDC) believed the only way to interrupt, and eventually eliminate, smallpox was to vacci-nate at least eighty percent of the total population, an approach termed "herd immunization."[73] However, the task in Africa failed under a heavy burden of logistical challenges.

On December 4, 1966, in an obscure corner of Nigeria's Ogoja Province, an entirely new strategy emerged, every bit as radical in thought and profound in effect as taking the handle off the Broad Street pump a hundred plus years earlier. Known as "surveillance and containment," the strategy demonstrated that smallpox could be treated and eliminated from large areas by immunizing as few as six percent of the people—if they were the right people at the right time! This astonishing possibility was demonstrated in anything but a tranquil environment, for this was Eastern Nigeria at the time when the region, which preferred to be known as Biafra, was embroiled in a brutal and eventually unsuc-cessful civil war.

As in the Broad Street pump story, the strategy rested on a combination of epidemiological creativity and rigor supported by the grounded intelligence of religious leaders able to draw on their religious health assets. Smallpox's Snow was Dr. William Foege, a long-serving and much awarded public health leader. But who was Foege's Whitehead? It was himself, in his alter ego as a Lutheran missionary in Nigeria, trained by the Epidemic Intelligence Service (EIS) of the CDC for his medical work, now doing what medical missionaries did in tiny bush clinics far from big cities.

In dealing with smallpox, Foege's religious mind was also at work. Called from surgery to take a radio message from a more remote missionary who sus-pected the beginnings of a smallpox outbreak,[74] Foege went immediately to the village, confirmed the case, and then convened a group of missionaries. Think like a "virus bent on immortality," he asked them; anticipate where and how the virus would go next.[75] Standard medical opinion of the time held that smallpox was so contagious that only full immunization of the whole population would stop it, but Foege had learned that smallpox was contagious for only two weeks, and relatively slow moving.[76] Moreover, it was not particularly infectious, and infected people rarely transmitted the disease to more than a few others, mostly within the immediate household, a view confirmed by later studies in India where "at no time were more than 1 percent of villages involved with smallpox (20 out of 2,331)."[77] There was time to react, therefore, even to anticipate where the disease might spread next. A window of possibility existed for surrounding a particular disease outbreak by vaccination and preventing its spread—provided one had sufficient intelligence about the human networks involved.

The vital key to this window lay in understanding the human context in which the virus traveled. It required, in effect, drawing a map of the contagion that, much like Snow's cholera map, was informed by knowledge of the way peo-ple actually lived and moved on the map. This is why Foege turned immediately to other missionaries. He knew fourteen of them in the region, and arranged to "meet" them every evening on the radio, comparing information about other sightings of smallpox. Each, in turn, used their extended networks of friends and members to go into every village and marketplace looking for signs of the disease. When an infected person was found, a map of his or her likely social pathways was drawn, and everyone on it immunized. However laborious, it was far more tightly targeted, efficient, and faster, than trying to immunize the entire population, especially one at war. From the initial six cases, four more were found in the first week. In the second week the radio network discussed twelve more, and another nine in the third week. By the fourth week, there was silence; the disease had lost its foothold and had, indeed, been defeated.[78] This became the fundamental logic on which the global strategy to eliminate small-pox rested. Applied subsequently in India, which presented an entirely different order of complexities, the last case was reported only nine years after Foege made that first radio contact with his fellow medical missionaries.

The initial impetus to eliminate smallpox in Africa came from the Soviet Union in 1958, based on early success in Latin America, not any global religious body.[79] However, once Foege and his colleagues had developed, tested, and successfully implemented their strategy of surveillance-containment, it was taken further. As it was extended, the web of smallpox surveillance moved from the passive professional disease-reporting model to an "active surveillance system" attentive to the whole social network. As the definitive article in the *American Journal of Epidemiology* reports, "Widely dispersed informal surveillance systems" included "other health services (malaria, leprosy), other governmental personnel (teachers, rural mail carriers, agricultural project personnel), local authority figures (village and area chiefs), and volunteer agencies, such as missions."[80] Striking here, however, is that the role of religious missionary actors is reduced simply to that of volunteers. This is a simplistic view that hides the richly complex religious mind operating with a deep sensitivity to the healthworlds of thousands of individuals. That, in turn, includes a capacity to draw on extensive and credible connections, and a capability for adapting to rapidly changing circumstances that allowed for the possibility of actively fighting a disease previously seen as an inevitable cause of suffering and death.

To be sure, religion can be unhelpful. In a region with high coverage rates Foege himself cites an unexpected outbreak of smallpox, because a group refused for religious reasons to participate in the immunization programs.[81] Similarly, in Benin, the power of deities was identified with the disease itself, which supported a self-defeating myth about its inevitability and invincibility, and gave authority to local healers who hid the disease, often out of economic self-interest, or who undertook practices that unwittingly spread it.[82] The religious imagination, not always attuned to change or a new idea, in this case the elimination of disease, should not be romanticized. Nevertheless, under the right conditions, properly appreciated and fully utilized, the potential of the religious mind for transformative interventions in health is considerable.

It is not the usual story, but it is fair to say that the intellectual breakthrough that doomed smallpox forever reflected an ensemble of insights, tested on a network of assets relevant to health, that were religious in nature. The most critical insight here is that the breakthroughs in the surveillance and containment strategy drew upon medical missionaries whose vital intelligence and creative imagination rested on their sensitive and credible presence on the ground, where disease most affected those among whom they lived and worked. It resulted from their participatory knowledge of human networks at very granular levels.

RECONNECTIONS: RECOVERING THE ROLE OF RELIGIOUS HEALTH ASSETS

That a deadly and horribly disfiguring disease could permanently be removed from human experience by systematic action was an unthinkable thought until it happened. What else, previously unthinkable, might be possible? The elimination of polio, measles, or more obscure blights such as guinea worm? Or, most basically, health for all? That last question, the most radical, demands an expansive imagination. The histories of Alma-Ata and smallpox eradication show that it included the religious imagination, which had shifted the prioritization of centralized clinical medicine offered by hospitals to the kind of life-changing health science possible "at the end of the road," upstream, extended into the reality of the tiniest village. If smallpox inspired thoughts of eradicating other diseases, primary health care inspired thoughts of extending to all the most basic promises of science. Each offered hope at different ends of the same tunnel: the great majority of diseases are transmitted in ways that are not as easy to interrupt and contain as smallpox, and most of them thrive in a complex stew of social, economic, and political reality that favors some people and not others. The idea of health for all is thus a grand vision situated within the hope of altering social conditions towards greater justice *and* mercy.

The best conclusion to the history of primary health care would be to declare it the archetypal success story of public health, but it is not, as we have indicated. The ideal of comprehensive primary health care, dissipated because of political, economic, and technical battles, was largely reduced to a limited, selective strategy that, by default, left much of the earlier paradigm intact and much unchanged.[83] The 1993 World Bank Development Report model for "Investing in Health"[84] was also largely "driven by economic and political ideology. There is little provision for ensuring equity in access to services, especially for people living in absolute poverty or the indigent."[85] In short, that noble but naïve WHO slogan, "Health for All by the Year 2000," signifies less an achievement and more, by cold contrast with the reality, a crisis, if not a failure, in public health at the end of the twentieth century.[86]

However one locates this crisis—at the door of medicalization, professionalization, the lure and cost of high-tech innovation, a market rather than a common good ethic, or, more generally, the uneven dynamics of contemporary globalization—the twenty-first century began with a realization of the loss of the original and driving vision of public health expressed by nineteenth-century sanitary reformers or the Alma-Ata Declaration in 1978. One way of dealing with that loss is to recover an emphasis on social transformation in health, of the kind that Basil of Caesarea, Snow and Whitehead, and the CMC would readily recognize. Fresh movements focusing on equity in health or the social determinants of health attempt just that.[87] Similarly, many, including the WHO, now call for a revitalization of the principles of primary health care,[88] with greater emphasis on civil society and a special interest in alignment and partnership with faith-based organizations working in health.[89] Moreover, some key figures who married the religious mind with primary health care or smallpox eradication did not lose the connection between religion and the health of the public.

This included Foege. Named as director of the CDC under President Carter, partly because of his role in smallpox eradication, Foege participated at Alma-Ata within months of his appointment. He also attended a quiet meeting in advance of that event that included a series of spiritual reflections by a professor from Valparaiso University, Dr. Tom Droege, also linked to the CMC. Droege, primarily interested in the intimate spaces of pastoral counseling rather than global transformation, nevertheless emphasized that all disease, and all healing, are connected—in the mind of God, and in human reality. If the pathologies are intertwined with each other, he suggested, so too are the generative forces of healing, justice, and mercy. This inspired Foege's imagination, releasing him from the impossible calculus of choosing eradication over primary care, physical over mental health, or public over private religious action.

Thus, in 1984, now at The Carter Center, Foege led a landmark conference on "Closing the Gap," which posed a simple question: "What can we already do to prevent unnecessary deaths and disability, and how can we get on with it?"[90] A full answer would require the active, creative participation of many people and institutions in society, and it would require great imagination. However, with what was already known, roughly two thirds of deaths before age sixty-five could be prevented (postponed, really, but that is a quibble).[91] Closing the gap would require the mobilization of the same broad social complexity as did active surveillance in Nigeria. The challenge is the social imagination, not technical innovation.

In 1988, three hundred religious leaders met at The Carter Center to consider the moral possibilities from this newly understood opportunity. Former president Carter, Foege, Surgeon General C. Everett Koop (secretary of Health and Human Services), Martin Marty (University of Chicago historian and public theologian), and Droege all spoke. The discussion focused on the social mobilization of religious networks, explicitly noting how the ideology of privatization undercut much religious imagination relevant to health: "One of the most perplexing problems for people who want to live out their faith traditions," said James Wind, "is the modern conditioned reflex that automatically turns religious beliefs, ethical questions and health-related realities into private matters. What is more, congregations have been understood and often understand themselves as zones of privacy, where religion is kept at a safe distance from the 'real world' of politics, economics, and the dominant social structures."[92] Could the opportunity for prevention join with the traditional religious moral commitment to mercy? If yes, what would that look like?

To work at this question, The Carter Center, funded by the Robert Wood Johnson Foundation, established the Interfaith Health Program (IHP) in 1992. Its mandate was to engage in what Foege called *reverse epidemiology*: "Where others look for early signs of pathology and the underlying pathogen, we look for effective community building and the underlying dynamic. Where most look for interventions that can stop the spread of disease, we are committed to interventions leading to an epidemic of good health."[93] The IHP, informed by a religious imagination that understood health through the broad lens of social determinants, took a comprehensive view of the possibilities for the faith networks to create healthy and whole communities, working to "develop conceptual frameworks that illuminate the most effective ways to describe the strengths of the faith community and how they can be aligned with the resources of the health/public health sector to achieve these shared goals."[94] Droege, retired but now associate director of IHP, pointed out that even if health leaders recognized that future improvements in health would come about only as people assume greater responsibility for their health and that of their communities: "This is a spiritual problem calling for changes in behavior, not a medical problem calling for a scientific breakthrough."[95]

Subsequently, the IHP established numerous faith health consortia across the United States and in Africa and Europe, trained lay congregational health promoters, played a catalytic role in developing Whole Community Collaboratives and, with the backing of the CDC, set up the Institute for Public Health and Faith Collaborations that trained "teams of health and religious leaders to address community-scale, underlying systemic conditions associated with health disparities."[96] At a further Carter Center meeting hosted by the IHP in 2002, inspired by the idea that "all assets and strengths of faith and health groups ought to be aligned with the most relevant public health knowledge and the most mature faith,"[97] another key initiative emerged, the significant and now widely known international collaborative of the African Religious Health Assets Programme (ARHAP).[98]

An interdisciplinary grouping of faculty and students from several African universities, Emory University, colleagues in Europe, and well-placed practitioners, in partnership with the Vesper Society in California, ARHAP was launched in December 2002 in Geneva. Here its founders also met with leaders of Christian Health Associations of Africa, and from here, the WHO later commissioned ARHAP to provide more than anecdotal evidence about the nature and significance of religious health assets.[99] Much of this book draws on these strands of activity. Taken together, they represent a growing body of work, matched to renewed interest from global public health actors, that reconnects the history of religion and the health of the public.

A close reading of that history reminds us that a half century ago a relatively small group of people, bridging the health sciences and faith, asked some basic questions about what might be possible. The unprecedented disarray from World War II and the reconstruction of global societies that followed, together with the rise of innovative science and technologies and the possibility of global action and coordination, required new thinking in health. Those people saw the opportunity in its novel complexity, and they understood the interdependence of ideas of science, theology, justice, prevention, healing, economics, and politics. They also had many connections to each other across the religious, disciplinary, institutional and guild boundaries that often constrain others, a key factor in the quality of their leadership.

Some of what they envisaged did alter dominant paradigms, if less than needed, and some of their effort helped achieve things almost hard to imagine, if only on certain diseases. Usually this is explained in wholly secular terms. Too seldom understood is the visionary capacity of those founding thinkers, a capacity resting partly on their deep connection to the lifeworlds of the people for whom it was all meant, partly on their imaginative transcendence of the limits of reigning orthodoxies, whether scientific or religious.

Fifty years of history is long enough to see a trajectory, but short enough to see the integrating threads of individual histories and organizations. This book stands in the intellectual trajectory whose history we have sketched in stories that are iconic for modern public health, taking the view that all of the key ideas that emerged then still matter, and that none can be left aside. Trees and ideas have seasons. There is good reason, in a different time and with additional insights, to think that a reconnection of religion with the health of the public faces a new spring. However, it will require an adaptive logic and practice in the face of complexity and unpredictability, one that works by putting together things that seem unlikely, even unthinkable within an established and secured existing logic.[100]

What challenges us is that the earlier ensemble of ideas lost coherence and energy as the fractures across disciplines and fields evolved into distanced and separate practices. This fracturing was neither necessary nor inevitable. What protects us from a sense of vast intellectual overreaching in this book is that this has all been thought before. That history encourages us to believe that seemingly intractable situations or apparent dead ends may, instead, be opportunities for transformation, and it recalls an integrative paradigm that we argue is both necessary and possible to renew.

3

RELIGIOUS HEALTH ASSETS: WHAT RELIGION BRINGS TO HEALTH OF THE PUBLIC

An integrative paradigm for religion in the health of the public begins in our thinking with the idea of religious health assets (RHAs). This gives the name to the work over the last several years of the international collaborative we helped found, the African Religious Health Assets Programme (ARHAP). Wherever we encountered others, the first puzzle, quite understandably, was what we meant by "RHAs" and why we were using this term. Explaining this, and laying the foundation for the interconnected ideas that follow, is our task here.

SHACKS AND SHACKLES: HEALTH IN THE ECOLOGY OF PLACE

Near the foot of Africa lies the peninsula known as the "Cape of Storms," a fifty-kilometer-long chain of mountains poking into the cold Atlantic Benguela current. Driving from the wealthy Atlantic coastal suburbs of Camps Bay and Llandudno into the beautiful Hout Bay valley, a stunning view of the bay unfolds, two peaks standing guard over the ends of a shimmering white beach. Looking left, the valley curls up toward the back of Table Mountain over which lies downtown Cape Town. Following the valley contour, a contradictory scene confronts one, a sprawling, tightly congested, and incongruous settlement of tin shacks and low cost houses spreading up to the last habitable space below the mountain crags. An occasional blackened area reminds one of huts destroyed by fires from a tipped paraffin stove or a fallen candle. The scene mars the panoramic beauty of the valley; it is aesthetically and ethically ugly. This is Imizamo Yethu, known as "IY" or "Mandela Park," home of the bulk of Hout Bay's black population, well over fifteen thousand people (no one knows for sure).

Most are there because work is nearby, or resources accessible that are scarce or missing in the distant rural areas from which the majority come. Some are refugees from Namibia, Nigeria, Malawi, and elsewhere in Africa. Very few trace their presence beyond a generation. Under Apartheid, Hout Bay was a largely white residential valley. Racialized social engineering moved black and "colored" populations from desirable parts of the valley into meager, cramped council housing on the slopes behind the fishing harbor or into shacks on sand dunes. The separation largely remains, along with the associated differences in wealth, privilege, and power. Recently, numbers of other, affluent, immigrants have arrived from Europe and elsewhere, people able to buy a second house in South Africa or acquire a property unaffordable in their native land. Hout Bay, containing a fractured population, is a global microcosm.

Mandela Park can be frightening; one sees open sewerage, scattered feces of animals, trash filling small gullies where children might play, and drug dens and drinking places whose customers are often unemployed young men with insufficient schooling, stilling their despair or simply living in anomie. Cases of sexually transmitted infections (STIs), HIV and AIDS, TB, hepatitis A and B, alcoholism, meningitis, and gastroenteritis have increased, and there is an alarming rise in mental illnesses. The place is a major health hazard. When winter rains come, sullied water cascades down the slopes into the stream that bisects the valley and ends at the beach, producing levels of pollution that far exceed even lenient public health standards and making swimming a hazardous affair.[1] IY is the result of racialized social engineering and, affecting the ecology of the entire valley and all who live in it, it is a symptom, an indicator, of the unhealthiness of the society within which it is located—a prime example of the link between individual health, and the social and environmental determinants of health.

Still, IY has a first rate health clinic served by dedicated professionals and supported by volunteers in an active Community Health Forum. The valley also has an excellent private medical center whose doctors often offer their services pro bono to individuals from Mandela Park, perhaps through an employer. Emergency services are readily accessible and highly efficient, referrals to public hospitals on the other side of the mountain relatively easily handled, and treatments generally free for low- or no-income patients. Altruistic professionals of all kinds offer assistance, while religious groups also do their bit. IY should be a success story, but it is not.

There are many ways to analyze this puzzle, and here too IY is not short-changed. It is a favorite location for university researchers and graduate students, NGOs and government departments, to the point where locals are sick of being the subjects of investigations that, in their daily experience, change little. Why do local governance and service delivery continue to fail over years? Think of all the contradictions.[2]

First, IY signifies deep inequalities, a toxic social illness.[3] A settlement it may be, but a settled community it is not. Besides the sea of affluence around it, within IY people compete intensely for jobs and services, factional interests abound, divisions between landlords and tenants are common, the presence of syndicated gangs is rife, street children prey on others, and an active, often abusive sex industry thrives. Not surprisingly, issues of security and aspiration, of identity and diversity, and of agency and access tax everyone. To seek health here faces one with a profound conundrum: the conditions that require intervention to achieve healthy outcomes are precisely those that thwart such interventions.

Second, the municipality can clear only a fraction of around nine thousand tons of human waste a week. Toilet facilities range from a few, shared water-borne stations to buckets that often overflow, producing greywater pollution, and dirty drains. An insufficient supply of fresh water exacerbates the situation. Public services generally are seriously limited, and residents see little reason to pay for them.

Third, increased services in Hout Bay pull people into the area from places that are worse off, exacerbating the problems whose systemic nature transcends local solutions. The city thus shifted toward a policy of "containment," simply trying to prevent new people from moving in, a policy that has also failed.[4] A high level of administrative and professional segmentation and duplication in the health sector complicates matters,[5] in turn hindering the work of organizations of civil society.

Fourth, IY is not a power-empty space.[6] Regular conflict between political or civic groups over control of local power structures occurs, while foreign migrants set up their own arrangements to protect themselves. Public agencies, thoroughly aware of these dynamics, are nevertheless bereft of means or ideas for dealing with them.[7]

All of this affects health issues. Earlier principles of primary health care that included a strong commitment to broad-based community involvement[8] are now largely reduced to the single issue of improving the quality of care. Similarly, earlier ideas of "empowerment" and "participation" have been replaced by supply-side thinking about health "users,"[9] a client-centered philosophy far less amenable to civic engagement or local agency. A policy of rational management has replaced the goal of local empowerment. These two contrasting approaches—one external, formal, and expert driven; and the other local, informal, and experience driven—create "an inevitable tension between participation and accountability...[and]...the need to technically manage the health system on a day-to-day basis...."[10]

The story of IY shows that environmental health challenges are not primarily technical, financial, or institutional matters. They are tied up with diverse human, social, and political conditions that inhibit or undercut financial, technical, or service delivery interventions. The human, social, or political side of the equation, of course, is not simple. Hidden agendas abound, and coded, indirect discourse rather than open encounter is common for people who live in a potentially hostile and risky environment.[11] The story of IY also reflects a general incoherence of purpose and vision, a fundamental disharmony in ways of conceiving issues, aims and goals, and a basic breakdown in relationships. What, then, would enable necessary minimum of social coherence to enable a durable transformation of the conditions described?

Most basic is trust, "...a crucial resource in the attempt to build a national health system that fulfils the expectations of equity, accessibility and quality,"[12] vital to any attempt to "liberate and mobilize human agency, to release creative, uninhibited, innovative, entrepreneurial activism towards other people," and thus increase the chances of cooperation and enhanced mobilization of resources and capacities.[13]

Trust, however, must be "generalized"—shown toward others who are strangers[14]—if it is to help create and maintain support for common social goods such as the health of the public. How does one achieve this? Froestad identifies four main challenges to the generalization of trust: domination, patronage, segmentation, and marginalization.[15] Following Offe,[16] he distinguishes between "civic communitarian" or "bottom-up" solutions to generating trust (associational interactions of citizens), and republican or "top-down" solutions (setting up trustworthy institutions). A choice between the two, says Froestad, should be avoided; better to conceive of trust as an interplay between them.[17]

Trust is "the belief that others, through their action or inaction, will contribute to my/our well-being and refrain from inflicting damage upon me/us."[18] Trust given is a risk taken, to be confirmed (or not) by an experience of trustworthiness. It is thus "a phenomenon of social reciprocity,"[19] which Gilson believes to be directly relevant to the health of the public, for "Health systems are inherently relational and so many of the most critical challenges for health systems are relationship problems."[20]

If so, then trust cannot be achieved through the instrumental rationalities of the economy or the state, but only through communicative rationality that pays attention to the discursive will formation of all citizens.[21] This includes taking seriously the validity claims of all relevant actors, especially those most affected by a particular condition or specific intervention. That, in turn, requires an appreciation of the lifeworlds of citizens, and how they utilize the assets, tangible and intangible, that they hold.

Therefore, into the heart of our work on religion and health over the last years, we have introduced the idea of RHAs. Initially a peculiar term, it is easy to stumble over. How is an asset for health religious? Why use the term "asset"?

CHANGING THE LANGUAGE: FROM DEFICITS TO ASSETS

Standard development perspectives would define IY as in need. Most literature on development, and the great majority of strategies, assume that needs are the conceptual starting points for any intervention or theory of intervention. Health is no exception.

What if we think differently? The goal of any developmental intervention, health included, is a sustainable overall improvement in the life of the target population. Two crucial measures of the quality of life are the extent to which individuals develop as persons in their capacities and capabilities, and how much this is mirrored in the community within which they live and find well-being. If we focus primarily on what individuals and communities lack or fail at, and what they need, then we face a major contradiction: we base action on the idea that one can empower people by building on what they do *not* have. This has two negative consequences. First, it ignores the strengths and resources that people do have, without which they would not survive at all. Second, it inherently invokes a dependency relationship because someone else must provide what is not there.

Undoing this contradiction means changing one's view of what is necessary. It means paying attention to what people have and building on that. It means ensuring that any external intervention enhances their capacities and capabilities by which they may better leverage what they do have or, where a need has to be met externally, use more effectively what is provided.

Such an approach has an element of justice, if we mean by that at least the importance of respecting human dignity: it requires that one take seriously the human beings for whom an intervention is intended, including their lifeworlds. These lifeworlds are often deeply imbued with religion, a faith, or a spirituality of some kind, including grand institutionalized traditions such as Judaism, Islam, Christianity, Hinduism, and Buddhism, and other, less institutionalized forms of "indigenous" traditions that are expressions of the life of a community.

Herein lies a particular challenge. Paying attention to lifeworlds requires something more than the decontextualized or ahistorical measures and metrics governing most policy frameworks of states and international agencies, for which the legibility of human behavior is the most fundamental requirement.[22] Indicators, cost-benefit calculations, cartography, demography, and the like may be necessary for modern, large-scale societies, but their tools, methods, and intellectual frameworks generally produce only a thin description of the human beings who actually populate society. How, then, do we aim for a useful but thick description of human beings?

We begin with Kretzmann and McKnight's idea of asset based community development (ABCD),[23] which places an emphasis on assets already available to people in their situation upon which one may construct an acceptable, sustainable intervention.[24] This represents a profound, paradigmatic shift toward taking seriously the local experiences, knowledge, and understandings of the people for whom development is intended. Its "three simple, interrelated characteristics" include: start with what is present rather than with what is absent in the community; place the stress upon "the primacy of local definition, investment, creativity, hope and control"[25]; and, focus on the human relationships that create and sustain the networks that can build the asset base of the community.[26]

A second, complementary theoretical frame is "appreciative inquiry," which addresses the role of the "outsider" in any intervention. Outsiders quickly encounter multiple, often competing interests, patterns of thinking, ways of behaving, and forms of legitimacy and authority; all have an immediate bearing on whether any proposed strategy is likely to succeed or not. People do resist interventions when they feel their own experience, wisdom, and contextually derived knowledge are insufficiently respected. Illusions, skewed or coded discourse, and disguised behavior all express what Scott calls "the arts of resistance" in the face of external power or authority.[27]

Appreciative inquiry also signals a shift from literal to participatory knowledge,[28] from an expert-determined understanding to a mutually exploratory one that seeks to connect memory, vision, discovery, and planned action.[29] Against the incapacitation common to those confronted with an overwhelming sense of deficit, appreciative inquiry evokes what Elliot calls the heliotropic principle of organizations—a move "toward what gives them life and energy."[30]

ARHAP uses these ideas in identifying and enumerating RHAs and in trying to understand what kinds of agency move these assets from rest into action.[31] The specific tools are less relevant, but the shift in language is critical. It changes the way one frames everything, including practice. Words are powerful, as Humpty Dumpty reminds us in his conversation with Alice: "The question is, which is to be the master—that's all."[32] The label "RHA" is an invention, with a serious purpose and rationale: to question existing conventions, to establish a different master for the requisite cognitive framework, to allow for further thought, to break open new thoughts.[33] The idea has raised two common critical responses, one on religion, and the other on the economic language of assets.

Health scientists do not often think of religion as an asset; they more likely think of it as a liability. A medic whose patient, on religious grounds, refuses or subverts treatment, is understandably upset; health professionals confronted with pervasive patterns of stigmatization through religious dogmas that undermine effective responses to HIV scream in frustration. Secularist ideologies, even if weakening, add to this disdain for the religious. One can write tomes about the negative effects of religion, and many have.[34] That religion may be a liability for health is clear enough. Its liabilities must be plainly addressed and either sidelined or confronted. At the same time, given the vast positive contributions to health that religious people or entities make to the health of the public, paying attention to the liabilities of religion is not enough. It is, we think, both disrespectful and strategically irresponsible to ignore those religious assets that can be discerned, built upon, and supported.

What about assets? Using the language of market economics to talk about the health of the public invokes potential contradictions, especially as their health cannot be reduced to cost-benefit calculations or rational choice theory. We take that as a permanent warning. Nevertheless, we retain the term for one major reason—the shift it signals from the needs or deficits-based approach to health that has largely been inadequate, toward an appreciation of what people have upon which we may build—including such intangible "assets" as dignity, trust, and compassion.

The term "RHAs," then, reflects first, a heuristic intention to press open the boundaries of contemporary discourse about religion and health, and second, an interest in investigating the phenomena that might count as religious assets, and of finding ways of understanding their significance for health in general and the health of the public in particular.

WHAT ARE RHAS?

Proton beam therapy saves the lives of people for whom there is no other hope, focusing enormous energy at subatomic scale to defeat disease in previously remote reaches of the brain. The equipment takes up about four acres, costs roughly one hundred and fifty million dollars, and is complex enough that even attending physicians find it hard to grasp exactly what it does. Most life-saving techniques and technologies are not at all like this. The real problems and opportunities of twenty-first-century health policy are at the other end of the spectrum—not subatomic, but at the level of families, congregations, and communities.

Think of a father in Memphis, admitted to an extended care hospital with eleven bedsores acquired in a bad nursing home. His distraught son and daughter, shocked that this could happen to a man who had led an honorable life, wondered about suing somebody—but simply held his hand. Nurses tended his wounds, which gradually healed, but now his family faced the hard work of navigating the next stage in his journey. With harsh insurance limitations, on what, upon whom could he depend for help outside the hospital walls? Who cares? What nursing home will receive him to sustain his healing? His widely scattered family may visit, talk, pray, and read to him—crucial healing experiences all— but who will help his family to help him find his strength and his capacity to be an agent is his own life?

Cost and payment are the relatively easy policy questions; the hard issues involve things that cannot simply be bought, but can only be nurtured. Three words usually left out of policy debates are critical: journey, cycle, and assets. The first two are fairly obvious: health is a journey, not just a disconnected list of expensive medical events; and the relationship with the medical system, given that most conditions can be managed over time, is less a series of events than a cycle. The third requires noticing the assets we have to work with in any person's journey of health.

This father's family discovered a wealth of religious assets around them, mostly intangible but real. They are long-term members of a covenanting community in the Congregational Health Network (CHN), an innovative extension of care, otherwise confined to hospital walls, that is now part of the Methodist Le Bonheur Healthcare system in Memphis. Their pastor is an experienced chaplain who, over time, has developed extensive caring capacities. In his congregation, every member is part of a small group tended by a trained volunteer, one of small group is a friend of this family. Such deep social assets, Ellen Idler believes, explain why participation in a congregation over time is powerfully associated with life span health.[35]

However, the story only starts with the congregation. The administrator of the extended care hospital attends a related church and, besides her professional skills, because of her own experience of pastoral care, she is deeply sensitive to the family and the supportive role of the congregation. The nurses tending the father's wounds were glad to welcome the pastor and the volunteer ministers into the healing relationship, praying with them naturally and gratefully. All these assets were already present, some reimbursed, others not, some material, others spiritual. But for the critical role of the CHN "navigator" who works for the hospital, doing the mundane labor of identifying, connecting, and aligning its human webs of trust and caring, those assets would remain disconnected and ineffective.

Not all places have the abundance of religious assets one finds in Memphis, but faith of some sort is endemic and ubiquitous wherever human communities grow. If faith can be toxic, it can also be generative. Participation with a worshipping community, for example, is often associated with a quality life span and good health. RHAs generally are increasingly recognized as potentially crucial components of a comprehensive, sustainable strategy for advancing health. To mobilize them, however requires new, sophisticated understandings of the interwoven logic of faith and health, new ways of linking social and scientific approaches, and a new set of leadership capacities to make it work.

This goes beyond technique, management, or instrumental science. Much hangs on who actually lives on any map of RHAs, and how they live. Because we are dealing with living, acting human beings, one needs, figuratively speaking, a three-dimensional map, one that integrates science with the lifeworlds of human beings. Seeing the assets is good, aligning them better, and sustaining a web of trust to hold and enhance them the best. But how does one "see" a RHA, especially if many are intangible?

ARHAP's earliest definition described RHAs as "a kind of endogenous resource that may be leveraged for dealing with health crises as part of public health policy and practice."[36] Because this is not very precise, a strong interdisciplinary working group sought a clearer view, generating an impressively long list of tangible assets (such as religious hospitals, chaplains, traditional healers, and care groups), and intangible assets (such as prayer, rituals, and networks). The question was how to organize them usefully, and the result was a matrix built around two basic distinctions: tangible or intangible RHAs, and proximate or distal health outcomes.

The matrix has the virtue of bringing into view intangible phenomena, not often considered, that may well be vital to health. The proximate-distal divide is more complicated for, as Nancy Krieger points out: "[It] inherently cleaves levels rather than connects them, thereby obscuring the intermingling of ecosystems, economics, politics, history, and specific exposures and processes at every level, macro to micro, from societal to inside the body."[37] For this reason, we are adamant that the notion of RHAs should be read in conjunction with its other necessary companion concepts in this book, and not as a standalone concept, when it could easily fall prey to the obscurations Krieger identifies. The four-quadrant matrix in figure 3.1 represents a useful starting point for thinking about RHAs. Its axes should be seen as continuous (reality is not neatly boxed), and used primarily as a heuristic tool.

The RHA matrix plays three crucial roles. First, it alerts us to the complexity of religion in the context of health, usefully discriminating between different kinds of religious assets. It thus alerts us to a different way of seeing health and religion, which impacts on one's analysis of the reality before one.[38] Above all, it calls attention to what is so often missed in inventing strategies for public health, the diverse and widespread ways in which religion is part of the picture.

Second, it alerts us to phenomena normally not "counted" or measured in health data, or regarded as of evident significance for science or polity. Yet intangible assets like motivation, trust, or a principled orientation to the suffering,[39] are likely to foster the health of individuals and communities. Hard to measure directly, like goodwill in financial accounting, intangible assets probably can be discerned through proxy indicators, and may well be a vital element of many positive health outcomes.

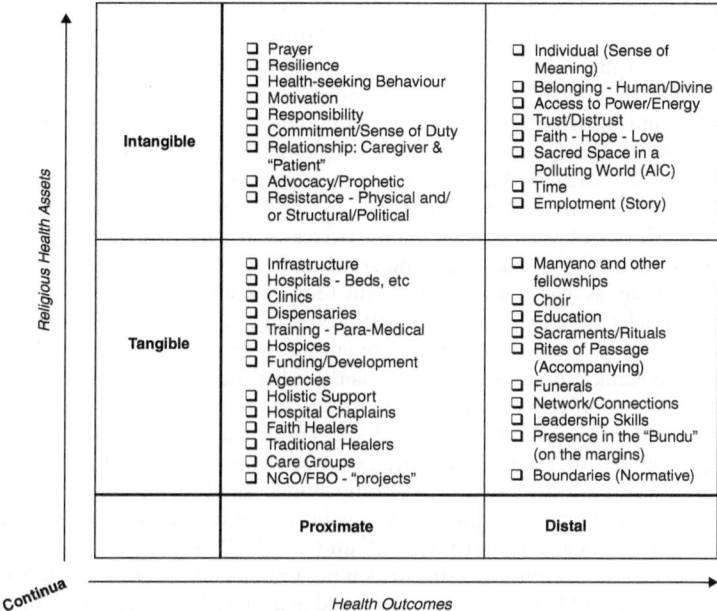

		Proximate	Distal
Religious Health Assets	**Intangible**	❏ Prayer ❏ Resilience ❏ Health-seeking Behaviour ❏ Motivation ❏ Responsibility ❏ Commitment/Sense of Duty ❏ Relationship: Caregiver & "Patient" ❏ Advocacy/Prophetic ❏ Resistance - Physical and/ or Structural/Political	❏ Individual (Sense of Meaning) ❏ Belonging - Human/Divine ❏ Access to Power/Energy ❏ Trust/Distrust ❏ Faith - Hope - Love ❏ Sacred Space in a Polluting World (AIC) ❏ Time ❏ Emplotment (Story)
	Tangible	❏ Infrastructure ❏ Hospitals - Beds, etc ❏ Clinics ❏ Dispensaries ❏ Training - Para-Medical ❏ Hospices ❏ Funding/Development Agencies ❏ Holistic Support ❏ Hospital Chaplains ❏ Faith Healers ❏ Traditional Healers ❏ Care Groups ❏ NGO/FBO - "projects"	❏ Manyano and other fellowships ❏ Choir ❏ Education ❏ Sacraments/Rituals ❏ Rites of Passage (Accompanying) ❏ Funerals ❏ Network/Connections ❏ Leadership Skills ❏ Presence in the "Bundu" (on the margins) ❏ Boundaries (Normative)

Continua → Health Outcomes

Figure 3.1   Religious health assets matrix.

Third, the matrix points to the internal sources of belief and action, their own self-understandings and worldviews, that drive the generative impulses in religious or faith-based communities relevant to the health of the public, and which explains their motivations, commitments, attitudes, actions, and relational or associational strengths.

In general, RHAs are better grasped as living organisms than material objects. They remain passive, "at rest," however, unless they are used or animated (in the French sense of *animateur*, the one who drives or galvanizes something). This introduces the question of agency, to which we also turn in due course.

The Tangible and the Intangible

Tangible RHAs are most easily identifiable and include care groups, congregational programs, NGO-styled bodies, campaigns, events, healing movements, religious hospitals, clinics, dispensaries, and intermediary organizations that provide medicines or specialized technical expertise. We know from some limited inventories of RHAs in Africa that religious organizations are widely active in African health. For example, one six-country study indicates that some form of support for AIDS-related orphans is present in 539 of 563 faith-based organizations (FBOs) surveyed (including 401 local congregations), and that they use more than 7,000 volunteers to help more than 139,000 orphans and vulnerable children.[40] Often recognized or accounted for in national public health systems and polity are formal facilities—hospitals, clinics, and dispensaries run or funded by religious bodies.[41] Most other tangible assets are misunderstood, overestimated, undervalued, unrecognized, or unaccounted for, invisible, and no one knows their combined scale and contribution to public health. At the least, then, grasping how religion generates fitting assets for health demands some better appreciation of the tangible assets religious communities have accumulated and built.

Important as that is, it would still only touch the surface, for even less is known of the broader range of intangible health-promoting religious assets. Understanding them is also necessary,[42] for they represent much of the volitional, motivational, and mobilizing capacities of religious faith, belief, behavior, and ties, themselves rooted in vital affective, symbolic, and relational dimensions of human life that might contribute to health. They push us to understand more about local knowledge about health, the trust so crucial to effectiveness, people's life span journeys of health, and existing patterns of accompaniment on this journey.

Understanding intangible RHAs has been part of the work of ARHAP on the eastern seaboard of South Africa,[43] and, for the World Health Organization, in Zambia and Lesotho.[44] In this work it became clear that people on the ground frequently regard best practice to be linked heavily to less visible, intangible elements, and in several workshops, for example, "compassion" and "love" were rated as most important, by both providers and health seekers, to enduring health.[45] It would be simpler to ignore such data, of course. Intangible assets are not readily susceptible to metrics, being impossible to quantify directly and largely qualitative in nature, and so they are very difficult to take into account in determining how and whether they positively affect health outcomes. Moreover, qualitative data is often regarded skeptically, which is not helped by an overreach of theoretical claims based on such data.[46]

Despite these difficulties, the task of properly understanding intangibles remains and, indeed, RHAs will not be well understood without them, for to concentrate on the tangibles alone would be to miss many crucial dynamics that play a role in whether or not a particular tangible (e.g., a clinic) actually works as a positive asset for health.

The Question of Agency

Assets, we have noted, remain "at rest" and are of no practical benefit unless they are utilized, that is, acted upon. Habitual acts may leverage particular assets, but being essentially nonreflective, they change nothing. Positive change or transformation in health requires more than habitual action. It requires agency.[47]

What is agency, how is it exercised, and what motivates or inhibits it? A common theory of agency views it largely in relation to a principal who contracts with an agent for particular purposes.[48] The agent, in turn, "acts for" the principal. This exchange-relations idea of agency drawn primarily from economics and contractual law contains, anthropologically speaking, a thin view of the human being. It also assumes an asymmetry of power (principal over agent) with an associated disparity in information, interests, ends, and risks. Here the principal controls the relationship, defining the nature of the exchange, and monitoring (policing) the agent, whose satisfactory performance depends upon measurable "deliverables" or "outcomes." These four elements—contract, asymmetry, deliverables, and control—are ubiquitous in the global political economy of our time. However, as Shapiro notes, it is an acontextual, ahistorical, and static view of agency, so that "blind to the asymmetries of power that course through these relationships, classic agency theory . . . is profoundly conservative, even dangerous."[49]

Another understanding of agency lies at the heart of the idea of RHAs, more like yeast as the agent that causes bread to rise. It is the cause whose action produces an effect, the "power to act" that resides in what it means to be human. Constraints on the human power to act mark what Ricoeur calls the beginning of "the reign of suffering,"[50] a powerful clue to understanding what makes for health or illness. This view on agency preempts the idea that outside agencies are the key to transformation. It emphasizes the importance of paying attention to the power (or lack of it) to act by the intended recipients of any health intervention.[51]

Health providers and leaders of health systems are continually second-guessing how those for whom their services are delivered, the recipients, will respond. Even well conceived and implemented interventions may falter when intended recipients (agents in our sense) respond in ways that frustrate or ignore their planned parameters. A more effective relationship between providers and users thus probably needs at least two key aims be met: embedding health provision and care in mutually determined relations of trust; and, appropriately addressing the usual asymmetry of power between providers and users, which at least means paying attention to what users value and what assets for health they hold that can be strengthened.

The first, trust, is not easy to establish for many reasons; yet trust (or its lack) is often diagnostic of the likely impact of any health intervention. Enhancing agency ("the power to act") and ensuring that institutional structures are set up accordingly is likely to increase trust, however. Here one may invoke (with suitable caution) the value and strength of religious ties, virtues, and values embodied in local contexts and communities, those positive qualities of religion that rest in lifeworlds that endure over time. Then it becomes possible to think about how to root interventions in local contexts durably, sustainably, and in ways that enhance the agency of those whose health is at issue.

RELATED IDEAS

The concept of RHAs can usefully be related to, or distinguished from, other current concepts. One, human capabilities, is of particular importance to us; another, spiritual capacity, is as here defined our invention, the subject of an ongoing research program in which ARHAP has partnered with several other institutions to probe male interpersonal violence.

Human Capabilities

An assets-based approach is highly compatible with Sen's and Nussbaum's important idea of human capabilities,[52] which is contrasted with the idea of human functioning. A functionalist approach tends to imply an accommodation to the way things are, whereas a capability approach points toward the way things could be. Where patriarchy is very strong or poverty particularly deep, for example, a "happy" acceptance of the way things are may be crucial to one's continued functioning, and challenging the status quo pointless or too costly; change is not preferred.[53] A raised consciousness about what "could be" in the same circumstances may lead to "unhappiness" with the way things are, and a preference for change. So preferences are not the real issue. They could be conservative or transformative, and they tell us little about what ought to be. Basing social order on preferences (or "rational choice") rather than capabilities thus inherently sidesteps the normative and ethical foundations of the good. A capabilities approach, however, which identifies several capabilities that are central to full human being,[54] emphasizes one's "power to act." It has the virtue of respecting persons, their preferences, and their quality of life,[55] while simultaneously valuing a concern for justice.

Applying these thoughts, it is clear that mapping or identifying RHAs only in relation to how they function in a person or community's life changes little or nothing, an unhappy thought in the face of the crises in the health of the public we face. This has nothing to do with the character of any particular RHA, and everything to do with neglect of the ethical demand for the good, which must necessarily ground any substantive notion of health and well-being. For that, we need a framework that, while appreciating the *informed* desire of the part of the relevant subject(s), places it within a vision of the *substantive* good.

ARHAP's approach to assessing and leveraging RHAs begins with a focus on "informed desire," by exploring the knowledge, wisdom, and experience of the intended recipients of health interventions. Its key research tools (Participatory Inquiry on Religious Health Assets, Networks and Agency, or PIRHANA)[56] produce data on such informed desire. A mapping of that desire, however, still needs to be placed within some notion of the substantive good. Otherwise mapping and assessing RHAs becomes merely another functionalist activity with little impact on transforming the conditions of the health of the public, of contributing to what is necessary to achieve health and well-being for all.

Community Capacity and Spiritual Capital

Health professionals and scholars are not unaware of the potential importance of community assets or human capabilities. Neither idea is far from the "community capacity" model inspired by the 1988 Institute of Medicine report on *The Future of Public Health*,[57] which "issued a call for public health organizations to reorient their activities to ensure conditions for health and give prominence to the community as not only the logical setting but also the catalyst for health promotion."[58] Related to this is the "ecological approach" to health that takes seriously "the interdependence of people, institutions, services, and the broader social and political environment."[59] Similarly, the "community capacity" model links population health status to ecological factors, community capacity, and health and human services systems.[60] Chaskin's influential definition of community capacity in fact closely approximates our RHAs approach:[61]

> Community capacity is the interaction of human capital, organization resources, and social capital existing within a given community that can be leveraged to solve collective problems and improve or maintain the well being of that community. It may operate through informal social processes and/or organized efforts by individuals, organizations, and social networks that exist among them and between them and the larger systems of which the community is a part.

An ecological model linked with a notion of community capacity to some extent addresses the link between assets, agency, and social context. However, at least as conveyed by the literature, it does not deal with the question of asymmetries of power, which is foregrounded by the key idea of human capabilities, and it does not consider the "vulnerability context" of a community—shocks, stresses, and seasonality; policy, laws, and institutions; and, culture, religion, and customs—that constrain the opportunities and choices people have.[62]

If the notion of community capacity has some relevance to the concept of RHAs, another that has been seen as relevant is spiritual capital.[63] A highly elastic concept, it has been linked to the ideas of both human and religious capital.[64] Generally interpreted within an economic paradigm, it links religion to patterns of consumption as a way of explaining how religion functions in society. Similarly Verter, relating spiritual capital to Bourdieu's notion of cultural capital, defines it as the "Spiritual knowledge, competencies, and preferences [which] may be understood as valuable assets in the economy of symbolic goods."[65] Berger and Hefner invoke Max Weber's analysis of the "spirit of capitalism" in Protestantism.[66] In every case, the primary interest is in the implications of varieties of spiritual capital for markets and democracy.

Woodberry, however, takes a somewhat different tack. The advantage of the metaphor of spiritual capital, he believes, is that it helps us "see religion as an investment and as a distinct end...that cannot be reduced to money or sex or power....[It is a resource] that people draw on to meet various challenges—sickness, political oppression, ethical choices, or social problems."[67] He warns at the same time against a reductionist view on human behavior, noting that religion is not just a means to particular ends, particularly personal profit, but "also concerned about shaping which ends people seek."[68]

Spiritual Capacity

"Spiritual capacity" might be treated as one among many "intangible RHAs," but it is better understood as a metareality that animates them all. It has, ipso facto, something to do with human spirit and spirituality. That does not mean that we are forced into a secular view, for it is not incompatible with any faith in some transcendent givenness or radical otherness. Similarly, seeing it as a generalized human capacity does not mean that it appears everywhere in the same form, for it will always be embodied in particular conceptions of faith and experiences of history and place, expressed in specific symbols and images, languages and discourses, practices and actions, relationships and institutions.

Spiritual capacity, then, is embodied in human persons and their communities as a dynamic life force, and it should be possible to identify where and how that is so. One could probe spiritual capacity by enumerating its concrete cultural and historical expressions and trying to identify some common denominator, but that would present one with a multitude of diverse, empirical, contingent, and changing forms of spirituality that mark people's experiences and practices—a bewildering sea of possibilities.

We begin instead with the insight that the human person has the astonishing capacity to imagine something that does not exist in nature and to bring it into being (a hoe, an x-ray machine, or a liver transplant, for example). We add to the world what is not already there. We do this with things of nature (governed by its laws) and with social and living arrangements (governed by the moral law or that which "ought" to be). In Judeo-Christian tradition, this is one meaning of the claim that we are created in "the image of God."

Even if *actuality* necessarily constrains us (to build a bridge, we must abide by the laws of gravitational and tensile forces), this transcendent capacity means that we are not bound by the way things are. We are also creatures of *possibility*, able to envisage the way something could be and to actualize it, de novo. This is the root and power of our *creative freedom*, and it obviously includes destructive possibilities. Our sense of transcendence also allows us to grasp the possibility of transcendent reality generally, which both animates our desires and expresses our hopes. This is what religious traditions seek to articulate in their own way.

Spirit is thus rooted in creative freedom—never in isolation from others— and *spirituality* is the way we express that truth (in incredibly diverse ways). However, if the human capacity for creative freedom can be turned to destructive ends, then we are faced with the question of freedom for what purpose, to what ends? Answering that question gives rise to communities of spirit who share similar ways of expressing it materially, relationally, ritually, and symbolically.

Instead of speaking about "spiritual capital," then, we speak of "spiritual capacity." There are probably many other indicators of "spiritual capacity" to consider, but four are worth considering as a start. The first draws on Victor Frankl's reflections on survival in a Nazi concentration camp, where he developed his idea of the *Trotzkraft des Geistes*, which might be translated as "the Nevertheless-power of the Spirit."[69] It is a refusal to be constrained by the actual when new possibilities for generative life can be envisaged and acted upon. Partially echoed in the idea of "resilience," it can also be linked to religious concepts such as the Islamic notion of *fitra*, the innate capacity for envisioning "goodness," embodied in the power of imagination, resistance, and freedom.

The second is awareness of world/self, which can readily be related to the Buddhist tradition of "mindfulness," for example. It represents an embodiment of a capacity for reflexivity and inclusivity. The third goes one-step further in the direction of dignity and respect as the key indicators of spirit. Clearly related to and enhanced by "awareness," it suggests more directly a capacity for morality, both in intention and in action, with the "ought" that we profess or embody. It would be linked to our transcendent purposes and ends expressed in the enhancement of creative freedom, of justice, and of well-being—as general principles applied to all and not merely as individual aspirations or inclinations. Fourth, in accordance with a holistic, ecological sense of life as suggested by notions such as *bophelo*, such a morality, being inclusive and expansive, has to do with a regard not just for selves, but also for the world in general, including the material and environmental conditions that govern our lives together.

Finally, like the idea of RHAs, even as it prevents us from ignoring that which causes death, including the significant disparities in health and inequities in health provision that affect the great majority of the world's populations negatively, it pushes us to consider health from the point of view of that which enhances life.

EXPLORING RHAS AND THEIR VALUE

An obvious question about RHAs is how to determine which of them are worth serious attention, for, inevitably, not all RHAs are equally valuable for enhancing the health of the public. The value for positive health outcomes of any particular RHA compared to another or against "secular" health assets no doubt needs further exploration. Here we do no more than introduce certain points of view that may help to guide such exploration and discernment in future.

"Levels, Pathways, and Power"

RHAs occupy certain social spaces and particular places, varying in level and changing over time. Here we follow a clue from Nancy Krieger's critique of proximal-distal ways of thinking, that understanding RHAs well requires us to develop "explicit language about levels, pathways, and power."[70]

Among the important pathways—intangible configurations of space—relevant to many RHAs are the larger networks within which they are embedded, the way in which they represent ties to others. Using the idea of social capital, these ties bond, bridge, or link people, and they may do so in ways that fill what are otherwise "social holes."[71] Asymmetric, historically shaped relations of power, however, affect social capital. Bonding ties, for instance, are important to people's sense of identity, belonging, and stability, though they can work against well-being when they become exclusive or reactionary. Bridging and linking social capital[72] often appear to be vital ingredients in successful community programs and projects in the interplay of various local and extra-local resources.[73] ARHAP's study of a comprehensive integrated faith-based program on HIV and AIDS in South Africa is a case in point.[74]

The effect of various forms of social capital upon health remains uncertain,[75] but the idea does contribute to the key insight that social relationships matter, and that they matter for any effective and sustainable delivery of public health services.[76] Consider, for example, the role of good grassroots or membership-based intermediary organizations that transcend the boundaries of closed or isolated groups, projects, and programs, filling the social holes that otherwise reinforce closure or isolation and, at their best, strengthening the capacities of local people and groups while serving as a buffer between them and the demands and agendas of external agencies.[77] Or the role of "boundary leaders," people able successfully to operate between the boundaries that define groups, disciplines, and the like, and who thereby assist others to make connections or enhance strengths, and often understand the interstitial spaces inhabited by so many people—undocumented migrants, refugees, or women in highly constrained patriarchal relations, for example—where daunting challenges to health and well-being are commonplace.[78]

Levels, pathways, and power matter, therefore, and draw attention to how hierarchies, systems, or structures impact on health. Being aware of this will shape the way we think about RHAs, and affect what methods or tools we use to map or assess them. It would be nice if we could keep our map of them constant as we design interventions around them, meeting the desire of planners and policy makers for controlled legibility, but clearly, to expect this is to work with an illusion. RHAs, we have said, cannot be understood without the human agency that moves them from being at rest into something useful. We might in fact speak of the dynamic life of RHAs, rooted in the actions of people who hold or leverage them. No longer viewed statically, it quickly becomes apparent that they will shift and change over time.

We might call this the RHA principle of indeterminacy. The analogy to Heisenberg's theory in physics is not trivial; like wave and particle descriptions of light, one cannot define the social world of RHAs with any clarity except in terms of their dual nature as both objective and subjective realities. One has to understand the level at which they work, the pathways through which they work, and the power-laden relationships within which they are placed, as well as what animates them. The goal cannot be the reductionist one of legibility alone, but must also include comprehensiveness, a grasp of the full complexity of RHAs—combining good science with adequate social intelligence.

Norms and Principles

Experimental science must bracket social or religious norms and principles as a methodological necessity if it is to understand the order of nature. Public health, however, surely goes beyond the orders of nature and must deal with orders of representation, with how and why people see things and act in a particular way. This applies to RHAs as much as any other. Understanding RHAs requires, then, that we pay attention to and take account of the norms and principles that animate them (for good or ill), which are highly likely to be linked with religious claims, axioms, and principles, embodying or expressing a religious worldview.

The normative considerations about community and society within which RHAs are likely to be rooted may, and often do, trump utilitarian positions or thin, reductionist views of human beings. One such norm, in most religious frames, is an orientation to the fullness of life, which we might call an orientation to comprehensive well-being. As Nancy Ammerman puts it, "Not all religious organizations are thriving, but the sector as a whole exhibits remarkable vitality.... This vitality flies in the face of a long tradition of sociological theorizing."[79]

Of course, some norms of principles in religious or faith traditions may be inimical to the health of persons or of the public. Stigma about sexually transmitted diseases, grounded in oppressive gendered beliefs and practices, is one obvious example. Taking such positions into account might then mean confronting and rejecting them. However, emancipatory trajectories are also widely present in religions and faith traditions, which is why Ammerman finds it important to comment on their vitality. Among the normative trajectories that are most important in this respect are those that highlight inclusion as opposed to exclusion,[80] that allow for progressive innovation within traditions (as in "prophetic" or "liberation" theologies),[81] that help one move from pathological to vital practices, that support one in the life span journey of health, and that build on the strengths of congregations—all issues we consider in later chapters.

Measurement and Legibility

Measurement is important in public health and policy processes. How can we determine, with some measure of reliability, where RHAs are, which ones matter most, and what they are good for? Raising these questions immediately confronts one with some well-known tensions.

"Quants" versus "quals," for instance. Quantitative procedures dominate public health science. Mathematical extrapolations, comparisons, and projections of one kind or another, based on various sampling methods and statistical tools, produce the metrics that largely govern how, to whom, and by whom available resources for health intervention will be allocated. Vast amounts of money and energy go into producing these metrics, and indicators such as infant mortality, immunization rates, and leading causes of death provide a powerful arsenal for understanding and advancing public health.

Nevertheless, despite a rapidly escalating body of data, we know that the arsenal frequently fails to address specific pathologies or to strengthen the general health of the public. Exciting advances seem to be paralleled by depressing retreats, and much data simply show us how big the problems are. However, qualitative approaches and their methods are seen as "soft" by comparison and, perhaps with reason, often as methodologically suspect.[82] If quantitative data tends to skim the surface of social reality at the cost of in-depth understanding, then qualitative data tends to mine limited realities at the cost of generalizability.

The tension between quals and quants is like the difference between paying careful attention to the roots that keep a tree alive, and viewing this one tree primarily as a statistic in a forest to be harvested. The one way of seeing focuses on the processes of life, the other on its control and organization. Any self-respecting scientist knows that both ways of seeing are inescapably partial. The challenge lies in finding one's way back from any particular partial view into a synoptic one that brings together differential insights and methods to illuminate better what is always but one reality.[83] RHAs exquisitely pose that challenge: they cannot be grasped at all, as it happens, without grasping their form and their dynamic, their measurable effects and their intangible sources of power and durability.

A related tension is that between the legible and the illegible, a distinction we take from James Scott's study of the way in which nation-states see reality.[84] Why do state schemes so often fail, he asks? One central reason is the state's need to make reality legible, to be able to apply metrics, measures, and coordinates to people, products, and places, in order to manage and, often, control them. This is the nature of state logic, a requirement of its function. Thankfully, life is never wholly legible; it is messy, given to unpredictable twists and turns, and readily escapes neat management and control. The intelligence appropriate to the state turns out to be less than fully intelligent, and so schemes fail.

Similarly, when it comes to understanding RHAs one must be cautious of models or metrics that pay attention only to what is legible and not that which is illegible. Both aspects are an integral and permanent dimension of the whole, and grasping the whole is the challenge for anyone committed to the health of the public.

A LAST WORD

While RHAs may be relatively cheap, they are not free. However, hardly any significant health care technology costs under a million dollars these days, and many a lot more. The investments needed to align and animate RHAs are a mere fraction of that. The entire CHN annual budget of Methodist Le Bonheur Healthcare, which engages over four hundred congregations in greater Memphis with measurable positive health outcomes, amounts roughly to the annual wage of a good cardiac surgeon.

Like any other assets, understanding and mobilizing RHAs takes attention, skill, systematic study, and careful work sustained over time. Engaging them is similar in scale and implications as investment in electronic medical records—the holy, and very expensive, grail of much current health care policy. Having everything wired together would close many of the cracks through which people, medicine, orders, and even logic tends to fall. The electronic medical record is probably essential for that reason—but it is expensive, difficult, disruptive, and, so far, connecting only those medical assets that lie inside the hospital walls.

The vision of RHAs helps us see how much more we have to work with. The promise lies in linking the electronic webs with the social webs; the scientific technology assets with the religious social assets. It is not proton beam therapy. However, its impact on the health of patients, families, and communities may be much more important, and it makes clear that we do not have to choose between science and faith. We simply have to find ways to use all of the assets, all of the time, and for all of the families in every community.

4

LEADING CAUSES OF LIFE:
PATHOLOGY IN ITS PLACE

Life is what it is about
I want no truck with death.

Pablo Neruda

I have set before you life and death, blessings and cursings;
therefore, choose life, that both you and your descendants may live.

Deuteronomy 30:19

In the US Civil War the battle of Shiloh, remarkable for its raw violence, the ignorance of its generals, and the age of its soldiers, turned the Tennessee River east of Memphis red with young blood. One general, leading a ten thousand strong Union division, took two days to find the road leading to the main battlefield, though the sound of distant gunfire was always present. Thick underbrush and the gentle roll of the terrain meant that thousands of men, many teenagers, lost their lives, dying without ever seeing their enemy. Most soldiers perished from lack of water or inadequate treatment of relatively minor wounds in desperate camps a few dozen miles removed from the battlefield while their generals dithered about what to do next. Others lived to fight again, but hundreds simply chose to walk away and keep walking, refusing to be party to such deadly meaninglessness.

In fact, any story of the American South ignores a narrative thread of meaningless violence only at risk of the truth, and that is still true today. Thousands of men the age of their Shiloh predecessors struggle now to find their way on urban streets, where meaningless violence and racial profiling remain mingled. About a third of young people in Memphis fail to finish high school, and many that do finish high school have such low skills that employment is unlikely.

So we write this book in sharp awareness of multigenerational patterns of struggle, violence, and failure. However, it is not about the all-too-obvious pathologies. There is much left to say about such troubles, but where do we learn something new? We argue that the answer lies in focusing on the idea of life.

LIFE AS A LANGUAGE

Life has a language relevant to health, and the notion of "leading causes of life" helps illuminate its core structure. To highlight these causes is not to ignore the many threats to life that normally capture the mind of public health practitioners, but to give complementary attention toward human health and how it spreads. Viruses are opportunistic, unpredictable, persistent, and occasionally deadly to their human hosts; they seem to have all the high cards. Nevertheless, humans actually carry on quite a respectable fight, using a set of life strategies. For instance, we do not reproduce very often, but we do so in the context of complex bonds of nurture, dependency, and affection that persist "in sickness and in health," for which these bonds are directly relevant. We can learn from viruses, but we have different capacities that allow us as a species to thrive.

We need to think about life with the same precision and rigor we use to analyze and beat back or postpone death. Death is simple compared to life. A short walk across any hospital campus crosses paths with many different diseases and injuries in the lives of people and families. Although there are thousands of names for it, in death something basically stops working. The breaking is simple; that which is broken—life—is highly complex, with many facets that exist in exquisitely rich relationship with each other. We live in connections, thrive in webs of meaning that make reality coherent, flourish in working together on things that matter, bloom in our experience of giving and receiving blessing across generations, and prosper as we are drawn toward hope. You can see all that going on in the lives of patients and families, if you know how to look. Not mere ideals, these causes of life are another approach to systematically pursuing population-scale strategies for health. They may offer a better logic for dealing with what Kreuter et al. call the "wicked problems" that seem to defy resolution.[1]

It turns out, for example, that the public health interventions that save the vast majority of life span years result from fairly simple, population-wide actions—clean water, sanitation, good food, and shelter. These are better understood as life processes than antideath processes. They reflect things that contribute to life of the whole community. In addition, they suggest that the right strategic tool is one designed to look for life, that the right analytic logic is one based on causes of life.

Life logic is curious about the way new things emerge that prove to be better adapted—fit—for thriving. That living beings are able to generate adaptive novelty is the key to how life goes beyond merely slowing the entropic drift toward death. Every living thing finally dies, of course, even the writers and readers of this book, sad to say. However, life finds a way to go on. Adaptation incorporates entropy and death, but it provides an overarching frame within which to comprehend them better. Jonas Salk, similarly, thinks of the point of discontinuity or inflection when a living being—or a species—must find a new strategy fitting to its situation if it is to transcend conditions that threaten it.[2] It does not help very much to look first for that which is running down, but rather for that which is emerging, opening new possibilities, and breaking through encroaching boundaries. Life always looks for what is next. And humans have more to work with in this regard than bacteria: imagination.

PURSUING AN EPIDEMIC OF LIFE

The closer one moves toward any human system, the more one sees its organic and emergent qualities; the less it seems a construct to be managed, the more it is to be nurtured, or healed. Salk, a philosophical but not a religious man, observed that it may be possible for health to spread among humans somewhat like epidemics. One might, he thought, be able to provoke an epidemic of health.[3]

If health is multifaceted enough to escape mere management or technique, perhaps it may emerge in another way entirely, rather like a positive infection in the body politic. This demands giving up the pretense or possibility of instrumentally organizing, even beneficently, the complex dynamics that make for the health of the public. In order to explore whether this might be possible, Heather Wood Ion, long a colleague and friend of Salk's, convened a group of diverse thinkers, including virologist Nathan Wolfe, who, like Salk, is deeply moral if not very religious. Pressed to say what humans could learn from viruses, Wolfe suggested that the most direct connection is that both must continually adapt to a shifting array of challenges for their survival. Moreover, human life might be moving into a world fundamentally hostile to our survival owing to what Friedman calls "global weirding,"[4] a way of describing the complex environmental changes in the chemistry of our air and water. Viral life assumes change and is built entirely on constant adaptation: "It depends on generating novelty," says Wolfe. It generates adaptive novelty by sharing and blending its DNA, its essence, combining with another to produce a new virus that may be better adapted to its host, replicating and thriving. Analogously, a human community generous with its essence—knowledge more than DNA—may also generate novelty, adapt and thrive even in the face of entirely unprecedented challenges.

If an epidemic of health depends on communicative generosity, then a healthy political economy might be nurtured by the presence of religious, spiritual, and faithful imagination. Perhaps the most relevant religious health assets are not clinics, hospitals, public health initiatives, or thousands of places of worship, but the most intangible asset of all—imagination. What would it mean to combine our essences, what forms of relationship informed by what ways of knowing might nurture a healthy body politic?

Here we touch on another vital element in life logic, the role of the human imagination in envisioning the possible and giving form to it in actuality. No matter what the circumstances, life seeks transformation, as we literally observe in those who face death but still come to terms with it, finding even there the strange presence of a life dynamic. In Christian thinking this is expressed in the seemingly contradictory claim that life ("resurrection") emerges from death ("cross"); it also happens to be a principle of evolutionary theory governing the conditions of the emergence of new forms of life.

Moving the focus of public health toward the language of life is harder than it may seem. It is easily treated as merely "inspiring" when, in fact, it has concrete operational implications. What makes it harder is that we already have a great store of thinking and expensive facilities devoted to resisting death and dying. Seeking life seems slightly off the point, which is exactly the point. Here, then, we sketch a model of the Leading Causes of Life (LCL) that offers a conceptual frame for understanding the logic of life.

THE GENERATIVE DYNAMIC OF LIFE: ANTONOVSKY'S LEGACY

A century after Shiloh, sociologist David Williams, at a conference on racial disparity in infant mortality held at the University of Wisconsin Medical School, reflected on the ways in which race and health in America produced very predictable outcomes generation after generation. Williams laid out ten things one needs to understand about the depth and durability of this pathology. There was little more to be said afterward, no room for curiosity except for one question: how, then, is there any life at all? Gunderson, assigned with the awkward task of following Williams to the microphone, for the first time introduced the phrase, "the leading causes of life."[5]

The moment called for a new paradigm of thought, but its beginning was not necessarily very impressive. The phrase named a nearly empty intellectual space, a question rather than an answer. The hypothesis that there *are* LCL, as clearly as there are leading causes of death, called for intellectual work, a moment of informed unknowing provoked by an obvious fact: life does find a way, it does emerge, and it is sustained in places one would not predict it when reasoning simply on the basis of pathological models. It is at least as important to understand how life works, as understanding how death tears it down. How do we describe this? What dynamic drives a process that is not entirely entropic?

Aaron Antonovsky, author of a fully elaborated theory of salutogenesis—that which generates healing and health—was one who began the search.[6] He held no romantic view of the human journey through travail and stress. Rather, his deep sense of pervasive chaos made him curious about the apparently contradictory fact that most people, nevertheless, find a life marked by health and meaning. Probing the health of a cohort of women who had survived the loss of families in Nazi death camps and who, as emigrants to Israel, had experienced three wars there, he was amazed when almost one-third (29 percent) reported themselves doing well.[7] Doing *well?* How is that possible? That, and not why others were *not* doing well, was the surprise. If stress and struggle are normal, then the mystery worthy of attention lies not in pathology, but in health.

Antonovsky's theory of salutogenesis focused on a "sense of coherence" (SOC) as the primary variable that enables one to predict how a person would navigate their way through life in the face of significant stressors and difficulties. People with a high SOC had a way of "seeing the world...as predictable and comprehensible,"[8] not chaotic or incoherent, however difficult. "The sense of coherence," he later wrote, "is a global orientation that expresses the extent to which one has a pervasive, enduring though dynamic feeling of confidence that 1) the stimuli deriving from one's internal and external environments in the course of living are structured, predictable and explicable; 2) the resources are available to one to meet the demands posed by these stimuli; and 3) these demands are challenges worthy of investment and engagement."[9] On this basis, he created his SOC scale, which he believed could predict health.

His theory remained in need of development, and he died young following a brief illness. He had published only two small books on salutogenesis, and a mere ten editions of a newsletter aimed at building a research network around the theory. However, between 1992 and 2003 his curiosity generated an expanding body of literature, at least 450 articles and 13 PhD dissertations, showing that "The SOC scale seems to be a reliable, valid, and cross culturally applicable instrument measuring how people manage stressful situations and stay well."[10]

Antonovsky clearly thought the most interesting and fruitful direction for health research lay in the unexplored end of the continuum of pathology and life. Just two years before his death, the Interfaith Health Program (IHP), as noted earlier,[11] had been launched at The Carter Center with a similar curiosity around faith and the health of communities, supported by Droege's seminal paper.[12] Public health had long had a sense for the complex ways that *suffering* was multifactorial and developmental over time or through generations, and Droege's decisive insight was that *healing* was similarly interconnected. As we have noted, this influenced Foege, CEO of the Center and by then a major leader in a number of frame-breaking global public health efforts, including smallpox polio eradication, global immunization, and treating violence, injury, and trauma as public health phenomena. Foege wondered what would happen if the IHP searched for unexpected outbreaks of positive phenomena, and understood the patterns that produced them by focusing on the obviously large resting assets of faith communities and their leaders that seemed to be relevant to the health of the public.[13]

This was radically opposite to the normal curiosity about how faith might apply to the manifold problems identified and prioritized by public health scholars and practitioners. Recognizing this dramatic gap, however, is not the same as having a strong theory on which to build programs to bridge it. Typically, most people think of a gap as something missing. The IHP thought of it as mountain people do—the low, safe way through a mountain range. IHP looked for the gaps between: (1) what was known in one field and where it was useful in another; (2) commitments already made, and further relevant implications of these; (3) a model that worked in one place that might be adapted to another; (4) people one already knew and those others relevant to the current challenge; and (5) current actions and their longer term implications.[14] IHP had no underpinning theory yet, but its curiosity was headed in a useful direction.

That led to twenty meetings with local leaders in faith and health activities across the United States, convened around two questions: (1) "What do you think is working that might be replicated elsewhere?"; (2) "What is *not* working for lack of a clear vision of what might be possible?" Like the later work of the African Religious Health Assets Programme (ARHAP) in southern Africa, these gatherings brought together leaders involved in the practice of health, and not primarily researchers. The range of their activities could be mapped as displayed in figure 4.1.

Almost anywhere that one group of leaders raised a problem, another had already found an encouraging way forward. Few of the initiatives had been evaluated to scientific standards, but they had been able to attract sustained investment for their local community.[15] The map depicts their diversity, as well as indicates an ever-increasingly complex web of interrelated activities that not only proliferate, but also evolve, morph, and mingle, like memes and DNA. They represent a dynamic map of life.

Like Darwin, we may ask what unifying logic accounts for all the differentiated forms of changing life. If one exists, it cannot rest primarily on our growing ability to describe problems and pathologies. The increasing precision with which we can describe our fears—cancer, say— accounts for some of the ways we respond to threats to life, offering possibilities for combating those threats. However, participation in any of the numerous public cancer walks that fill the calendar discloses a surprising fact that they are lively, indeed, full of life. The soup kitchen or clinic for the poor may be drawn to hunger or disease, but the social phenomena that arise at the intersection between need and response

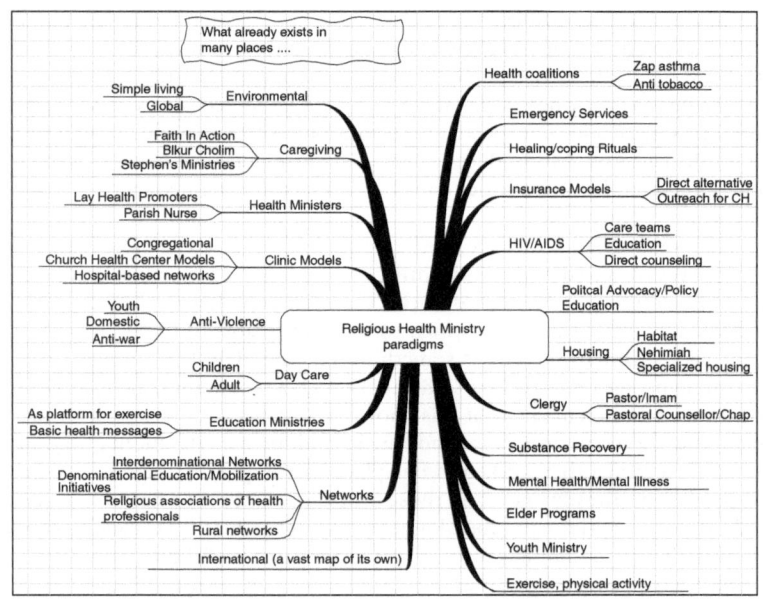

Figure 4.1   Mapping religious health activities.

are themselves marked by life through relationships that bring energy to all involved. They go beyond the personal. Moreover, rather than being entropic they signal the opposite, an emergent and vital complexity.

To answer the question posed by Antonovsky and the IHP of what accounts for the life in the presence of struggle, one needs a theory not about the unsurprising nature of personal suffering, but about the surprising character of societal life. If public health, through a focus on pathology, tends to "see like a dying person," we want to see like a living one.

CAUSES OF LIFE

The first step to an adequate theory of the causes of life is to see that life is generative and much more complex than death. Life works by adapting to a constantly shifting and unpredictable array of challenges and opportunities. The ending we call death is simpler to grasp because it *is* simpler than the decades of flexible adaptation that distinguishes the human response to life. Humans adapt—Antonovsky says, "cope"—to ameliorate the challenges they experience, such as loss of affection, disease, or cataclysmic war. Often doing so strengthens their capacity to live. Antonovsky thus observes that stresses, though disturbing at the time, are not always negative for life span health. For him the difference is a SOC, or its lack.

In his last book, Antonovsky points to the possible future development of the field of salutogenesis, of which his theory is one stream.[16] He notes that a SOC neither develops at an entirely individual level, nor is it a uniquely personal attribute. Yet, astonishingly for a Jewish sociologist working in Israel with survivors of the Holocaust, he misses that a SOC is mostly something acquired and adapted from one's community or social network, an aspect poorly developed in his theory. Does the theory add up to anything more than a set of tools for assessing and encouraging adaptive personal life strategies? Could it have *public* significance?

The follow-on from the World Health Organization (WHO) Alma-Ata meeting was the 1984 Ottawa Conference that marked the global launch of the "health promotion" movement. Antonovsky attended the regional premeeting in Scandinavia, but his thought was not yet sufficiently developed to have visible effect on that conference. As the IHP learned a few years later, having a clutter of promising practices may create a movement, but it cannot sustain one. A movement needs a theory.

Lindstrom and Eriksson suggest that the field of health promotion still lacks a sustaining, integrating theory, and that Antonovsky remains the best foundation on which to build one. Reflecting on this some twenty years after the Ottawa Charter, they argue that the contemporary evidence base for the salutogenic framework supports the Charter's philosophical and practical intentions, especially regarding the maintenance and development of health and the quality of life.[17] Elsewhere, they note that the recent history of public health reflects an evolving, underlying concept of health that has moved from a relatively static opposition between health and disease toward a dynamic, emergent phenomenon of well-being. This includes a "shift from the biomedical paradigm towards social and psychological perspectives," a much broader use of "theories and strategies from other fields of science than medicine," and the introduction of theories focused "on health as a resource for everyday life and health promotion." All support "the realization of the Ottawa Charter in terms of salutogenesis and quality of life."[18]

Our premise is that instead of placing first importance on pathologies, notwithstanding the need to understand them, the primary issue to be addressed is that which is generative of health. We name it *life*.[19] There is a good bit of "found science" to support this approach, once one knows where to look. Many health promoting practices dealing with transitional conditions that have been explained using a mechanical, silo'd, and linear logic are more usefully explained using the organic, multifactorial, and fractal logic of the LCL, especially when the intervention involves any form of human variable.

Even Antonovsky's advanced model of the SOC is improved by moving it into the LCL approach. His three core concepts of comprehensibility, manageability, and meaningfulness partially match the notions of coherence, agency, and connection in the LCL model, but the model adds at least two other critical concepts. The first is intergenerativity (originally named "blessing"),[20] and the second is hope, a concept able to articulate Antonovsky's untheorized awareness that anticipation and expectation fostered health. The LCL theory also allows us to consider the role of a further, rich aspect of human life with enormous practical value, that of imagination.

THE SCIENCE OF POSITIVE LIVING

One well of "found science" from which LCL theory is able to draw comes from the deep water of positive psychology. Here we turn first to sociologist Corey Keyes, who has labored productively to develop the concept of "flourishing" in relation to mental health. Keyes and others such as Martin Seligman had by the early years of the twenty-first century pushed their ideas on positive psychology well into the mainstream of the American Psychological Association.[21] Keyes' model developed a way of measuring two transversal continua (not one, as in Antonovsky): one tracks pathology, running from "no negative symptoms" to terminal problems, the other a trajectory of thriving that runs from languishing (no positive signs) to full and abundant flourishing.[22]

We adapt and generalize the model to offer a similar view on the LCL.[23] The overlapping area of the two continua (figure 4.2) can be described in terms of countering pathological phenomena, using the language of coping, risk avoidance, resilience, resistance, and prevention. Pargament even connects this to the positive value of religion.[24] The LCL model goes further by noticing the generative life processes that are also at work. Thus, resilience or a capacity to cope may be seen as a byproduct of a generative process that itself needs support.

Many activities regarded as public health successes, such as those that claim a health benefit by preventing something (smoking, obesity, drug abuse,

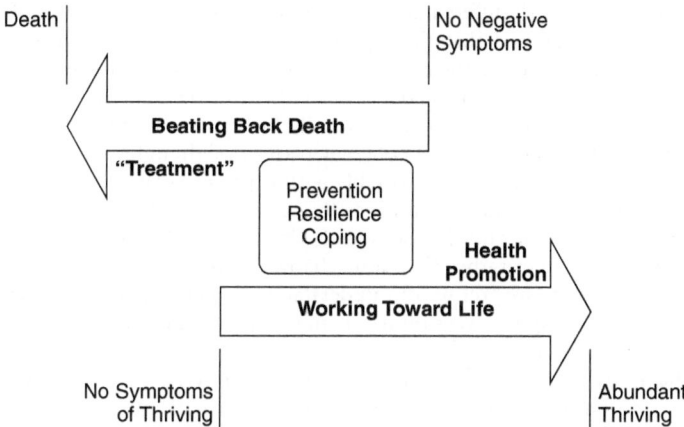

Figure 4.2   Death-thriving continua.

unsafe sex, or bad driving), often achieve the effect by means that borrow heavily from the life-oriented phenomena commonly and naturally used in a faith group. Lowered risk behavior is best understood as resulting not from changing health risk choices, but from the positive choice to move toward life, a human drive to transcend the given pulled by aspirations for the more fulfilling. This is true not just of preventive public health interventions, but also of many that depend on a complex, long-term set of positive actions sustained over time.[25]

The challenge for any theory of health built on the dynamic of life, or for researchers trying to work with it, is considerably more complex than relatively simple, linear, entropic, and pathological logic. Life finds its way; the task is to describe it appropriately so that it may be nurtured. There is no reason, in principle, why medicine, with the vast amounts of energy and money that it wields, should focus less on supporting life than it does working against death.

Here we call attention to another conceptual development that Antonovsky anticipated but could not quite explain. At a meeting of scholars sharing their research in early SOC days, Antonovsky heard a physicist ask how "We can understand the emergence of order in systems, given the powerful, immanent and diverse forces constantly pressing toward chaos."[26] Antonovsky, stirred up, embraced the idea that "For every scientist, physical, biological, or social, no less than for the philosopher or theologian...the problem of chaos is omnipresent," linking this thought to Johann Georg Hamann's view that "Nature is no ordered whole: so-called sensible men are blinkered beings who walk with a firm tread because they are blind to the true and profoundly disturbing character of reality....; if they glimpsed it as it is—a wild dance—they would go out of their minds."[27] Antonovsky thus rejected a brittle, rule-based, and control-oriented model of human coping, in favor of the notion of developmental adaptivity.

Whether dealing with differentiated social structures or with problems of system functioning, he argued that the capacity "to carve out a coherent pattern of interaction with reality, is the core problem at the frontier of all science."[28]

Antonovsky's body of thought is difficult to bring into the heart of public health precisely because he was brutally honest about the chaotic context in which it tries to carve out a coherent pattern of thought and practice. His perception of reality fits uncomfortably with expansive commitments to a fully rationalized, self-evident, and universally extended health science. One is not surprised, then, that this Jewish sociologist pondered whether God is best understood as a poet rather than a mechanic: "His works are full of allusion, puns, despair and love. Yet we can understand a poem. My own work has been devoted to studying the ways human beings cope with the reality of the poem that is social existence."[29]

The LCL theory embraces Antonovsky's clear view of the banal cruelty of chaos in human affairs, but we see equally, and with him, that humans do more than cope; they live lives rich in meaning and purpose, generation after generation. Emerging from within an African context, LCL theory is shaped partly by historical traumas and multiple pandemics where the compelling mystery is that life nevertheless finds a way. Our concern is to better understand that mystery, for the sake of medicine and for the health of the public. Not just poetry, the model is best seen as one version of the emerging sciences of complexity.

A MODEL OF THE CAUSES OF LIFE

Tom Munnecke—software designer, philosopher, and social entrepreneur—believes that "transformational ensembles" can change the world, or more precisely, that they are what change it.[30] This delightful term expresses the minimum set of factors capable of sustaining transformation. It is also a useful way of understanding the LCL, which we now describe. However, first, what does it actually mean to describe them as causes?

No one experiences causes directly, but only through their effects, to which we attribute a cause within some frame of thought. To suggest that there are causes of life, therefore, is to exercise a synthetic judgment. The phenomena are real enough, but to understand them we must add explanation and a theory. The causes of life are therefore not self-evident substances or essences, but are found in how we explain certain recurring functions and relations in the phenomena we observe.[31] This is as true of health or social life as it is of particle physics. The adequacy of these explanations is determined by the extent to which their framing theory does (or does not) grasp the rich complexity of experience in providing the simplest but most meaningful, comprehensive, and complete understanding of that experience.

We call them causes of life, then, because they appear, in varying contexts and conditions, to express adequately what people experience as generative of human life. Each cause is sufficiently discrete to cover a range of crucial experiences, and each, relative to the others, expands our understanding of those experiences.[32] There is more than one cause of life but not innumerable causes, and those we can discretely define are not isolated from each other but interrelated—they work as an ensemble. What then is the ensemble of the LCL?

First Cause: Meaningful Life—Coherence

Coherence enables us to make sense of life, to see it as comprehensible and not filled merely with wholly random events and inexplicable forces. Clearly, Antonovsky saw this as the vital element of salutogenesis. Another influential figure who thought along similar lines was Viktor Frankl, a Jewish psychiatrist who survived Auschwitz.[33] His theory of logotherapy expressed a positive view of what generates mental health, in contrast to the largely negative thrust of Freudian psychoanalysis. Frankl identified three psychological reactions to incarceration: shock first, often followed by apathy, and later, depersonalization, moral deformity, bitterness, and (if one survived) disillusionment. From within a situation of horrific suffering and death, he argued that meaning of life was key, and that the meaning of life could be found in every moment of living. Convinced that this was the only way to "explain the apparent paradox that some prisoners of a less hardy make-up often seemed to survive camp life better than did those of a robust nature,"[34] he often cited Nietzsche's words: "He who has a *why* to live can bear with almost any *how*."[35]

Coherence is so vital to human beings that they rightly fear incoherence as a fundamental threat, one reason why religion (or anything that replaces it) is so commonly linked to violence. If the story holding a person's life together frays at the edges and starts to unravel, incoherence gains strength, and the threat to life is quickly felt. We could even think of a hospital in this way—a place that frequently feels utterly incoherent to those who enter it, a disorienting condition of fear and vulnerability. Conversely, many indications suggest that a SOC gives a people the capacity to be agents in their own healing: to have reasons to take their medicine, do their exercise, and generate their own life. Thus Pennebaker's work utilizing the art of self-disclosure or "storytelling" to build that SOC in enhancing health shows that there is a clear positive impact on the human immune system even seven months later.[36] Coherence may not be enough, but it frequently tilts the balance—not least because it provides a way of seeing and trusting the connections across which life might flow via those who hold one up until one is healed, but also because it provides with the opportunity, later, to return the favor.

Second Cause: Supported Life—Connection

Walking down a particular block near Uptown Memphis, one comes across Roxie's—from one angle a dumpy, code-violating corner store and grill that any public health officer would think of as a risk vector, a likely pathway for disease or injury. However, Roxie's is actually a life vector, a connecting point for many kinds of relationships across which sizzle vital stuff such as food, hope, and intelligence. It is a multirelevant place of connection, of just the kind that humans prefer. Such connections, which also exist in community centers or congregations and a host of other places, are often generative of life. Humans are social creatures. Capable of only brief episodes of solitude, human life thrives on our complex social connections to each other.

Healthy, generative human communities are connected in ways that enable them to adapt to changing threats and opportunities as a whole. The Roseto community study in the 1960s–70s underlined how this supportive mechanism protected men from heart disease, by looking beyond the individual metrics and lives to "...a social structure that reflected remarkable cohesiveness...sense of unconditional support, strong family ties, respect for elders and one in which...no one was ever abandoned."[37] Unfortunately, this protective mechanism no longer held as traditional social networks frayed in Roseto, resulting in a typically unhealthy human community that found itself incapable of adapting to reality: its connections lost their generative and complex nature.

The Sesotho notion of *bophelo*, the ecology of relations that make up human connectivity in its full complexity, makes clear just how deep and extensive connection is in support of life as a whole. In this view, a person cannot be understood abstracted from family, community, nation, or land and creation.[38] Even to describe them as connected implies that they could be separated, but they are more like a diamond with facets than a machine with parts. Any disconnection at any point represents a fissure in the whole; any particular violation of the whole, therefore, is as deadly as a malignant virus attacking other elements of the whole, including individual persons.

Language often hides this complexity by neatly sorting us into discrete categories: man, woman, husband, wife, brother, sister, cousins, uncle, aunt, neighbor, member, and citizen. Yet, neurological evidence suggests that our minds are designed for the task of recognizing, initiating, managing, and responding to highly complex social relationships that define our life.[39] Indeed, scientists believe that the human brain can recognize the face of one person among thousands in less than a quarter of a second.[40] This is clearly an adaptive strategy in the evolutionary process, suggests Greg Fricchione, head of psychiatry at Women's and Children's Hospitals at Harvard University, in reading human experience as a tension between attachment (connection) and separation.[41] The importance of connection has also been conceptualized in the theory of social capital through the notion of ties to others,[42] which recognizes that connection is more than a nice thought. Seeing the world as a weave of thick or thin, strong or weak relationships has implications for understanding the health of the public.[43] Developing greater intelligence on how these relationships work is critical to understanding how people seek their own health and life, a point we will pursue in the next chapter.

Connection is also linked directly to two other elements of the transformational ensemble of the LCL model, intergenerativity (or memory), and hope (or anticipation). Psychoanalysis has taught us that memory and anticipation can be pathological, but primarily, memory helps us define those attachments that will enhance our capacity to thrive, while anticipation enables us to recognize a possible future with enough clarity to move toward it. And both rest strongly on the extent to which we are able to exercise our agency.

Third Cause: Active Life—Agency

One vital way of understanding human life is in terms of verbs: we go here or there, now or later, fast or slow; we lift, reach, touch, hold, dig, study, watch, fight, love, seek, build, invent, and make things. Our agency, or lack of it, is definitive of the quality of our lives, so much so that it allows a sociologist such as Zygmunt Baumann, in his Gifford Lectures, to define the new class divide in a globalized world as those who can exercise agency through mobility, and those who cannot and are thus readily marginalized from its centers of power and influence.[44]

We have already spoken of agency in relation to religious health assets, relating it to the dynamic idea of human capabilities,[45] and it requires no leap of imagination to see how a rich mix of human capabilities enhances life, just as their lack diminishes it. Agency is "the power to do" or to act, not unlike Bandura's concept of self-efficacy in relation to coping.[46]

As human beings we cannot not act. The clinical description of a "vegetative state" shows by contrast how important agency is for a view of human life. Conversely, the wise nurse on a cancer ward nurtures the agency of the patients, finding ways for them to express choice, even if only between cereal and oatmeal for breakfast. The physical therapist pulls the patients onto their feet after a shockingly brief period of passive rest because the human body is designed to grow on its own capacity to do, or it atrophies. If this is true for muscles and bone, how much more for the spirit, the mind, and for life in general?

Conversely, to undermine human agency diminishes life. In *The Careless Society*, McKnight documents how professional helpers can undermine the agency of communities by creating relations of dependency, which then gives the helper greater agency than the helped.[47] The United Nations International Children's Emergency Fund (UNICEF) works hard to avoid making this deadly mistake, as do the best of clergy, the most successful of physicians, and community organizers.

One can see agency clearly where the largest agencies did not expect it, amid the overwhelming swell of AIDS orphans in Africa. The obvious answer to this challenge—rapidly establish orphanages—is improbable amid already broken African economies. UNICEF and others launched a small study in six countries to evaluate what might be done.[48] They learned that small groups of village women had already moved quietly, on a large scale, to deal with the challenge. On an average, in thousands of villages, each group of women (usually members of a small church) takes care of about a hundred children without any encouragement, training, or funding from donors or health agencies that were thought to be indispensable for such work. The carers might not be able to explain the etiology of the HIV virus or how it spreads, but they feed, shelter, and find ways to clothe and protect the kids. They give them a chance at life.

Such agency creates the possibility of more agency, generating space for the other causes of life too. However, it takes both courage and art to foster the agency of those who otherwise are expected to be grateful for what is done for them. One might even say that agency is a sacred, generative well of life to be tended with reverence.

Fourth Cause: Anticipatory Life—Hope

Of all the LCL, hope most requires an adjective: "informed" hope. Hope is grounded in life itself, which led existential philosopher Gabriel Marcel to speak of children as the biological basis of hope.[49] However, informed hope has to do with what philosopher Ernst Bloch called anticipatory consciousness.[50] Bloch linked the idea of hope to history and society,[51] and to the arts and music.[52] Hope is not wishful thinking, which cannot issue in action toward a healthy future.[53] A philosophy of hope, he said, "will have conscience of tomorrow, commitment to the future, knowledge of hope, or it will have no more knowledge."[54]

This is more than an abstract philosophical idea. Anticipatory consciousness can in fact be grounded in neurobiology. As Schachter et al. discovered reviewing numerous scientific studies, "imagining the future depends on much of the same neural machinery that is needed for remembering the past"; the hope that energizes human beings is lodged, indeed, in what we might call our "prospective brain."[55] Of course, we need both past and future to live in the present, but the point is that humans live out of their expectations, and not just their histories. We anticipate, expect, weigh the likelihood, and then act as if that is what is unfolding. To the extent that our action is informed or reflective, rather than just instinctive, reactive, or impulsive, human hope is about a "riskable" expectation. It might even be called a "memory of the future," a phrase coined by David Ingvar.[56]

The risks animated by hope are most viable when they are tested against the hopes of others to whom a person is connected, sometimes in ways that are not obvious. Embedded within the complex set of interconnections that make up the social life of persons, informed hope is not only a condition of being human. It is also an imperative, because any action we take in anticipation of a different future or possibility reverberates in the lives of others around us. This is what makes us responsible for our actions and accountable for their outcomes.[57] Moreover, this is pertinent to religion, as Ted Karpf says so pointedly: "The best of religion tells you stories of past that inform the present and inspire for the future. That is the social function of religion. It speaks deeply, to the bones across time. It inspires curiosity, inspiration, and responsibility."[58]

Hope is then linked to agency in a double manner: as anticipatory practice and as responsible action. "Against the idea that we are headed over the cliff into some abyss (collapse) or that we are about to run into a solid and immovable brick wall (limits)," says David Harvey, it is better that we "construe ourselves as embedded within an on-going flow of living processes that we can individually and collectively affect through our actions."[59] These living processes he calls the "web of life." Similarly, we speak of "webs of transformation"[60] as animated by hope.

All of these thoughts invoke the human imagination, as all the authors to whom we refer recognize. The immensely powerful capacity to imagine something new and to devise ways to bring it into being marks our lives as human and not merely biological. We add something to what we experience that was not there before. We invent, we make, and we create what did not exist. We are able to transcend what is given to us, and this is a capacity we already begin to learn as children, when we call it play.[61] In one sense, then, imagination is not only a cause of life; but it also permeates every cause of life.

Of course, the power of imagination and human creativity can be turned to destructive ends, given human freedom. But then we are dealing with pathologies rather than causes of life, and they are of course two sides of the same coin. The key point, however, is that most health interventions still focus largely and shortsightedly on only one side, pathology. It is our view that where both sides of the coin have been embraced, we might expect better outcomes.

Fifth Cause: Adaptive Life—Intergenerativity

Every significant moment of life is part of a journey of constant adaptive movement by humans through various social spaces, frequently marked by discrete passages of life. Relevant science can be found that has carefully examined many of these passages, such as transitions of age, circumstance, wellness, or relationship. Here we probe one such passage, an archetypal one: life at the end of life in the passage toward imminent death. The question is whether the LCL theory offers some explanatory power for understanding this passage or illuminate ways of approaching it that could lead to better experiences and outcomes.

Methodist Le Bonheur Healthcare in Memphis runs the largest hospice in the region, daily caring for about two hundred people faced with the last weeks of their lives. Hospice care, whether in Africa or Memphis, is a rare time in the medical journey, when one can expect to see all the components of the system arrayed in relative respect for the patient and family. This is one time when the medical system behaves itself, listens to patients, creates space for shared roles with extended family, social networks, community, and volunteers, as one expects. It welcomes the presence of chaplains and other less-trained religious helpers, and includes symbols of all sorts to aid the passage to death and the process of regaining a SOC at the end of life. One might wish that one did not have to die to experience a well-behaved medical system; still, the end of life is a time when one can see a life as a whole—or, at least, how one life is part of a larger whole. It is here that the concept of intergenerativity becomes most obvious.

Intergenerativity, inherently, is not about one life, yet it can be highly relevant to one life. "As my mother approached her own death," Gunderson remembers, "she was blessed by a high level of mental and spiritual acuity even as her body broke down." He was able to talk directly to her about her funeral for which he, the youngest but only ordained member of the family, would be primarily responsible. She decided which grandchildren would read which scriptures. They both wept as he read the various passages aloud and the nature of the service emerged. When the day came, he preached his own mother's sermon, finally breaking down, shifting from preacher to grieving son, leaving the pulpit, and joining his brothers, sister, wife, and daughters as a family that would live on. His younger daughter, only seven, put her hand on his knee and whispered, "Daddy, you've been a good son today." He was in right relationship—a generative relationship—to his mother, to all she carried of her family with her, to those around him, and to those that will live beyond him. Had Gunderson's immune system been tested using PN1 measures at that point,[62] he would probably have scored optimally.

LCL theory adds nothing to the event itself, but it does introduce an understanding of the highly complex generativity of further life inherent in what otherwise is an oversimplified view of an ending of life. The end of one life is also a time when the family's SOC is challenged. LCL theory sees life as inherently intergenerational, not just from the old to the young, but the other way, too; not just between generations that can see and touch each other, but across the span of those whose lives influence each other over time and space. It thus even offers a different view on some pathologies, such as what community psychologists refer to as "historical trauma" (Native Americans, the Khoisan in southern Africa, or war generations of Germany).[63] In addition, it can inform interventions beyond the individual person.

For example, ARHAP scholars have employed their participatory research model to help the Hospice Palliative Care Association of South Africa extend their services by aligning them with community health assets, many embedded in the religious networks of those communities.[64] This has become necessary because the HIV pandemic and AIDS sufferers place extraordinary new demands upon hospices. AIDS is no longer necessarily terminal; but people do die and, all too often, the hospice ends up with their children. Both realities go far beyond the traditional capacity of hospices. The driving need is to identify community assets to support palliative care and get them into alignment with the hospice, quickly and sustainably. From one angle, this merely extends the medical system one "service line" further than before, nothing unusual in the world of health. However, from another perspective, the participatory action process itself draws the local community to its own life by systematically bringing into view its unconnected connections across generations, its opportunities for a broader expression of agency inspired by both the living and the dead, its active engagement in supporting and blessing crucial life passages, and thus, its capacities for exercising decency even in the face of overwhelming need.

To call this, as Antonovsky might, a community finding its SOC is a great advance from the extended service line language of the medical system. Nevertheless, more than coherence, it brings intergenerativity into view as an animated expression of the agency of a much larger part of the community relevant to end of life. Moreover, it challenges the model of services delivery as the determining criteria by which to understand the health system.

DISORDER FIGHTS BACK

The logic of the LCL stumbles over the lived reality vividly evident in many villages and townships of Africa or on the streets and in the hospitals of Memphis.

Like religion, it holds together not only the story of life or creation in ritual and narrative, but also the mystery of death, loss, and suffering that evokes only lament. There may be, as David Bohm argues, an unfolding order implicit in the very fabric of reality.[65] However, how does one explain the inexplicable, ongoing unfolding of disorder? One cannot illuminate the scale and interwoven constrictions of suffering simply by saying that life has not yet fully emerged. Disorder, felt and named in the language of disease, injury, and disability, is not just a lack of health; it appears to fight back against the implicate order, often winning. Dr. Martin Luther King, Jr. did not simply fall short of full maturity; he was shot down on his way to dinner with friends before leading another march. He expected the new order he saw and announced but, like Moses, he sensed that he himself would not get there. Disorder is part of every human system with effects that are unpredictable and turbulent. We have to deal with the interplay between emergent new order and the reality of disorder.

Religions, nearly all, have some way of naming the disorder that fights back. Sometimes it is seen as animate with intentionality, purpose, and power, and named as demons, Satan, fallen angels, or malevolent forces. Many African religions speak of dangerous spirits and displeased ancestors. Indeed, one could sort various religions according to the different ways they name and explain the relationship between order and disorder.

The LCL paradigm does not directly address the frequent failure of life to order human experience at personal, family, social, and even political scale. One need not stand on the battlefields of Shiloh—or before Rwandan churches filled with skulls, or in the killing fields of Cambodia—to realize that positive, adaptive causal theory falls short of a fully adequate explanation for human experience, any more than disease theory adequately explains everything. It is not enough simply to hold the two stories in tension, one of healing and life, generative imagination or emergent order, and the other of disease and death, formless void or active disorder.

If causal complexity rests, as Kant following Hume insisted, on the fact that we can only name effects and not causes, then our naming of its parts must always be open ended. Bohm called this "participatory" knowing, which does not collapse the unlimited into a limited and inherently partial, thus inaccurate, knowing.[66] Such rigorous methodological humility is required if we are to acknowledge the continued presence of turbulent disorder as an inherent part of what we call life. The two things are not complementary but entangled. Martin Luther King, who saw this clearly, spoke of history arcing toward justice slowly, over many life spans. He was probably neither surprised at the bullet, nor believed the arc was broken by it, as he fell to floor on the balcony of the Lorraine Hotel.

RETHINKING SICKLE CELL ANEMIA: LIFE LOGIC AT WORK

Disorder and order are visible not just in the contemplation of realities of obvious awe, but also in the patterns of life found amid diseases of troubling etiology, traveling mysteriously complex and painful journeys. Sickle cell anemia is certainly one of those diseases, so embedded in African, thus African American, experience that it has names that lead us to the edge of mystery. To grasp some of the implications of the LCL model, then, to see how it might lead to action that is more adequate, let us consider what sickle cell anemia looks like in Memphis.

Sickle cell anemia is not infectious. Transmitted genetically, it is unaffected by behavior or choice. Named after the sickle shape that red blood corpuscles assume as the condition advances, it originates in Africa where it is thought to have evolved by conferring some resistance to endemic malaria. With its pattern of episodic, variable, and unpredictable but wrenching pain, and limited to people of African descent, it was not even universally considered a real disease until midway through the twentieth century. It gained global attention as one of the archetypal molecular diseases only when new tools of molecular research found sickle cell to be a perfect candidate for scientific investigation.

The first sickle cell clinic in the United States was opened in 1958 at the public hospital in Memphis, now known as the Regional Medical Center at Memphis (the Med).[67] This made sense for reasons that are not pretty: a lack of alternative sources of medical care ensured that researchers would have access to an effectively endless supply of African American patients who could be diagnosed early in their life and kept in treatment throughout their life, as they "graduated" from children's care at Le Bonheur and St. Jude's hospitals to the adult wards. World-class molecular researchers came to Memphis to conduct extensive research on sickle cell anemia and associated medical conditions. The research engine that ran on the fuel of available patients expanded throughout the medical center of Memphis, lifting the University of Tennessee with it.

That story belongs to another book. For our purposes, it is enough to note that Memphis has a long history of engagement with people living with the excruciating pain of sickle cell. A new chapter in that engagement was the acceptance by Methodist Le Bonheur Healthcare of responsibility for adult treatment. With the roughly two thousand adult sickle patients now coming to a faith-based university hospital instead of the Med, for the most part this is simply a change in destination, not in paradigm.

Using a simple outline of best treatment practice, we ask if the LCL theory could add anything to what is already known about how to care for those experiencing a sickle cell crisis. If we treat the engagement between a patient and a medical delivery system as part of a process, not just an event, what would advance life and, simultaneously, improve treatment outcomes?

Sickle cell is a curious and oddly brutal disease. The life of someone living with sickle cell is marked by unpredictable cycles or "crises" of extreme pain coursing throughout the body. The best evidence-based practice in treating a sickle patient, largely limited to pain management, usually involves a combination of powerful medications. Any adult sickle cell patient knows which medicines, in what combination, are most effective in controlling their crisis events.

However, the emergency room (ER) clinician, faced with an adult complaining of severe pain and wanting narcotics, showing no broken bones or obvious medical condition, has a problem figuring out whether this is just a drug-seeker, someone living with sickle cell, or something else. Any sickle patient has stories of being treated as a drug-seeker, at best given an unhelpfully low dosage painkiller and then being put into observation: even the Le Bonheur hospital finance committee chair's son was treated this way in a university hospital ER in California where he was attending a conference on sickle cell. Many adults living in the unpredictable chaos of sickle cell are also unable to hold down a good job with insurance. This adds sizeable negative economic implications to treating someone who might inappropriately be abusing the limited resources of the hospital.

The decision to treat or wait also has big consequences for all concerned. If appropriately treated and controlled within two hours of onset, the painful crisis can be limited to eight or twelve hours per episode as an outpatient. If not controlled within that period, it will likely end up being a three to five-day inpatient admission. As many adult sickle patients lack insurance (if male, even under government programs), their care will be unreimbursed, a loss for the hospital.

LCL theory notices that more than medicine determines the likelihood of getting that two hour window right. Many decisions are involved, and the most important ones are not necessarily made by an overworked ER clinician in a hurry, but by those making daily life decisions rather than medical ones. What affects the decision to come to the ER at the early onset of the crisis?

The decision to navigate to the ER is a choice to expend one's agency, knowing it may well end with a demeaning, incoherent, and ineffective result given one's profoundly disruptive dependency on a hospital that regards one as a financial burden. Other burdens rest on family or friends who inevitably need to be involved by providing transportation and attending to the details of one's life while in a hospital for a few days. As every crisis event is unpredictable, the sensible thing to do is usually to wait until the visit to the ER simply cannot be avoided—exactly the opposite of what "evidence-based medicine" recommends. Then ER staff may have only minutes to get the diagnosis right before the two-hour window passes, making more likely the five-day inpatient stay that everyone dreads.

LCL theory suggests many opportunities for dramatically improved management of this situation, beginning with noticing that sickle cell sufferers—who are, after all, alive—have many mediating connections beyond the ER. They are not just patients, but members of one or another social association. Probably at least 70 percent of the two thousand people living with sickle cell in the range of Memphis are known and cared for by somebody in one of Methodist Le Bonheur's hundreds of Congregational Health Network (CHN) congregations. Those congregations are connected with many other mediating networks that penetrate every neighborhood and social network, reaching far beyond those who show up to weekly worship.

The link of a sickle cell person to any CHN congregation can be registered in the hospital computer, enabling those at the admissions desk to connect the two meaningfully. This simple act changes an unknown person who may look like a drug seeker into a human being who is part of an existing, covenantal relationship with the hospital through the CHN. It allows one to trigger an automatic visit from a chaplain and, if desired, a request to the congregation to come alongside and share in the care. Alternatively, the sickle cell person may remember to call their congregational liaison, trained to either accompany them to the ER or arrange for someone else from the congregation to meet them there.

An experience that is normally fraught with appropriate fear and embarrassment, besides great pain, can now be expected to take place with some assurance of respect, understanding, and community. The pain will not be less, but since a decision to come quickly is much easier and a diagnosis will not be confused by suspicion, that two hour window is likely to be more successfully navigated, with the person returning home later the same day. Correct diagnosis within the window can mean the difference between giving away eight hours of outpatient care (roughly $1,500) or five days of inpatient care (roughly $20,000). Naturally, the chief financial officer enjoys the fact that the hospital has avoided $18,500 of unreimbursed expenses, but that is by far the crudest measurement of what has actually happened.

Antonovsky would also quickly note the dramatic improvement in the patient's SOC, which draws from an encounter that is indeed more coherent for everyone involved—the congregation, ER staff, hospital administration, spiritual care staff, friends, and family. All experience themselves as participants in the event, with an opportunity to share in the successful passage through a crisis of one they care about, in a way that reinforces everyone's sense of coherence, connection, and agency. Rather than diminishing the life force, as Antonovsky predicted, the stressful passage actually builds the consciousness that a person has of her or his extended social networks, and of the resources necessary to deal with a circumstance that cannot be predicted or avoided.

HEALTH AS LIFE EVENT

LCL theory shows that life is not just a useful tool to enhance what is really a medical event, but that the medical exchange of services is really a life event. Many events poorly understood merely as medical transactions also offer opportunities to medicine if understood as life processes. Quality, efficacy, and even efficiency may indeed be improved by recognizing the life processes that enfold medical processes, as we see clearly in the case of sickle cell anemia.

The LCL enhance each other as they swirl in a living ensemble among and between persons and social bodies. Making the life process visible feeds another powerful component, the human and social imagination that sees beyond what is to what might be. Images of what might be emerge naturally from gaining a clearer image of what is already underway.

The LCL is a theory, but it is also visible in practices that arise out of the confluence of faith and health. Better viewed as a potent set of questions rather than of self-contained answers, LCL theory gives leaders operating in the context of complex, fluid, and turbulent community challenges a way to envisage the life of the whole. Part of a larger suite of ideas emerging at the intersection of faith and health at a public scale, it is also part of a larger scientific curiosity about how order emerges, is sustained, and moves toward higher order in complex systems.

As Bohm argued, reality is only properly understood in terms of the assumption of total connectedness. Reality is a single phenomenon and must be engaged more as a song than a construction project.[68] In this, Bohm sees no distinction between physical and life sciences: "It may indeed be said that life is enfolded in the totality and that, even when it is not manifest, it is somehow "implicit" in what we generally call a situation in which there is no life."[69] Reflecting on change as a kind of movement through the passage of life, he suggests, "Movement is comprehended in terms of a series of inter-penetrating and inter-mingling elements in different degrees of enfoldment all present together. The activity of this movement then presents no difficulty, because it is an outcome of this whole enfolded order, and is determined by relationships of co-present elements...."[70]

The LCL model looks at the scale of human communities seen within the horizon of generations; it sees the wholeness and not the pieces, the passages, and the journey. Understanding and engaging living phenomena through the logic of life keeps one's view on what counts for health, and enables leaders and social networks to enhance it.

5

Seeking Health: Persons, Bodies, and Choices

The invisible message of the interaction between professional and client is, "You will be better because I know better."...Through the propagation of belief in authoritative expertise, professionals cut through the fabric of community and sow clienthood where citizenship once grew.

John McKnight, *The Careless Society*[1]

A Gardener's Mind, a Mother's Despair

For three years, he came to the family home every week to mow, rake, and maintain the garden for which two professionals had little time. Leonard,[2] a young Xhosa man, itinerant, uncomfortable speaking English, living in a shack with his brother, and unable to find full time employment, lived precariously. Yet honorable, trustworthy, diligent, and always friendly—even if cannily—he was easy to deal with.

One day, Leonard arrived looking ill and in pain, eyes swollen and infected. His employers took him to their private doctor who prescribed antibiotic ointment, a painkiller, and rest. The infection receded, only to reappear some weeks later, and required to be treated again. Then, he uncharacteristically requested a fair-sized loan from his employers that he could never repay; it turned out that Leonard was seeking other treatment too—the money was for a *sangoma*. Sometimes mistakenly regarded as a "witchdoctor," the sangoma is a health provider who might use traditional medicines (such as a herbalist), but more generally, employs a mix of psychosomatic and spiritual treatments, with a particular sensitivity to relational realities that may impact upon health or ill-health. The sangoma is a holistic healer—a psychologist, family therapist, community counselor, behavioral expert, nutritionist, and more.

Gradually Leonard's health declined, increasingly provoking the concern of his employers. He started requesting the use of the toilet with worrying frequency, and more startlingly he began to arrive at inordinately early hours, even in the dark. He had never had a timepiece, but punctuality had not been an issue before. Progressively more confused, even about which day it was, Leonard also became increasingly scared of people, fearful of returning to his shack lest others might see him. One of his employers, knowing from her work in the field that such symptoms define a late stage of Acquired Immune Deficiency Syndrome (AIDS), pleaded with him to go with her to test for the human immunodeficiency virus (HIV)—not to the local clinic, for he feared for his anonymity, the stigma being too strong, the shame implicit, but to a removed nongovernmental organization (NGO) specializing in such matters. There Leonard was counseled by Xhosa-speaking professionals, tested, and diagnosed positive for HIV. The obvious next step was to determine Leonard's CD4 cell count; his symptoms were, after all, threatening. This was too big a step for Leonard. At first willing, he quickly withdrew, refusing all entreaties, and instead asked for leave and money to return to his home village in the distant Eastern Cape. His employers thought he was going home to die.

The story does not end there, though. Weeks later, he unexpectedly appeared again. Moreover, he had not returned home at all, but had gone to another nearby township where, for the duration, he had been treated by another sangoma, and a herbalist. He looked better, and the treatments had made him feel healthier, but the HIV virus hides deep and was almost certainly still there. Would he now go for a CD4 count to check? His answer is not unusual: "No, I am well! The people were wrong, I don't have HIV, and I never did!" The sangoma had clearly assured him that he was well and thus, intentionally or not, led him to conclude that the entire health system on which his employers depended was suspect, perhaps wholly untrustworthy. His mental frame of reference for understanding and defining his health and well-being had shifted.

Naturally, this changed frame of reference did not appear de novo. It was always there, lurking offstage, as Scott would say.[3] Suppressed in public, it was alive in private, creating a membrane between the world of biomedical science ("white ways") and his traditional cultural referents. In initially agreeing to be tested, this membrane was still permeable; now it had hardened into a wall. This kind of dissonance in the worlds of health seekers is not peculiar to exotic African contexts or to HIV. It happens everywhere. Moreover, it sometimes leads to fatalistic behavior when there simply seems to be no way out, as another story will illustrate.

Ruby, an African American female, was born in 1925 in the Mississippi Delta.[4] Daughter of a sharecropping family, eldest of twelve children, she was the great hope for her family; she was "smart." "Colored" children in the Delta area mostly received no formal schooling, or they worked with decades-old textbooks and substandard teaching from poorly paid women; however, Ruby could count long before her cousins and began reading before age six. Three of her siblings died in infancy, so she was her mother's hope for a better life, and her grandmother Ms. Addie doted on her; they would find a way to send her up river to her Great Aunt in Chicago, to a real school so she could become "somebody" and help her family.

Often hungry, Ruby found it hard to concentrate on learning. Like many children born to sharecroppers, before going to school she had to plant, hoe, and pick cotton while the season lasted. Sharecropper's life was hard, thick with racism, and marked by a fatalism born of a life that seemed permanently stuck in heartbreaking work and abject poverty. Ruby's family lived in a three-room shack north of Mound Bayou, the first area deeded to freed slaves—an undesirable, swampy, and mosquito-ridden area so thickly humid that simply to breathe was like drinking liquid air. Sharecropping meant working steadily from sun up to sundown with little to show for it. It was like legalized robbery—the landowner took everything. One could buy shoes and clothes from the "company store," but prices were set by the landowner who made sure you had little money left.

This landowner's wife, however, was fond of Ruby and taught her to read. Ruby read all she could find: old catalogs or newspapers used as toilet paper, discarded magazines, and even labels on cans in the store. However, her father drank too much, spending money that should have fed the kids. Ruby did not mind much, except when her father's inebriation led to rage and beating of her mother; then she covered her ears and tried to imagine life in Chicago. Meanwhile Ms. Addie's health declined and her weight dropped. Beaten shoes on swollen feet caused blisters, her feet stung and tingled, and walking got harder. The old female root doctor who lived nearby provided herb poultices to put on Ms. Addie's feet and now and again, when the family could afford it, she soaked her feet in Epsom salts. Animals were afforded better quality care than sharecroppers on the farm, while physicians charged them exorbitant prices, and therefore sharecroppers seldom asked for health care. However, eventually the blisters on Ms. Addie's toes turned red, then black, and a doctor was called. He took one look, shook his head, and said the toe must go. She had what the elderly called "high sugar." Over time, Ruby watched in horror as Ms. Addie lost toes, feet, and limbs. When she died, Ms. Addie was happy to go, telling Ruby, "Baby, cry when you are born and laugh when you die, because you are going Home to God and out of the misery of this awful life."

Ruby was stunned, her mother heartbroken, depressed, and barely productive. Ruby pined, grew disenchanted with learning, and looked for ways to escape the poverty and bleakness. Weary of everything, having given up on an education that seemed futile, she met a young man named Anthony. Fine-looking, a few years older, and earning some money at a local cotton gin, Anthony owned a store-bought shirt, pair of pants, and shoes that were not hand-me-downs, which he wore every Sunday to church. A smooth talker, he impregnated Ruby not long after Ms. Addie's death, but Ruby could not tell her barely functioning mother. Instead, she attempted to hide reality, tight wrapping her belly before going to pick cotton, until one day she passed out in the fields. Her mother just sighed and said, "Girl, you were our only hope. You ain't gonna have no better life now."

Anthony did marry Ruby, but because of Ruby's belly wrapping their first-born child was "mildly retarded," the doctor said. With two more children following, Anthony started drinking like Ruby's father, and after a couple of beatings, Ruby had had enough. Her cousin in Memphis found her a house-cleaning job and offered to have her and the children move in for a while. Ruby jumped at the chance.

TRICKY EQUATIONS: HEALTH
SEEKER AND PROVIDER

The stories of Leonard and Ruby not only illustrate the disturbing realities of the political economy of health, but they also raise fundamental questions regarding the relationship of health seeker to health provider. Health providers tend to assume that they know best, and so their relationship to health seekers is frequently marked by deeply hierarchical and asymmetric structures of power/knowledge.[5] Many believe that science, matched by a sufficiently educated or informed public, will bring the holy grail of health for all.

Increasingly providers and scientists acknowledge the inadequacy of their assumptions, but the standard views still permeate practice and theory. Even deeply gracious physicians who genuinely respect their patients bemoan, perhaps even rage at, what they see as the ignorance of people like Leonard resulting from cultural backwardness or poor education. The frustration can be understood, even sympathized with; though Leonard's education is poor, merely railing against behavior that is anchored in a way of seeing and being that matters to him changes little. Further education may do little to alter behavior and action, especially if it takes the standard view that discounts alternative or "other" ways of knowing and being—for they often remain potent and they are not necessarily wrong.

Intervention and practice, advice and behavior, prescription and choice, are all lodged within a complex and complicated reality filled with contested and conflicting approaches to health, as our two stories illustrate. We need to understand better this complexity and its dissonances. Willy-nilly it shapes how persons act, and greater intelligence about it should lead to better practice and outcomes. This requires a reorientation of perspective. Health provision is never a one-way street, as every health provider knows, and the health seeker is a crucial part of the equation. But is it really an equation? Are the terms of the relationship between health provider and seeker equal, balanced, or symmetrical?

The modern health provider, generally wielding vast amounts of energy, time, and resources, has a long-established and highly respected role, often deeply institutionalized in weighty structures and influential guilds. This gives the provider an inordinately powerful role in determining what should be done for whom, by whom, when, and where. Constraints—of medicines, personnel, finances, and so on—do not change that fact and, indeed, they may produce decisions that increase the gap between those who will receive and those who will not, worryingly embodying the aphorism that "unto those who have, more shall be given."

Health seekers usually must deal with whatever is placed before them, including an often overwhelming and incomprehensible body of knowledge that experts may wield against them, whether one thinks of clinical, biomedical, complementary, alternative, or indigenous providers. Globally, the availability of health care, access to it, and its affordability also test health seekers.

Few have sufficient means to get what they want when they need it, and most are faced with hard questions of cost. Trust, a rare commodity, is also no small issue.

Health seekers are not without power of their own. They weigh their odds, survey their options, consider their risks, shift their points of reference, assess and reassess what they will take as authoritative, and make choices accordingly, negotiating the terrain of health provision in complex, sometimes contradictory ways. They are in fact subjects who exercise their agency as best they can, even when they are confused, frightened, and in great need.

Yet the relationship between health provider and health seeker remains largely, often profoundly, asymmetrical. Neither power nor the knowledge that supports it, nor resources and means, are evenly distributed. One common result is a diminution of the role, the experience, the wisdom, and the acquired knowledge, "folk" or otherwise, of the health seeker in determining what is best for their health, and a corresponding amplification of the role of the health provider.

SOME SHIFTS IN PERSPECTIVE: QUALITY, RECIPROCITY, DECENCY

A relational view of health presses us to explore this asymmetry further. In some respects, asymmetry is inevitable. Special expertise, for example, is often desirable and sometimes vital. Urgent action sometimes requires a strict and efficient command structure, as emergency room (ER) personnel well know. However, many circumstances, perhaps the great majority (chronic conditions, for one), do not have to be characterized by an inequitable asymmetry in knowledge, power, or means. What would it mean to move toward less asymmetry and greater equity in the relationship between provider and seeker?

Rethinking this relationship requires some conceptual shifts from established, conventional thought and practice. Arising from the work of the African Religious Health Assets Programme (ARHAP), we introduce the notion of healthworlds, which conceptualizes how health seekers think, choose, and otherwise behave. Obviously, the need to understand health seekers and take them seriously is not a new issue in the world of the health sciences, so first we pay critical attention to other notions that already exist in this regard, particularly quality of care,[6] reciprocity,[7] and decent care,[8] to name three of the most noteworthy.

"Quality of Care"

Growing attention has been given to the notion of "quality of care" as a marker of health provision, and it has been related to religion and spirituality.[9] One archetypal report from the influential Institute of Medicine (IOM) in the United States cites the "quality chasm" as the most fundamental task to be tackled, noting that "the current care systems cannot do the job. Trying harder will not work. Changing systems of care will." Defining quality of care as the goal of health system reform, the IOM sets out six aims to achieve this goal. One focuses on patient-centered care—we would say health-seeker oriented care—which it characterizes as "providing care that is respectful of and responsive to individual patient preferences, needs, and values and ensuring that patient values guide all clinical decisions."[10]

The reference to values here and, to a lesser extent, to preferences, suggests a fairly strong role for the patient in determining the relationship to the provider. This is emphasized by the statement that patient values should "guide all clinical decisions," one potentially so radical that one wonders what was meant. It seems to challenge the asymmetric nature of the normal relationship, but does it? Two critical remarks are pertinent.

First, the language of "the patient" is a decisive limitation. A patient is only such, once she or he is placed within the care of the professional and, for all practical purposes, only so long as that care continues. Generally, the patient represents a case, a problem to be solved, limited in time to the attention required of the provider, and in the space controlled by that provider. There is no human history here other than the highly truncated, narrowly framed, and perhaps wrongly named "history" that goes with good diagnosis.[11] There is no intentionality aimed at a thick description of the human being who is the patient. However, a health seeker is not simply a patient; he or she lives in a journey of health, shaped by a history lodged in a cultural and social space, embroiled in a multiplicity of defining relationships with significant others, and dependent on a complex network of supports—and all frames their healthworld. This may not matter much to fix a broken arm or stitch a wound. But for other interventions, it might matter a great deal.

Second, none of the six aims advocated by the IOM,[12] including that of a patient-centered health system, suggest an attitude to the health seeker ("client," "customer") that could not just as easily be adopted by Wal-Mart. The determining paradigm remains largely individualist (the person as an isolated entity), exchange-based (the person as a consumer of care), and contractual (the person as a legal entity). Its anthropology is one of the individual actor making rational choices according to a scale of costs and benefits. The suggestion, therefore, that the values of the patient should "guide all clinical decisions" turns out to be based on a rather thin foundation, or better, a rather emaciated view of the patient as human being. While the idea of patient-centered health care is undoubtedly an advance, it moves only a few steps along a route that itself appears to be headed nowhere. In short, the underlying paradigm, the one that is in crisis, is fundamentally neither challenged nor changed.

"Reciprocity"

Another recent term that articulates a revised view of the relationship between health seeker and provider is reciprocity, also a promising idea. It sits within the tension between medical paternalism (deciding about the care of the other and asserting one's authority to do so) and patient autonomy (independent agents who decide for themselves whether they will accept treatment or not). Reciprocity may be defined as negotiation around treatment to mutual advantage.

In the context of public health, it highlights the tension between judgments of aggregate need (the most bang for the buck, for example) usually determined by epidemiological data, and the distribution of burdens, which cannot be aggregated. Denier defines this as the distinction between "statistical lives" and "identifiable lives," or between probabilities and persons.[13] Reciprocity seeks a balance between the two sides of the tension, which mostly means paying greater attention to identifiable subjects (communities) and their particular contexts. It also includes the idea of partnerships in public health, but usually the focus here is on how different health care agencies might work with each other or enter into partnerships with local communities. A positive development, it nevertheless skims the surface of our concern.

The literature on reciprocity still largely works within the paradigm of exchange relationships, governed by an instrumental logic and focused on calculations of cost-effectiveness. Its philosophical foundation remains the social contract.[14] In this frame, the relationship between health provider and health seeker is, willy-nilly, inherently predicated upon a formal, rule-governed, and, hence, objective trade-off. The terms of exchange—assumed to include parity of choice, opportunity, and means—may be at stake, but there is little that helps where parity does not exist, which happens to be common. One could seek to extend the idea of reciprocity beyond such limits, but because it remains caught up in the basic exchange paradigm, this is an uphill battle.

The point becomes clearer if we consider the difference between a contract and a covenant. The former assumes a juridical frame governed by the letter of the law and a theory of rights, the latter a moral frame governed by the nature of attestation, trust, and mutuality. That a contemporary practice can in fact be built upon a covenant rather than a contract is clear in the emerging agreements between a major hospital system and its surrounding communities, through the Congregational Health Network in Memphis, which we discuss later.[15]

Properly understood, reciprocity implies living well together in just institutions, as Paul Ricoeur argues in his philosophy of ethics in *Oneself as Another*.[16] There is no genuine reciprocity where justice is not present. Injustice, in this context, refers to a situation in which asymmetries of power, knowledge, information, and means generate suffering through the avoidable privileging of some and disadvantaging of others. Outside of the demand of justice, reciprocity easily becomes another name for a continuation of the status quo, providing the appearance of an ethical position but shortchanging the ethical demand.

These significant caveats notwithstanding, the language of reciprocity, as with that of quality of care, certainly represents an advance over past models. It has the great virtue of forcing attention onto the relationship between health provider and seeker. To make that relationship visible so as to take account of the health seeker is to be welcomed; just not at the expense of hiding the asymmetries of power and knowledge behind happy talk.

"Decent Care"

The idea of "decent care," developed within World Health Organizations (WHO) circles in the context of HIV, is influenced by the International Labor Organization's concept of "decent work." Loosely defined, it is "holistic care that not only addresses the recipient's needs and expectations but also respects his or her dignity and self-worth. Both the provider and the recipient of decent care should agree upon what it signifies."[17] A key implication is that "people living with HIV" (PLHIV) be drawn directly, at every level, into decisions about how the disease is to be tackled.

Decent care can be directly related to patient-centered care as far as it calls for an orientation to patient values.[18] Yet it goes further in two respects: it does not rest on the concept of the patient, which we have criticized above as too limited a view of the human person; and, it requires that a person's values (normative frames of reference), more than just guiding clinical decisions, should help determine why and how they are made.

The consultative process that gave form to the notion of decent care included people who represent some of the most powerful normative frames of reference: religious traditions and institutions, and PLHIV. Asked if the goal of decency makes sense of their understanding of health and well-being, and what their conception of decency would be, the goal was to find common ground around the notion of decency. The purpose was to help the WHO and the wider public health community rethink the participation of health seekers in decisions about health provision. The approach "enrolls the community in the problem-solving and support for care" and is seen as capable of restoring "the human face to the entire range of prevention, treatment, care and support services."[19]

At its heart, then, the idea of decency rests on an intrinsic orientation to a discursive or communicative logic rather than an instrumental one. It incorporates six core dimensions: dignity and agency (individual values); interdependence and solidarity (social values); and, subsidiarity and sustainability (systemic values).[20] A provider may contest particular norms and values of a health seeker, of course; decency suggests this is resolved not by sidelining or ignoring what does not fit the perspective of the provider, but in a process of parsing the claims to validity presented by all relevant parties, with a view to mutual learning.

The concept of decency is still young. Its practical implications and full theoretical reach still remain insufficiently articulated to be able to see how the idea might play itself out in practice, or how its elaboration might assist the development of new tools for assessing the extent to which decency is actually at work in any context. Nonetheless, the idea of decent care heads in a novel and potentially paradigm shifting direction, and it further helps us to recognize the growing impulse to rethink the relationship between health provider and health seeker.

Clearly, whatever language is applied, the turn to the health seeker is decisive. It rests on substantial indications both of a failure of systems as they currently work, and of the potential for improved health outcomes from such a turn. Paying special attention to the health seeker as a human person, approaching her or him based on the ideas of respect, dignity, reciprocity, or quality, provides an exacting indicator for any health intervention: how it deals with what counts for health and well-being in the view of the health seeker her- or himself. Practice is fraught with failure precisely at this point, for here subjectivity looms large. The intrusion of the subject is perhaps the single most difficult challenge for health science, or for science in general, for subjectivity with all its messiness—imprecision, diversity, ambiguity, unpredictability, and particularity—is exactly what the hard sciences seek to exclude.

Still, few believe anymore that good science alone is enough, though understanding the impact of subjectivity on health behavior and practice is not easy. The turn to the health seeker is an invitation to engage its messiness, requiring no less intelligence than does any exploration of anatomy, biochemistry, or neurology. Just as the immense possibilities of gene combination present a challenge of the highest order to researchers, to be met only by identifying basic patterns and processes that can bring some order to the complexity, so too do we need to find ways to bring order to our understanding of how health seekers perceive and act in the world.

Thus, sociologists and others have tried to recognize and identify patterns and processes that can be meaningfully generalized across populations by introducing the concepts of worldview and lifeworld, while cognitive scientists speak of "frames."[21] Some have recognized that religion (broadly understood) is one particularly potent and widespread way of framing one's story or existence in relation to health.

WHAT DO WE KNOW ABOUT HEALTH-SEEKING BEHAVIOR?

The contemporary counterpart to the ancient aphorism, "physician, know thyself!" might be, "Physician, know the one who seeks your help!" Even if physicians had the interest and the time, this is no simple task. Pinning down the behavior of health seekers is notoriously frustrating, though many attempts have been made using various theories and tools.

Confounding the issue is that concepts from various disciplines ("sick behavior" and the "sick role" in medical sociology,[22] "medical pluralism" in anthropology,[23] and "trust" in public health,[24] for example) are seldom integrated with one another, undermining any comprehensive view of health-seeking behavior. In one respect, the task may be hopeless: human beings with imagination, wit, and skills honed on the back of experience, some rooted generationally, never stop maneuvering or seeking to control their lives in ways only partially and tentatively predictable, in contexts that continually shift. Those charged with making decisions about health provision invariably therefore choose some simplified version of this reality as the basis for action. Bringing predictable order to such malleable diversity would require a massive synthesis of knowledge probably beyond our reasonable capacity. Even then, reason could not do it because contingency can only be grasped statistically via probability, and then only partially however sophisticated the mathematics.

Still, those who have made it their business to investigate health-seeking behavior have made some valuable gains. Perhaps small in the grand scheme, within their limits the theories and tools that have been advanced do in fact illuminate something of health-seeking behavior. Researchers of the Disease Control Priorities Project (DCPP) have provided an excellent overview of what has been achieved to date and how,[25] outlining the most influential tools and theoretical models on health-seeking behavior and health system response from the fields of cultural epidemiology, anthropology, social psychology, medical geography, and social economy. We draw extensively on this study here.

Probing the correlation between community knowledge and biomedical concepts, many studies of health-seeking behavior survey people's knowledge (K) about medicine or health, their attitudes (A) toward various interventions, and the kinds of practices (P) they adopt around a specific health problem. These "KAP surveys yield highly descriptive data, [but] without providing an explanation for why people do what they do."[26] Their most problematic theoretical assumption is that proper knowledge leads to appropriate behavior. Thus KAP surveys, while cheap, easily done, suited to large studies, and useful for assessing the distribution of desirable knowledge, remain rather limited as a tool for understanding health-seeking behavior.

Seeking a deeper understanding, anthropologists using qualitative methodologies have developed "focused ethnographic studies (FES)," combined with rapid assessment tools, to study health-seeking behavior. These methods, designed "to identify local illness concepts and categories,"[27] help to clarify the overlap between biomedical and local knowledge, and to understand how health system features, economic factors, and household decision-making processes impact upon behavior. Seen as a considerable advance over KAP models, there remains a strong emphasis in FES and rapid assessment approaches on cognitive factors to the detriment of other facts, including social determinants. They also rest heavily on explanatory models of behavior that focus on "aetiology, onset of symptoms, pathophysiology, course of sickness (severity and type of sick role) and treatment"[28]—in our view, an insufficiently defined categorization of the normative frameworks of reference that are relevant to the full picture of health-seeking behavior. However, the DCPP authors do point to the need to explore the "logic of interacting concepts" beyond an enumeration of illness categories, through which different sources of knowledge amalgamate, often syncretistically, in actual health-seeking behavior. Our notion of the healthworld, explained below, explicitly extends that understanding.

Other models outlined in the DCPP document that, taken together, capture the diverse investigations of health-seeking behavior, include: the Health Belief Model (perhaps best known in public health), the Theory of Planned Behavior model (an extension of the Theory of Reasoned Action, used in HIV studies), the Health Care Utilization Model (also called the socio-behavioral or Andersen model), the Four A's Model (availability, accessibility, affordability, acceptability), the Pathway Model (routes people follow in using different health care options), and ethnographic decision-making models (for predicting behavior).[29]

Just to name them is exhausting. It indicates something of the complexity of the field, and the difficulty of understanding health-seeking behavior or establishing theoretical coherence across the field. Fundamental weaknesses remain. All overestimate the capacity of individual choice, assume that individuals seek to maximize utility, undervalue emotional and "nonrational" behavior, and underestimate relations of power, symbolic life, and the role of historical processes in health-seeking behavior, while few "take into consideration health provider factors."[30] Generally acontextual, these models lack insight, inter alia, into gender disparities, poverty, economic inequalities, vulnerability contexts, and cultural and religious constructs.

In sum, the DCPP report demonstrates that "there are no cook-book instructions for the right approach to choose. Neither is understanding health-seeking behaviour a simple issue of choosing the right methods, qualitative or quantitative."[31] No way of researching the issues is more important than another. What might be needed, however, is a more adequate metaempirical foundation, a richer theory to guide the use of specific models and methods. That is just what we pursue here—using the interface between health and religion, broadly understood, as our not-so-arbitrary foil—to introduce a theory of the "healthworld."

Healthworlds: Ways of Seeing Health and Well-Being

Consider again the stories of Leonard and Ruby. Leonard lives in at least two worlds of perception and practice simultaneously, each with its specific cognitive logic, emotional content, and material foundations. Never wholly discrete, each interacts with the other differently according to circumstances and Leonard's judgments of what best meets his search for health. One world is governed by biomedical understandings of HIV, supported by a health system set up to manage things accordingly, including the NGO that provided counseling and accompaniment for his HIV test. The other world is governed by long-standing and honored Xhosa practices of health that have not disappeared, and should they be erased, it would be at the cost of a traumatic destruction of memory and place.

Perhaps Leonard personally sees little contradiction between the two frames, which he has probably harmonized in his own way. Nevertheless, as systems of health care, they are commonly in conflict. Overlaps are possible. Biomedical science, for example, is interested in indigenous medicinal knowledge, and psychologists have shown great interest in African understandings of the psyche. More likely, however, are serious mismatches between the two frames with grave implications for interventions and outcomes.

Recall that Leonard's employers strongly encouraged him to use available biomedical science, convinced that he was dying. Initially agreeing, subsequently vacillating, and finally choosing the worldview he trusted most, he rejected the biomedical analysis of his condition. His health-seeking behavior demonstrates how critical patterns of perception are to health choices, and how impotently unfitting a particular health intervention can be if they are not taken into account. The reality perhaps is not always as stark. Comparing Asian understandings of acupuncture to Western allopathic medicine, Kim argues that the different paradigms are more porous than generally imagined: "In practice they are always mingled and mixed without recourse to a sole worldview or epistemology."[32] Studies on health-seeking behavior do suggest that mixing is normal in "the mangle of practice."[33] A theory that helps grasp the workings of different worlds of perception would help to understanding this.

For this reason, ARHAP researchers have introduced the idea of the healthworld. It articulates a coherent, empirically relevant theory of the complex reality of health behavior and practice. It also enables one to see why religion—understood as a vital, framing set of ideas and practices that orient one toward reality and shape one's actions—is so thoroughly embedded in health perceptions and behaviors. If we think of Ruby's story, it also allows us to recognize that deprivation, depression, and despair are signals of a damaged and broken healthworld: diabetes, the medical condition that frames the story, is closely correlated with poverty and deprivation, powerfully revealing the impact on health-seeking behavior of the social determinants of health.[34] These, too, are relevant to the idea of the healthworld, which is only properly understood when located within a much wider theory of society and persons, of structure and action, of systemic forces and human agency. To that idea and the theory that supports it, we now turn.

The Concept of a Healthworld

The origins of the idea of the healthworld, proposed by Paul Germond who led the ARHAP team conducting research in Lesotho and theoretically developed since with Jim Cochrane,[35] lie in a failed attempt to probe how local people understand the link between religion and health. What immediately brought us up short was simply that the question, quite literally, was unthinkable: religion and health in the Sesotho language are inseparable; they are bound in a single concept. In modern European thought, Cartesian and Baconian influences have tended to separate mind (thought) from body (emotion, feeling), objective from subjective, privileging the former and bracketing the latter—especially in experimental method and natural science. The study of religion as an independent reality is part of this shift, and so is the separation of religion from health, which now become distinct, even disconnected categories. However, religion and health are intimately connected in Sesotho linguistic constructs, and only one word is adequate for both, *bophelo* (with equivalents elsewhere across southern and eastern Africa).

Minimally, bophelo means biological life; in its fullness, it describes the *telos* of comprehensive well-being in a fully healthy society. It thus invokes, in the mind of a Sesotho person, multiple intersecting experiential reference points: the human person, the family and homestead, the village, the nation, the ancestors, and the earth. "Ideally, each dimension should 'have bophelo' in full."[36] If any one dimension lacks in bophelo, it compromises the whole. Health, therefore, cannot be reduced to an individual person, let alone to a biological condition. It includes a rich, and decisive, web of extended relationships—to others (including those in the past upon whose contributions our own lives rest), to the *polis* or social ordering of life with others, and to the earth that sustains one. It is not far from the WHO's definition of health, in fact, though it includes another dimension, namely, spiritual health.

As noted, investigations of holistic understandings of health are not new. Medical anthropologists, in particular, have explored such understandings, uncovering many parallels to the Sesotho conception.[37] However, each such conception is linguistically and culturally specific, which tends to thwart a generalized concept. The idea of the healthworld aims precisely to establish a generalized concept.

Healthworld in a Lifeworld

The idea of a healthworld draws from Jürgen Habermas's discussion of the lifeworld in relation to system imperatives, in his theory of communicative action.[38] Others have linked his theory model to health,[39] but the notion of the healthworld is new. It reflects a particular ontological construct of the human being in the world in relation to the facts, norms, and experiences that guide human behavior.

The lifeworld is one of three basic contexts of social action identified by Habermas, others being the state (polity) and the economy (markets). As persons, we inhabit a lifeworld, but organizations of power (the state) and money (business) inhabits us, so to speak. As social structures with some command over our lives, they express system imperatives. Their logic is fundamentally instrumental, their particular goals (administration of a society, management of an economy) purposive rational, that is, oriented toward technical and operational ends of order and material stability.

We cannot escape these system imperatives, nor set aside their logic. However, as human beings and not robots (perfect expressions of system logic), we live—rich, diverse, and complex—emotional, relational, historical, and cultural lives expressed in countless ways. This includes symbolic, ritual, and aesthetic practices, associations of one kind or another, products of the imagination, play, and recreation. This is our lifeworld, and religion is very much part of it, often providing coherence and meaning where otherwise disorientation and anomie might prevail.

Influenced by existing lifeworlds, our own is constructed through our parents (or their surrogates) and others around us who transmit language, patterns of behavior, particular norms and values, and a framework for our identity. This occurs not only verbally, materially, and consciously (barely the latter at first), but also nonverbally, symbolically, and unconsciously.[40] Preinterpreted for us before we are born and a fundamental structure of being, the lifeworld consists of "a culturally transmitted and linguistically organized stock of interpretive patterns" that forms the taken-for-granted background of our everyday lives and shapes our convictions.[41] Its structural components include culture, society, and personality, mediated respectively by cultural reproduction, social integration, and socialization.[42] Unable to step out of it, it frames our horizon of action.

Over time, complexities increase, influences expand, their diversity grows, and we negotiate our way through it to make sense of our world and act accordingly. So even if lifeworlds retain powerfully influential deposits, they are also malleable. Elements of our lifeworld regularly move out of the background into our consciousness, at which point we may affirm and confirm, alter and adjust them—even, on rare occasions, reject them. Lifeworlds may therefore be highly stable, but not set in stone.

What brings the background aspects of the lifeworld to consciousness are what Habermas calls relevant action situations. What is not relevant to an action situation simply remains mute, though never entirely absent. Leonard's initial agreement to test for HIV, and his subsequent foregoing of biomedical interventions in favor of traditional healing approaches, illustrates this dynamic with exquisite precision. It also reveals the potency of lifeworld convictions around health and well-being. The desire for health and well-being, however, is powerful and anthropologically generalizable enough for Germond and Cochrane to believe that it frames more than a particular action situation. They argue that it identifies a fundamental region of the lifeworld, central enough to human being to warrant an independent concept: the healthworld.

Healthworld as a Region of the Lifeworld

The key to any healthworld in a person's life is its aim—comprehensive well-being. It represents the telos of life, that which animates one toward a goal of all-encompassing health. It is also affected negatively by the damaging or destructive effects of system imperatives driven by the instrumental logic of money or power.

Speaking in psychoanalytic terms, it is the drive for fulfillment in the face of the loss with which the neonate, sooner or later, has to come to terms, as a baby moves out of the phase of identification with the (m)other into recognition of its own, independent subjectivity. The lifeworld thus includes both loss and gain. The healthworld represents the drive to recover what was lost in a search for wholeness and completion. How readily, then, the healthworld expresses itself through religious symbols, images, narratives, rituals, and teachings, filled as they are with anticipations of wholeness and completion—liberation, redemption, salvation, *moksha*, and *nirvana*.

Remaining with the psychoanalytic perspective, we may also discern how a healthworld is connected to something more than individual existence. The undifferentiated self (in Lacanian terminology, the *moi*) from which the human infant frees itself gradually gives way to the fully present and conscious "I" (the *je*), the speaking, reflexive subject. However, this coming to an awareness of self (identity) only occurs in relationship to the (m)other and the larger other—the growing number of people, particularly significant others, to whom its identity is bound. There is no self apart from the other or, as Ricoeur would put it, no self without another.[43]

As the human subject (the "I," the je) matures, she or he expands her or his vision beyond the self, begins to recognize how one is bound up with others, grasps what this means for life together in family, community, and the wider society, and in the process, grants the claim of the other for recognition, reciprocity, and mutuality. That claim, however, is also what the self in principle demands from others, and this gives rise to a second irreducible region of the lifeworld, namely, the requirement of justice.[44]

The achievement of the telos that the healthworld projects, is thus not possible without justice, extended to all creatures and to the world that sustains one. Here we are very close to the conception of religion and health expressed in the Basotho view of bophelo. We are also close to the position reached by leaders from various religious traditions who, in discussing the idea of "decent care," determined that decency is most simply understood in terms of the golden rule, "do unto others as you would be done to," of which each religion had its version. Health and justice, like health and the religious impulse, are thus intrinsically related, a realization more prosaically (and narrowly) captured in current thinking about the social determinants of health.

Healthworld Debilitated

Reality, however, is filled with injustice at every turn, so the drive for health and well-being may be, and often is, frustrated. Indeed, injustice may occur with such frequency, depth, and personal impact that the healthworld is deeply impaired or disabled. Ruby's history carries exactly such an implication; here the telos that drives the healthworld has turned into an expectation of no change, to fatalism. One must expect the consequences for health to be devastating, that the best intentions from external agents seeking to change the health-seeking behavior of someone in such a context, would founder on the hard rock of injustice.

The regular experience of frustrated hopes of a better life, perhaps reinforced by an intergenerational history of such experiences, can probably only be met by an alternative experience, one that once more evokes the expectation of a different telos. Otherwise, there is unlikely to be any enduring shift in health outcomes, at population scale, of people such as Ruby and her family. Instead, as is well known in public health, one must expect that problems of alcoholism, diabetes, or interpersonal violence among such populations will remain endemic.

Healthworld Embodied

Experiences that impact upon healthworlds, and the perceptions that flow from healthworlds, are not only cognitive. They are also embodied, patterned in neural pathways, felt in the flesh, and written on the body, both metaphorically ("you look stressed, exhausted, crushed") and physically ("you have been battered"). In Pert's words, "The body is the unconscious mind."[45] Mind, body, and person—they are one. This, too, is a part of the concept of healthworld. It is not simply about the framing of norms, values, and attitudes in an action situation. Since it includes a drive toward the telos of greater health or comprehensive well-being, it also injects action-oriented behavior into a situation. The healthworld is thus linked to agency. People act in order to try to restore, maintain, or increase health, and this acting is what we mean when we speak of health-seeking behavior. There are three ways in which the healthworld places the body, embodiment, and, thus, materiality, at its center.

First, the healthworld expresses itself through corporeality, as the goal of well-being demands. However, if the self is irrevocably bound up with the existence of the (m)other, and others more generally, then corporeality is not atomic, restricted to an individual physical body. It includes the body of others who make up a community, the material environment within which bodies are located, and the emotions and human spirit that animate the body.

Second, the body experiences and records in itself the effects of power relations. Foucault, through his studies of mental health, the clinic, and prisons,[46] makes clear how much the exercise of power is material, physical, and corporal.[47] Power relations point to contestation over the human body, which directly affects healthworlds, as one might see in many ERs. This is also clear in the history of Ruby and Ms. Addie's "sugar" illness.

Third, the healthworld drives the desire to solve the problems of the body as individual and social, which is why indigenous diagnostic, treatment, and prevention regimes are so acutely attentive to the complex whole in which the individual body lives, moves, and has its being, always greater than the sum of its parts, and always intensely relational.

The notion of bophelo with which we began makes this all very clear. Here each person is understood in relation to distinct life phases, which add to the physical body a social dimension: from birth processes, through childhood to adulthood, into marriage, having children, the gradual attainment of seniority in the community, and finally, to death and a passage into the realm of the ancestors. Each stage is accompanied by ritual embodiments of what makes for health and well-being, including the transition from a child's to an adult's body through initiation rituals, and the physical modification of the body through circumcision, scarification, tattoos, and dietary regulations. Similarly, the mind, emotion, and spirit of the person is accessed, nurtured, and disciplined by an engagement and manipulation of the exterior body, through fasting, meditation, or other rituals of self-control directed at well-being.

However one looks at it, the embodied healthworld expresses itself in behavior and, in a dialectical dynamic, shapes and reshapes behavior, almost always in concert with others, present or imagined. Further, the relationships that constitute the healthworld include large-scale social and economic relationships[48] and have a direct bearing on the demographic reproduction of health and disease.[49] In sum, the healthworld cannot be separated from the other two constitutive realms of the lifeworld, namely, those that have to do with justice and freedom. As such, it thus offers a theory that incorporates the recognition of the social determinants of health, even as it allows us to see how perceptions, actions, embodiments, and relationships enter into health-seeking behavior. Finally, beyond mere utilitarian approaches or demographic impact, it provides the means to understand how religion impacts on public health.

The Use of Healthworlds

Because it describes patterns of perception that are lodged in cultural and social memories and processes, the idea of the healthworld helps us get beyond the impossible task of trying to understand the unique behavior of every health-seeking individual. That would clearly be useless in thinking about how to imagine public, civic, or communal practices and institutions for health. The patterns are in fact more general and identifiable, and their relative importance in any one context can be gauged.

Yet they are also fluid and mixed. Any one health seeker is likely to employ and deploy more than one healthworld pattern in reality, depending on what they are trying to resolve, what matters most to them in that regard (including the consequences for any relationships that are important to them), the resources available to them, and their accessibility and affordability. One should thus know something about the possible mix of healthworlds at work in any existing context[50]in order to take them into account in designing health systems and in shaping their imperatives and goals.

While the pattern of a generalizable healthworld may be usefully established theoretically, it should remain clear that in practice no one pattern appears as an entirely discrete phenomenon. The mix of healthworld patterns in any one person is dynamic, and shifts according to changing circumstances. Behavior change is thus possible. It is simply less likely if based on a denigration or denial of any functional healthworld that is valued by the health seeker.

CONCLUSION

We have attempted in this chapter to open up the question of health-seeking behavior as critical for any health intervention and the policies and the institutional practices that surround it. We have done so by briefly surveying other studies of the issues, and by introducing the concept of the healthworld. That concept provides a way of better understanding the issues, with a view to rethinking current policies and practices and constructing new ones appropriate to that understanding. The health seeker is the focus of our attention, but the health provider is part of that equation too.

Paying attention to the health seeker is not just a means of improving current ways of delivering health and building health systems. It is also a move beyond the instrumental, purposive-rational ways of thinking about them that mark the governing paradigm. Much of what passes for health care in the modern framework is in fact determined by system imperatives of money (economy) and power (polity), expressed in marketized and managerialized modes of thought and practice. This is so not because people committed to giving their time and energy to others in their search for health and well-being—nurses, doctors, attendants, counselors, and so on—do not care or understand what it means to be human, but in spite of them.

That is what it means to speak of a systemic imperative with a logic of its own. It is neither a conspiracy nor simply a matter of choices, even if all systems are ultimately the result of aggregate choices by human beings over time as they seek to master the world around them. Systems are not evil, they just are. However, systems easily overrun their capacity or, worse, exceed that for which they are intended: human thriving. As their power, range and extent grows, spurred by new technologies and knowledge in a shrinking world, institutionalized in varying kinds of bureaucracies, so too does their capacity to intrude upon, threaten, and damage lifeworlds. Habermas refers to this as the "colonization" of lifeworlds, a stark example of which is the commodification of anything and everything, including what used to be considered sacred, that is, set apart from the mundane and profane forces of production, distribution, and consumption. Everything now can be subsumed into the market and consumed. This is true of health care; and it is true of religion.

A focus on healthworlds is a reaffirmation of the importance of the lifeworld. Besides anything it may offer on how we work for the health of the public, it also represents a challenge to what we mean by health care. If we continue to invest more and more in the instrumental, purposive-rational, bureaucratic, and market-driven practices and processes attached to health care while ignoring the need to invest far more heavily in how these practices and processes square with the healthworlds of the persons for whom the health care is ostensibly meant, then we must expect that the problems of health systems and health providers will not only continue, but also probably intensify.

Change is not only a need or an option, but also a growing desire for many who work in and run health systems or institutions. Recent literature makes this clear, in studies, reports, and policy proposals, many of which we have mentioned here. We are on a journey whose end is not yet clear, but it is underway. If that is so for health providers, it is equally so for health seekers. While understanding healthworlds in itself is important, equally important is grasping that they are not fixed essences, rigid frames, or impermeable membranes. They accompany the journey that health seekers inevitably take from one point to another, from one way of thinking and acting through another, and from one challenge to another. That journey has to be better understood.

6

PEOPLE WHO CONGREGATE:
BUILDING ON STRENGTHS

Public health professionals are often surprised at how ubiquitously and actively congregations already engage in work relevant to the health of communities. Congregational leaders are equally as often surprised to learn how much of what they "naturally" do is relevant to the health of the public. As their activity in caring for individuals is so common, reflecting deeply held historical norms, they do not think of their work as advancing or sustaining community systems of health that they can deliberately improve.

Despite these disconnections, the fact is that both sets of people are interested in social-scale, complex, and dynamic patterns or determinants of health and well-being over life spans. To a remarkable degree, they flow within conversational range of each other, if all too often along parallel courses. Mostly missing is a common, mutually informing discourse about the knowledge that lives between them. The intent of this chapter is to serve that discourse.

A MAN, A WOMAN, AND A MOVEMENT

Stretching in low-hanging loops in the lot behind the church, yellow crime tape ran from the telephone pole to the old gym that the car had hit, after short, deliberate, and deadly acceleration. The deacons rewatched the tragedy unfolding in the fuzzy surveillance camera monitor as the police surveyed the grizzly scene where a man had killed himself. William Young, the pastor, watched too. He had known death in many ways, having served in Vietnam, witnessed the wars of an institutionalized mental asylum, and seen battles on the bitter streets of Memphis. However, this was a new kind of death, and he knew the image would burn in his memory and the consciousness of his congregation for many years. On the screen, the man nobody knew pulled his Oldsmobile up to the pole, tied a rope to it, went back to sit in the car for a few minutes, slid the rope around his neck, paused, and then drove out of this world into another.

Pastor Young and his congregation had seen another suicide seven years earlier. On Easter morning, under the cross in front of the church, a woman had shot herself. Young was affected personally. However, he was as a pastor of a particular kind of organization—a congregation, an entity that forms faith amid and in response to the wild and mysterious ways that life and death, futility and transcendence, weave into each other. He and his congregation took this seriously. The congregation is called "The Healing Center," virtually in defiance of the tides of death and disarray that surround it. Its mystery is that it does have strengths to heal. Not looking away from that terrible death on its back lot, the congregation found the man's family and his story. The spot he chose for his final act was not coincidental. Recently divorced after a troubled marriage, that back lot was where he had long ago played as a child and where he had met his wife. The Young's and other church members attended the funeral, participating in lament and honoring the bonds of humanity, spirit, and sorrow. With this event, the Healing Center's resolve was mobilized.

It is provocatively peculiar that a fragile congregation in the wrong part of Memphis would find in those deaths not a sacrilege but a window of possibility. Aware of hundreds of other similar stories, within two years after the first woman's death, The Healing Center had hosted a national convening of clergy and health professionals to probe the link between the black church and suicide. Further meetings spawned even wider hopeful dialogue in other congregations, in Washington and state capitols, and with the World Council of Churches. This energy builds very practical patterns of early intervention for those seeking what Young calls "emotional fitness," which reflects a brilliant reframing from deficiency to strength. The State of Tennessee gave The Healing Center $250,000 to pilot a neighborhood-level collaboration with twelve other congregations in Memphis to offer safe, trusted peer counseling and screening for emotional fitness. Since then, more than six hundred people have been referred into the more formal professional mental health system, which most probably would not have happened otherwise. A house of worship they could trust to treat them as humans, members, and neighbors was their pathway. The Healing Center, drawing on faith communities, opened up space to create what is now a global-best-practice model to prevent suicide.

In its work on suicide prevention, The Healing Center embodies an optimally functioning congregation. What is the nature of such an entity? What, of significance for the health of the public, are its strengths? Hundreds of thousands of congregations or "faith-forming entities" (FFEs) are found in neighborhoods everywhere, in Memphis and Africa, India and South America. Similar to other kinds of organizations, congregations are unlike them, too. Looking at any single one, such as The Healing Center, merely as a social service entity or affinity group obscures as much as it discloses. Lost is the peculiar mystery of how a congregation functions over time, how it is generative and resilient amid contexts rife with challenges only hinted at by the dramatic stories of suicide on the grounds of The Healing Center.

The Healing Center is one of over 350 congregations that partner with Methodist Le Bonheur Healthcare (MLH) to build a system of caring that incorporates but extends beyond the hospital. Called the Congregational Health Network (CHN), it blends what pastors understand about the life of their neighbors and what the hospital understands about their medical conditions.

Violence, a leading cause of death among the young and, quietly, among privileged white men too (suicide), accounts for a very large fraction of what is seen in emergency rooms (ERs). The hospital helps survivors of violence, but knows almost nothing about the causes or modalities that would prevent it. Pastoral intelligence recognizes that the answer to violence, self-inflicted or otherwise, intimate or anonymous, uncontrolled or utilitarian, requires more than "personal," individualized therapy. The answer looks more like a youth choir than an ensemble of professional therapists or surgeons.

At the heart of this book, we see faith and life span health as social in every dimension. The life of any one person of faith such as William Young is a fruit of a multigenerational congregate history, however much of his unique leadership gifts express that history in the particular neighborhoods, institutions, and interwoven lives of the people among whom he moves. A congregation, not just its leaders, has deeply woven strengths. In their own right, congregations are thus seminal religious health assets.

Many pastors, professors, and disillusioned church members, let alone skeptics of religion such as Hitchens or Dawkins,[1] can tell us of the obvious and chronic weaknesses of these same congregations. Anyone who has ever observed, much less served in, been employed by, or led a congregation knows that religious people can be feeble, distractible, and capable of stupidity and meanness. Perhaps surprising to some, the scriptures or traditions of many religious faiths also capture this. To acknowledge the weakness or failures of FFEs is one thing; simply to ignore their strengths or accomplishments is entirely another. We need a logic model that, despite the obvious frailties, brings into view the strengths in the social structure of FFEs that persist and generate new possibilities, even healthy ones, decade after century after millennia.

The frailties of FFEs can be explained as weaknesses of leadership, training, or management. Moreover, the social sciences find it recreationally easy to dissect many congregations for their awkward fit with modernity, perhaps offering to repair their failings with their expertise. Their shortcomings may also be represented as a side effect of an inadequate self-understanding of positive or emancipatory trajectories in a particular religious or faith tradition. None of this adequately accounts for the persistence and equally present life-enhancing contribution of FFEs. Yet, precisely this capacity is the most interesting and useful thing to know, if the assets of congregations are to be aligned for the health of the whole community.

We argue that FFEs are best understood, analyzed, and engaged in terms of their strengths. They enable and express social life in permeable webs of trust. They often function as religious health assets for the wider environment in which they find their life. They nurture people, raising up boundary leaders on journeys of life. They usually know well, and often do something about, the interface between faith and health in ways that are replicated and adapted over generations in serving the health of people.

The strengths of congregations are holistic and fractal, and though often expressed through individuals, they are not contained in one person, not even the clerical leader. The *social* entity in this case is seminal, whereas the personal is derivative or expressive of it. Just as personal health primarily proceeds from the social even if expressed in personal choices, experiences, and outcomes, so too with the strengths of the congregation. A competent, appropriate, and brilliant leader such as William Young remains more like a gardener than either an architect or a mason.

WORKING FROM STRENGTHS

People who congregate around religious or faith traditions tend to establish associations that evidence quite specific and identifiable patterns of strengths relevant to the health of communities. In themselves, and taken together, these strengths enable those who lead congregations (often also others outside them) to build their capacity to act in ways that generate assets rather than liabilities for health. At least eight such strengths can be meaningfully distinguished: the strength to accompany, to convene, to connect, to "story," to give sanctuary, to bless, to pray, and to endure.

In introducing these eight strengths, we wish to avoid the all too common oversimplification of how congregations function in relation to the health of the public. The strengths are characteristic, but they are not part of a recipe book. They are nonlinear and organic. A congregation is thus not best understood as a structured institution with bylaws, offices, and rules, but as a field of constantly changing, living patterns of complex human relationships, held in place by marks of attraction that are themselves qualities of life.

History of the Congregational Strengths Model

The eightfold model of congregational strengths has a particular history in the early years of the Interfaith Health Program at The Carter Center, funded by the Robert Wood Johnson Foundation in discussion with the Centers for Disease Control and Prevention (CDC). In the 1990s, public health professionals were continually expanding their curiosity to include health conditions far from the classic focus on infections and more rooted in human behavior, including the determinants of behavior that demand social, political, and environmental explanations. This inevitably drove a renewed appreciation for the potential role in applying evidence-based preventative science to the enduring health challenges of communities that community partners could and should play, one being faith entities. Dr. Foege in fact believed that the convergence of faith and public health could make possible a very particular vision:

> It is not impossible to dream of thousands of congregations working alongside public health, sharing an understanding that health is a seamless whole—physical, mental, social, spiritual—that poverty and illiteracy and addiction and prejudice and pollution and violence and hopelessness and fatalism are forms of brokenness, diseases that require the deployment of both their assets in building whole, healthy communities.[2]

The challenge was and is more complex than simply activating religious networks and their hundreds of thousands of congregations. The issue is how the particular, often peculiar, social form of religious body we call a "congregation" could be understood and linked in a useful and sustained way to public, science-driven health agencies. These agencies, because they tend to think instrumentally and functionally, "like a state,"[3] usually do not grasp the way congregations actually work to make their particular contributions.

The idea of the strengths of congregations was thus a clear and determined attempt to probe beneath the functional approach and its polity or legal apparatuses, and to explore the ways in which this social form offered assets relevant to the health of communities complementary to those of public agencies. The eight strengths were thus conceived in relation to heightened concerns about the reach and effectiveness of formal health systems and health services. While framed in the context of US public health policies and practices, they are clearly not specific to American congregations, nor indeed to any one religious or faith tradition. They are likely to apply in some form or another wherever people congregate in the name of their faith.

Understanding the Congregation

The systematic study of congregations has engaged the minds of some of the most well-known students of religion. An early figure was Richard H. Niebuhr,[4] but more recently, Wind and Lewis have written a landmark multivolume study on *American Congregations*.[5] The field has provided a generation of scholars with tools of analysis that have illuminated many aspects of congregational reality, but generally, it lacks a satisfying paradigmatic framework with which to work. Some approaches are appreciative (Ammerman),[6] others objectively curious (Thumma and Bird's analysis of megachurches),[7] still others baldly utilitarian (Cnaan and Boddie, who see congregations as social service providers with useful credibility, or Bennet and Hale's analysis of "medical religious partnerships").[8] From its inception, much of this scholarship has been seen as "practical," complementary (at best) to the more traditional focus on the systematic study of the theological ideas of faith.

In *Deeply Woven Roots*, Gunderson wrote about the role of faith in forming and sustaining healthy human communities, arguing in theological terms that "[i]f there is any hope at all, it is that God intends the renewal of the whole world. Congregations are a tool for that greater purpose, not themselves the point."[9] Eschewing a functionalist or utilitarian approach, therefore, he challenged familiar views of the congregation as a weak, frail, and complicated link in the logic chain of health, and articulated fully for the first time his approach to "a new understanding of how faith groups are integral to communities, not separate; how their strengths integrate with those of other institutions to weave the roots of community for health."[10]

Unpacking the key social strengths of congregations that are relevant to the health of communities required a novel weaving of streams of thought present in the fields of religion and public health, and produced the eightfold strengths model. It challenges premature conclusions about congregations, including by public health agencies, that see their value only in terms of useful techniques, messages, and activities, often simplistically reducing them merely to places for healthy spirituality or venues for the delivery of health messages.

Congregations are formed by people of faith, but people of faith are formed by and through congregations. In that sense, it is best to think of congregations as FFEs, a critical insight not captured by nomenclature such as the widely used term "faith-based organizations" (FBOs). Calling them "faith-forming" forces one to focus on the primary dynamic that produces what matters in congregations—those texts, rituals, beliefs, stories, songs, memories, expectations, and the like that shape both individual members, and the ethos and practice of the group. FFEs are the seminal religious health assets from which other forms of assets derive, some highly structured (clinics, social service agencies) and others far less so (prayer circles, orphan care groups).

In every society, alongside a proliferation of other social forms, the presence of an intricate array of FFEs persists. People continue to congregate—come together—for reasons of faith and spirituality, and congregations remain relevant to the health of vast numbers of individuals, families, neighborhoods, and their societies. This is true even if the "solid modernity" characteristic of earlier industrial society has become what Bauman calls "liquid modernity,"[11] filled with the rapidly morphing and moving forms of association, technologies and modes of communication characteristic of contemporary social and political organizational patterns. The strengths of congregations remain the same.

The idea that FFEs have strengths suggests how an alignment between religion and public health might be approached. Understanding these strengths also suggests what not to do, or why organizational practices imported from secular settings will likely be useless or, worse, damaging to the faith-forming entity and detrimental to the community outcomes to which their vitality and strengths are relevant. To draw on FFEs for getting things done means understanding the way that they live and have their effect.

The Eight Strengths of Congregations

Accompanying

People gather, they congregate. In the most basic sense, the gathered people accompany each other through their journey of life, even to its end. They show up in times of dependency, celebration, lament, learning, and loss. The acts of accompaniment are a part of membership. Membership is usually bound by an explicit covenant bond, spoken and marked by rituals of entry. Less formal ways of membership grow organically through patterns of association that also build webs of relationship and accompaniment. One experiences accompaniment as the fruit of human association, as an affirmation of commonality, not dependency; one of the company, one is accompanied. The faith-forming entity has the peculiar strength of generating such associations across bounds of race, blood, class, party, and even distance that are crucial to the health of the community.[12] As Ammerman and Farnsley put it:

> Religious congregations, including the small groups they house and sponsor, are then a space of sociability where real commitments are made (even if temporary and partial) and where persons are thereby formed and transformed. Congregations are not best described merely as the product of individual choices. They are social realities sui generis. While people may shop for the congregation that best fits their individual tastes, the resulting group is usually not merely a collection of individual consumers but a community, a public, a collective, a piece of the larger societal whole.[13]

Congregations are not merely aggregations of autonomous individuals making rational choices designed to secure individual benefits; they are socially created and sustained over generations. To be sure, especially in "liquid modernity," congregations are not always associated with specific geographical spaces in which all their members live. Easy to notice in stable, archetypal small communities, congregations are also the most visible form of accompaniment in the radically new kinds of translocal and transcultural networks of new immigrants growing on the suburban edges of liquid cities such as Atlanta or Cape Town.[14] Even messages and presentations absorbed privately via the Internet, cassette tapes, videos, or other contemporary media connect one to social spaces in which people gather. This is evident even where cultures and livelihoods are most at risk or turbulently fragile, on the borderlands where two or more life-worlds mingle and multiple or hybrid identities are formed. Thus, in the Atlanta suburb of Doraville residents use their churches as places to negotiate their way in a broader context of segregation. The newest residents, facing multiple forms of discrimination, turn to churches not only for refuge but also as a place that provides space and the symbolic and material elements with which to engage a public sphere from which they are often excluded. Simultaneously, they often maintain links with the places they left, their churches becoming pathways for the "formation and maintenance of transnational, transregional, and translocal ties that shape the ways in which they negotiate the city's often inhospitable landscapes."[15]

However malleable, such congregations establish networks of relationships that hold many capacities, beyond that of the clergy. Luz Maria, for example, is an undocumented Mexican immigrant to Atlanta who cleans homes for a living. However, her vocation is her work as organizer of the Mission's chapter of St. Vincent de Paul. Her dedication to this work has earned her the status of unofficial matriarch of the church. "Here," she says, "it feels like the town square [*plaza del pueblo*]. We come, we get to know each other, we mingle with each other. We listen to the word of God, but we also develop friendships.... It's like a vision of a plaza where people from all countries encounter each other."[16] Luz Maria's role is not only healthy for all the reasons the Leading Causes of Life (LCL) theory would suggest, but it is also an expression of congregational strength, best understood in terms of being in the company of people who are not simply servicing each other, but walking together, participating in each other's lives as they journey through life.

Congregational accompaniment is powerful precisely because it is not professionalized, but built on the efficacy and intelligence of nonprofessional leaders and actors, protecting community agency in the process. This is not trivial. McKnight, in *The Careless Society*, points to the ironic trap of poor communities held down first by circumstances, and then again by the weight of trained and paid professionals who minister or administer to them: "...the invisible message of the interaction between professional and client is, 'You will be better because I know better.'...Through the propagation of belief in authoritative expertise, professionals cut through the social fabric of community and sow clienthood where citizenship once grew."[17] Both the form and the function of congregations hold open the social space for people such as Luz Maria to bring life through the expectation that they will accompany others around them, and the belief that this is part of their membership of the religious community.

Convening

Getting people into one place where health issues can be discussed is not always easy, especially where civic or accessible venues are not readily available. However, to be able to convene groups of people is frequently important to the practice of public health and its professionals and practitioners. Very often, therefore, those outside the social network a congregation represents want to engage that network, and they will ask congregational leaders to convene a gathering. The authority of such leaders, however, is not simply individual, but deeply derivative of the social structure of the congregation itself. Congregations, Cnaan and Boddie note, provide a venue for the community "where people can interact with others whom they trust and care for."[18] They open up necessary space, often foreclosed in resource poor or politically repressed situations, where issues, local and beyond, can be discussed.

The story of Pastor Christian Führer's Nikolai Church in Leipzig is a stunning example of the power of convening. In February 1988, he invited fifty people advocating for the right to leave East Germany to hold their meeting at the church. About six hundred turned up, but then increasing numbers of people began to attend his regular prayer sessions. More followed at prayers and vigils until, in May 1989, the authorities decided to block any traffic going to the church. On October 9, despite this restraint, and notwithstanding beatings and arrests in Leipzig and other cities, at least seventy thousand people turned up to the Monday Demonstration chanting, "We are the people." Pastor Führer, with others, ensured that the protest was nonviolent, which confused the police, whose sharpshooters were everywhere waiting to unleash the violence that would break the movement. They received no useful advice from Berlin, so the march simply went ahead. With that, the authority of the rulers was broken. The next Monday, there were one hundred and twenty thousand people, and on November 9, the Berlin Wall fell.[19]

Certainly, many of those convening at the Nikolai Church were not active members of the congregation or even religious, but that is not the point. The capacity to convene is, even if, like any other strength, it may also be turned to purposes not always for the good. It is also not as rare as this iconic story might lead one to think. On the contrary, Cnaan and Boddie suggest, "The voluntary coming together of people as a group in a respectful and reflective manner distinguishes the congregation as a unit of social intervention from any other institution in the community."[20] FFEs or congregations may no longer be part of the command structure of society, of course: "Nobody has to come when the church calls or do what the mosque says. But amid the decline of many other unifying social structures, it can convene. It has capacity to bring together people across lines that frequently divide; such as profession, economics, race and self-interest."[21]

Convening, then, is a second strength of congregations, upon which many health education and health promotion programs working with faith communities depend. As part of an ensemble of interrelated strengths, it is particularly close to the strength of connection.

Connecting

Congregations, which tend to persist in time and space with greater resilience than many other social organizations, represent stable networks of connections independent of any individual members that pass through. They connect, too, to other existing pools of social capacity in other networks and organizations. The strength to connect is especially valuable at the level of community systems, not only enabling access to existing resources and services but also generating the social imagination needed to create new entities or social forms that do not yet exist.

If the power to convene brings people together, connecting is marked by creating links across which resources, assets, power, and knowledge flow. Sometimes the connections mature into wholly new organizations that become part of the community's organizational infrastructure, when it is easy to forget where the organization came from, how the meaning and purpose were formed, where the leadership was raised up. Once visible and stable, these connections are easy to name, products of what some call social capital,[22] a term that helps mark relational phenomena as valuable in the same way we speak of religious health assets. However, the economic language also distracts from the underlying generative dynamic that produces new connections among highly animate beings. Even on Wall Street, capital is just money until somebody has an idea for its use. If one wants to build a community, one does not start with social capital either: "A social infrastructure is just a skeleton until it has compassion and discernment. These are what breathe life into the connections, and they depend on the strength of congregations to nurture them."[23]

In many communities, congregations connect to each other and to larger networks of institutions through their leaders who form critical social webs. As Ammerman notes:

> The typical congregation can touch the lives of many people, but its most direct impact—beyond its own members—is likely to be limited to a relatively small and local circle where emergency assistance can be rendered, the precepts of faith shared and support and enrichment provided.... But when congregations want to reach beyond their own local community or want to do more than their own limited resources make possible, they work through other organizational channels.[24]

If some public health scientists emphasize the way religious communities create social friction, Ammerman shows that it is rare for congregations to stand alone: only 3 percent of congregations have no network of partners.[25] Most are permeable networks with multiple, flexible ways of linking people, ideas, resources, social, and political capital relevant to the functioning of the social whole of which they are a part. They also connect people, ideas, and practices across and in the borderlands or interstices of social and political structures, as Vásquez and Marquardt show, helping us see how "religion generates hybridity, opening, in the same ways borderlands do, liminal spaces of transcultural creativity and innovation. For no matter how rigid they might be and how hard the nation-state and elites work to maintain them, borders are always permeable."[26]

Denominations are and have been the most common form of network partnership among congregations for at least a century, according to Ammerman.[27] However, she notes, the average congregation supports about five service organizations beyond whatever the congregation does on its own or through denominational affiliates.[28] Moreover, 73 percent of the congregations in her study have at least one connection to an organization that works for the health, education, and cultural enrichment of people beyond their members.[29] Significantly, many of the community partners to which congregations connect are not explicitly religious, and many are impossible to classify neatly at all. In the US context, "almost no service organization is without a religious presence of some sort, nor is any organization—no matter how apparently religious—utterly without secular influences. Almost by definition, when charitable intentions take organizational form they are at once both sacred and secular."[30]

Connection creates new intelligence and new efficiencies relevant to health at community level. For example, Memphis has long been a destination for medical students, about one-third coming from other countries, and many have stayed. The neighborhood north of Summer Road is much like other working class areas but for one thing, the *Masjidjāmi*[31] and its stream of members from countries around the world. Many of its founders came to Memphis as students, built it, its school, and, subsequently, a free clinic open to all established with the Islamic Medical Society, all expressions of their faithfulness. In the constant ironies of faith-based health care, the clinic secretary is a redheaded Methodist who enjoys being in a faith-based ministry, while the *Masjid* medical professionals also connect with other faith-based institutions such as the MLH where many of its physicians serve on the staff.

The personal connections of faith woven into the Masjid create a safety net for hundreds of patients, including those without insurance who need hospital treatment and otherwise find access to good care difficult. This has led the MLH to waive its charges when a physician, acting out of their own faith, forgoes their charges, irrespective of which particular tradition generates that faith. Multiple kinds of connections are thus clearly a powerful strength of the Masjid congregation, enhancing the health of individuals, families and, indeed, the whole polis within it finds its life, and representing an intelligence that looks for synthesis and synergy, and that sees health as a whole.

Congregational connections also produce some efficiency of resource flows. People can get what they need because the resources are made visible and accessible across their networks. Some connections, assuming institutional form, link hundreds of congregations of all traditions, as with the Greater New Orleans Federation of Churches, a sophisticated structure that enables a broad network of congregations to offer extensive and ever-mutating programs for education, training, elder care, grief counseling, advocacy, adult literacy, food, shelter, a cable TV channel, health initiatives, and prison ministry.[32] A bridge that links "the spiritually concerned and the socially concerned," the Federation functions by "connecting the religious, social, political and economic communities of New Orleans in order to serve the needs of the whole city."[33] It extends, but does not replace, the smaller scale intimate connections that congregations develop and sustain, across which extensive caring is expressed.

Sometimes, connections are capable of withstanding a hurricane and help the community grow back when almost all is washed away. Cnaan and Boddie wrote about congregations three years before Katrina came ashore, scattering institutions and drowning buildings. Congregations survived that, providing a kind of trellis on which life could grow back, using their existing connections and their strength as life demanded. If accompaniment is the root asset for individuals, connection plays the same role for the health of social wholes.

Storying

One of the mysteries of health is why people continually make choices against the best data and advice. We are increasingly awash in data, information, and advice, much of it contradictory or highly contested. New communications technologies make it easy to find technical answers quickly. Often missing is the larger story within which we can understand ourselves.

To think of this as a story is crucial; it shifts us away from data to narrative, and pulls us toward the essential role of FFEs: "The challenge of where to find unifying, trustworthy stories confronts business, government and leaders of all kinds as they discover that it is quite literally true that where there is no vision the people perish."[34] As expressed in the concept of healthworlds, people make choices in the context of a larger, multiply-storied narrative that gives coherence to their world, locating them in relationship to other people, to time, to circumstances, and even to their own bodies. Ricoeur calls this "emplotment," the vital need to see ourselves as part of a narrative and historical weave within which we are able to interpret the world around us and our lives within it.[35] The strength of "storying," as always, is two-sided; religious leaders can use it simply to protect proprietary language or as tool of domination—as religious sacred writings often themselves point out! Yet, handled with humility, it can also be like water in the desert.

Nothing is more characteristic of FFEs, of how they express and nurture the other strengths, than their strength to story. As Ammerman's extensive work shows, congregational life is fundamentally grounded in stories: they incorporate past, present, and future; recount action; and build on relationships, current and intergenerational. Congregations "invite their members into the sorts of shared experiences that demand to be narrated," and make possible "a meeting ground where new, shared stories evolve."[36] Clergy are often asked by public health authorities to disseminate health messages that carry credibility by being spoken from the pulpit. However, the strength to story is much deeper and more powerful, if less predictable, because the stories with traction are those that arise out of the congregational life itself.

Nowhere is this more telling than in the history of the relationship between faith congregations and human immunodeficiency virus (HIV) and acquired immunodeficiency syndrome (AIDS). Canon Ted Karpf tells the story of a young man suffering from AIDS who came to his parish hall to ask if he could die there in safety. No other place would have him.[37] From this and similar experiences—well before most people had heard of AIDS, Karpf was burying members of his parish from it—he and his congregation built a narrative for the living that took him over the next decades into congregations in many other parts of the world, telling the story, encouraging others into it, and advocating for practical change to meet the pandemic. His story enables other stories that cohere, connect, and inspire: "Those of us who have worked daily with persons living with AIDS have seen nobility of spirit, courage of heart, power of the will, patience in the midst of suffering, and genuine holiness."[38]

The strength to story, then, is not just in the telling of them but also in hearing them, in participating in a larger story as it unfolds in the lives of anyone within caring distance. The congregation is a social space in which such stories find, give, and transform life. This does not hold true always though: Rosalyn Carter notes that the first word religious leaders should say to those living with mental illness is one of apology, because "congregations have often been the last bastion of the worst stigmas that persist in our society."[39]

Recognizing a strength, again, is not to ignore the weaknesses that are part of the ambiguity of congregations, or any form of community for that matter. Still, Wendell Berry argues, those who hope for community must dispense with childish wishes or complaints, among which he includes Mark Twain's stories of Mississippi life. It takes an adult familiar with the ambiguities and disappointments of lived social life to get the story right, to move beyond facile complaints: "What is wanting...is the tragic imagination that through communal form or ceremony, permits great loss to be recognized, suffered and borne, and that makes possible some sort of consolation and renewal. What is wanting is the return to the beloved community, or to the possibility of one. That would return us to a renewed and corrected awareness of our love and hope for one another."[40] Any true story of the relationship between those whose health is at stake and communities of faith is complex, tantalizing, disappointing, tragic, and hopeful, all at the same time.

Giving Sanctuary

FFEs usually have spaces we may call sanctuaries. They occupy both intangible social spaces, and tangible ones that stand for generations. Ancient cities such as Istanbul, Delhi, and Canterbury are defined by their grand religious sanctuaries, but even in many streets with almost no name at all, the faith-forming entity has the largest meeting space in the neighborhood. Space matters. However, what kind of space?

As the story of Canon Karpf above indicates, even those people most cruelly stigmatized have a reasonable expectation that a house of worship might be a safe place to enter and find protection. Though not always, they can. The space sends many important signals about whether it is safe for those on a life journey, safe for "difference." For example, the Episcopal Church of the Incarnation in Atlanta before the mid-1960s was located predominantly in a white area. Now, however, the area is predominantly black, with a distinctly mixed economic status. As the population changed, so did the churches. Some new ones were built, some old ones changed hands, and some, like Incarnation, were transformed, in the process creating an environment that gave people safe space, a sanctuary, where they can express their identities and their diversity. Now, throughout the Church of the Incarnation, "the walls are covered with pictures from different cultures, depicting Jesus as they see him."[41]

Sometimes even when confused about *what* to believe, people know *where* they believe, which holds them in social relationships where personal meaning can grow. Consider Gunderson's Bible study class, for example, where he teaches men and women who began to meet as young married couples more than five decades ago, in the same room. Almost everything in their world has changed, all of which they have witnessed together, washed in tears from time to time and just as often in laughter.[42] Then again, think of a socially active, black base ecclesial community in an informal shack settlement in KwaZulu Natal whose work was shaped by conversations held in a protected space—a space more than necessary in the face of threats of the white-ruled state and its local proxies.[43] Alternatively, reflect on the protected space *Masangane*, the Moravian-instituted group in Matatiele in the Eastern Cape of South Africa, offers to those who are shamed or attacked because of their status as people living with HIV, within which they recover their vitality, energy, and agency.

For words to become deeds, they need a place where they can come alive and be embodied; for stories to be embodied, they need a sanctuary, especially in risky or dangerous places or filled with costly consequences, such as Memphis during the Civil Rights movement, South Africa under Apartheid, or anyplace where HIV thrives.

Congregations as sanctuaries have both proximate and distal implications for health. Perhaps they offer valuable venues for dissemination of health information and health services—blood pressure checks, counseling, perhaps to model testing for HIV or prostate cancer. However, health messages and services only work because of the trust engendered by what has gone on before or still goes on in that space, where stories can safely be told and take form, and where people experience their membership in a community of meaning and accompaniment—a sanctuary built and sustained by repeated, mutually witnessed, personal, and social transformation. Whatever their ambiguities, an intrinsic strength of congregations is that they can and often do offer safe and trusted spaces upon which one may build.

Blessing

Many people in health professions or health education think that congregations and religious leaders have extensive powers of persuasion, even coercion, that direct behavior in ways that have direct and indirect deleterious health effects. Within the ambiguous jumble of religious life, such judgements can be justified. Religious condemnation is one culprit, HIV, for example, far too frequently being described as a punishment from God, a sign of poor faith, or a result of sin.

Nonetheless, unsurprisingly, we begin again with assets or strengths. As Ken Pargament has shown, a sense of condemnation is not good for health. He, Koenig, and others studied 596 people hospitalized for a variety of illnesses, all fifty-five or older, all saying either that they felt unloved, abandoned, or punished by God, or that the devil's work was responsible for their problems. Such negative beliefs put patients "at increased risk of death," 19 to 28 percent of them being more likely to die (during the two-year-study period) than the control group.[44]

The tethered opposite of condemnation is the strength to bless. Essentially, blessing another (or oneself if need be) means to affirm rather than condemn, and to offer one's presence, physically or in spirit, in support of that affirmation. Blessings are healthier than religious warnings, scolding, or negative rules. This embodied strength, close to but different from the power of forgiveness, is one root of the transformational evidence for the changes in identity, ideation, and behavior that is so crucial to life span health, especially in patterns of community. If those who seek to enlist FFEs in targeted campaigns or social programs to push people to do certain things ("get your H1N1 vaccine") or stop doing other things ("just say no") are often disappointed, they might better grasp the power to bless and its effects: "Blessing sets people free, free to change, to untangle from their bondage. But blessing never prescribes, dictates or manipulates."[45]One might, of course, ask what good such freedom is in the face of a killer virus or a threatening illness?

Think again of the bitter story of Ruby and Ms. Addie.[46] Eventually Ruby found her way into Memphis but, like her grandmother, she also took on the journey of diabetes. Having no health insurance, she had never been to a doctor barring her first pregnancy. In her late sixties her weight dropped, her feet began to sting, and bathroom trips became frequent. Now also with the "sugar," a kind nurse assured Ruby it could be "managed" if she controlled her diet and checked her sugar regularly; but Ruby simply sank into depression. Images of her beloved grandmother losing her legs paralyzed her with fear. Worse was giving up her beloved coconut pie, fried chicken, and corn bread, her only real treats. Deciding it was better to "go on Home to God early" like Ms. Addie, Ruby told no one of her diabetes, and did not change her behavior.

Several months later Ruby collapsed at work, her situation dire. Her daughter pleaded with her to survive for her grandchildren's college graduation and for her mildly disabled son John. Ruby learned to check her sugar levels, and later, encouraged by her pastor, joined diabetes classes through Memphis Healthy Churches. With peer encouragement, she remembered one of her first loves, reading, and reading everything she could about her "sugar," she felt hope, even walking the track close to her house and attending aerobic classes. In her mid seventies, Ruby felt better than she had in years, and when Christ Community Health Center opened in her neighborhood in 2007, it was a dream come true. Here medical support came with spiritual support, or what we would call a blessing. Ruby no longer thought about Ms. Addie with horror, just sadness and a resolve to help other people with diabetes live better. Overcoming her fatalism, she currently lives as well as anyone could at her age, managing what physicians call her chronic illness, but what she calls her life. If a health educator would honor her for self-management, the true story lies in how her multiple relationships blessed her, giving her strength and freedom to choose a path toward life.[47]

Another example is *Masangane,* a highly successful faith-initiated, comprehensive, integrated program for HIV and AIDS, working in a poor, largely rural part of South Africa. Its success depends upon many things, but among the most important is the support it gives to those it serves. Some of this support is material, to be sure, but most of it takes the form of a physical, emotional, and spiritual embrace of those who know they are HIV positive, encouragement for those who fear to be tested in the face of stigma and shame, and regular personal or group encounters where they are strengthened with messages of solidarity.[48]

Whereas Koenig suggests that religious beliefs help everyone, especially sustaining in astonishing ways those who often have "nowhere else to turn" nor "the resources available to survive,"[49] the strength of blessing is found not in disembodied, abstract faith, but faith mediated through the physical human relationships found in a faith-forming entity that provides for the social integrity of the blessing. Blessings that produce the liberty that produces health cannot be bought or sold, only given and accepted gracefully, where a community provides a place for embracing the full complexity of life, where one is welcome, forgiven, hoped for, and included.[50] Ruby's fatalism was overcome not solely through a health professional relationship, but through a congregational one.

Praying

"Congregations," Ammerman points out, "are fundamentally *religious* organizations. That is such a commonsense assertion, but the perception of what congregations are about is often distorted by all the talk about them as deliverers of social services, builders of social capital, mobilizers of political constituencies, or even producers of culture."[51] They nurture spirituality and faith by means of corporate worship and the rituals of their faith, they teach and educate people through the course of their members' lives, and most have some way of encouraging individual commitment to their faith.[52]

People of faith, when they congregate, are thus present to each other as individuals and as a social body sharing what they experience and understand as holy or sacred. "Prayer" is the simplest possible name for a very long, deep menu of means to evoke and celebrate the presence of the holy in their lives. It includes not only formal prayers offered by an ordained person in full-ecclesiastical regalia, but also the silent candlelit witness offered on the streets of Alameda County at the site of a handgun death, or by a mélange of people in front of St. George's Cathedral in Cape Town during the struggle against Apartheid.

Health education messaging in a congregation can focus too sharply on rational instructions, underestimating the critical importance of the social phenomenon. Similarly, prayer abstracted from its social embodiment or location in a healthworld is readily turned into a mere therapeutic technique, whether done well or badly. Much significant literature on the health effects of prayer reflects this reductionism, and most of it, in our opinion, lacks a theoretical context in which to understand the limited, even contested, association between prayer and health outcomes. The whole phenomenon is the message.

The actual practice of prayer nearly always emerges in some form where people congregate in faith. The faith entity creates the space in which prayer is made credible and thus accessible to individuals, even when they are not active members of a particular congregation. Pilgrimage sites, for example, may appear to be mainly special physical spaces, but they are also profoundly social in genesis and affect. The Sunday school class mentioned above of older people has met for decades in a bland room dominated by a cork bulletin board. The board is wholly unremarkable until one comes close enough to read the dozens of clippings, notes, pictures, articles, cards, and reminders of who the members are, how long they have traveled together, who they love enough to pray for—prayer directed not just toward God but toward each other, reminding them of who to visit, touch, call, and feed.

Prayer, precisely because it is a social practice at the boundary between physical and spiritual, private and public, fear and belief, hope and mystery, also illuminates the relationship, sometimes bizarre, between religion and liquid modern reality. Vásquez and Marquardt begin their exploration of globalization and the sacred with a story that takes place in a Florida strip mall in Clearwater, where people gather to observe what they perceive to be an in-breaking presence of the holy in the form of reflections on the windows of a building that are taken to represent the Madonna.[53] Here there is no normal congregation, and that makes a difference. Instead there were local residents, the "occasional curious out-of-towner," members of the national and international media, volunteers from a lay Catholic organization dedicated to interpreting and spreading "Mary's messages," transnational Mexican immigrants who saw Our Lady of Guadalupe, multinational pilgrims on their way from other pilgrimage sites such as Medjugorge and Conyers, and tourists on their way to Disney World in Orlando.[54] Prayer and its practices in the borderlands of the holy turn weird when abstracted from the faith-forming entity whose social bonds provide context.

The opposite story of healing prayer is found in the many congregations that open their doors for prayers of blessing to those whose daily work drains their spirit—teachers, nurses, and social service workers who live on the bleeding edge of social problems and tend to wear down. The Free Synagogue in Evanston, Illinois, for example, holds a monthly prayer and healing service for social service workers, Christian, Jewish, or otherwise. Focused on silence and meditation, it uses powerful, nearly universal symbols that mark the way toward the holy, usually beginning with the lighting of a candle and a brief meditation on the theme of light.[55] This is prayer as the most, not least, common denominator of those who live in service of others, and it is a strength of congregations.

Enduring

Among the most remarkable strengths of congregations is that they last, often much longer than any other kind of place of meeting or gathering. They are not only generational but also intergenerational. In Broad Street, Soho, London, the Reverend Whitehead's St. Luke's Parish still exists, even if with little similarity to his time (though there is a Dr. John Snow Pub!). Its practices and theology have inevitably shifted in multiple ways, yet the parish retains its congregational strengths, in potential if not always in practice. Congregations are durable.

Still, the nature of congregations is changing in many ways that also need to be understood to grasp how their strength to endure might display itself. A faith-forming entity no longer needs to be physically rooted in one place, though many still are. Many congregations today are spread across several spaces, some even virtual. Congregational studies have yet to come to terms with this fact, a consequence of the compression and dispersal of space and time, driven by new means of communication, or what we call globalization.[56]

In this context, Vásquez and Marquardt call for a deepened and extended stress in congregational studies on "lived religion," able to account for the increasingly common fluidity, conflict, and paradox within religious localities, where religion is regularly deterritorialized and reterritorialized. "It is not," they say, "that locality and face-to-face encounters do not matter anymore, but rather that they have become more unstable, stretched, and shot through with hybridity and disjunctures."[57] If many congregations look more like borderlands or flowing rivers rather than fixed entities, Vásquez and Marquardt also show that fluid, shifting, "liquid" congregations do not lose their capacity to endure.[58]

Congregations or FFEs are social spaces in which humans bring and live their actual lives. "Social" is not the opposite of "personal," for congregations still provide the space, real or virtual, within which the personal exists, changes, and adapts over time. Congregations are living fields of social soil, which, even better than "capital," hold and nurture ever emergent life, including the passing— even dying—of its temporary but intimately attached members. As Ammerman points out, congregations function in community to nurture the life of the social whole even when their structure passes away leaving its "social capital" to be reclaimed and invested in other social structures that emerge from the ecology of the community.[59] Like other forms of life, any particular faith entity is durable but not eternal. Even it's passing, however, is not an end, properly understood, for it usually sits within the strength predicated in the story of the faith it holds to, so that what truly lives in congregations is in fact more lasting than their particular embodiments.

STRENGTHS FOR THE JOURNEY: ACCOMPANYING THE PEOPLE

The core argument of this volume is that the social precedes, without replacing, the personal, in both faith and health. A second recurrent claim is that we are in motion, maturing in faith, evolving in health through space, time, and a thick fabric of relationships. To say that life is a journey is not a metaphor but a far more accurate description of what happens along the way from birth to death, and a better understanding of the social and geographical location and circumstances of both birth and death. Some traditions see the journey as circular and find meaning in the cycle, while others describe a linear path made meaningful by its *telos*. Both faith and health languages fail when used to describe events, interventions, medical management strategies, services, and "outcomes" as a disconnected clutter of singularities. They are best understood as parts of a sequence, a narrative, a fractal stream of causation and influence, a history of a journey.

Whatever the social and political context, the health sciences increasingly recognize that health is a life span phenomenon in which access to specific medical services form a small fraction of what determines the quality of health life along the way. While the traditional medical "history and physical" focuses on diseases and their proximate determinants, such as smoking and genetics, the best science now values the long-term effects of social location and deeply embedded identity, security, love, intimacy, confidence, and hope—all qualities better suited to describe a journey rather than a service.

That journey is rarely taken alone. FFEs are organized around the life stages of journeys that people predictably take—preschool, adolescence, young couples, older women, and so on—while many congregations also organize around disruptive life passages such as divorce, retirement, living with cancer, or substance dependence. The best-known rituals, weddings and funerals, draw people toward sacred spaces, even if they otherwise are removed from regular participation in the life of a congregation. These are landmarks on a journey of meaning.

What difference might it make to those living in the simple world of providing health services to realize that their activities are part of larger social journeys? Recently, examining national patterns among the elderly of their journey out of a hospital, researchers discovered that 19.6 percent of these journeys cycled right back into the hospital within thirty days, mostly because of a failure to follow simple medical advice and protocols, or because of missing social supports such as transportation to follow up medical appointments, or even because of more minor causes. The cost to Medicare for these unplanned rehospitalizations in one year (2004) was $17.4 billion.[60]

Just as an individual gains the possibility of efficacy by way of a trustworthy narrative of the journey through life, so too an organization providing some kind of service gains power by seeing the story of those it intends to help. Concretely, a service provider such as a hospital gains intelligence beyond its limited competence by paying attention to the journey of its patients before and after they enter its space. Yet, such science-based institutions pay remarkably little attention to where their patients come from and go to, or the unpredictable behavior of patients outside the hospital around their own healing. Hospitals are so confused, says Dr. David Hilton, that they mistakenly refer to patients as "inpatients" when they are actually out of—estranged from—their normal way of life.[61] The hospital is "out," not the patient, just as a fish is not normally "in" the boat. Health for both depends on a quick return to their normal environment.

A hospital or clinic tuned to the wider context of the humans who pass through it would pay special attention to the journey of their patients, with a special curiosity about the critical weeks before and after admission. This would make any need for hospital care identifiable earlier, increase the chances of manageable care in the development of any disease or illness, and render the visit less costly and fraught with fear. It would include paying attention to their pathways back to the social networks where their healing could be completed. On either end, the provider of specific services would necessarily be interested in how to align itself with other organizations in their patients' lives that offer relevant services and advice, creating mutually supporting processes and better meeting their own goals.

Trying to pull any one living thread from the tangled journey only illuminates how interwoven they are in reality. We must see the whole system, not its parts, in order to begin to understand those parts. Here, it is much easier to live in this weave than to map it, or even name all the threads. If, as one example, one can identify congregationally related patients, one can pay attention to the relationship between the patients admitted to one the hospitals and congregations in their specific neighborhoods.

This requires a conscious relationship between congregation and hospital, as is increasingly happening at MLH in Memphis as more congregations and their members "sign up" into the CHN. Early CHN data, comparing its members with others who are not part of the CHN program, matched for diagnosis, gender, age, and race, show dramatically positive gains for CHN patients. The differences extend to such fundamental things as mortality, cost, and premature readmission—three of the golden rings pursued by hundreds of millions of dollars invested in electronic technology and platoons of highly qualified specialists. CHN patients come in the same door as others, sadly mostly through the ER, see the same doctors and have a comparable length of stay; no difference there. The significant difference is that CHN patients are more systematically connected to the network that primarily cares for them— their faith-forming community—where they are accompanied, where care teams can be convened, and where they find the social webs within which they find what they need.[62] This is one place where we see how FFEs embody a story of membership that is not just about dependency and frailty, but includes safe sanctuary, from hospital to home, relieving basic fears of isolation and violation. They also offer the confidence of liberating blessing at a time of traumatizing vulnerability and, of course, they pray, marking the journey as a sacred one in life and not just a slow entropic decline. These strengths not only echo the causes of life, but also make them accessible, participatory, and practical.

Such basic strengths of the faith-forming entity or congregation are evident in patterns that cross lines of theology, class, and culture. They are visible in African villages and in poor and rich, black and white and brown parts of Memphis. They are evident in entities echoing with the Koran, Isaiah, Revelation, and oral lore of African traditional religions. Indeed, one of the most important implications of the eightfold model of strengths is that it helps those standing in one stream of faith (or none!) to see another stream as an asset for health without stripping it down to instrumental manipulation. Leaders who are able to do so find the greater depth of field keeps more of the assets in focus and thus amenable to alignment. Imagination moves beyond simplistic functionalism toward vitality, even in breaking, broken, and broken-open communities. Such leaders are more comfortable with the dynamic fluid complexity common to turbulent human systems. We call those people boundary leaders, and that is our next subject.

7

BOUNDARY LEADERSHIP: EMBODYING
COMPLEXITY IN TURBULENCE

UNDERSTANDING BOUNDARY
LEADERS: KOTZE AND KING

Mowbray, an otherwise innocuous suburb of Cape Town, is a transport hub, a place of transition. Here all sorts of workers, mostly from distant townships, are on their way into or out of the city, getting off the train and onto a bus as they travel. Here, food and goods are sold on the sidewalk, crowds pushing this way and that under the careful and constant eye of police, commerce and conflict amid the noise, and replete with smells and energy of a thriving society.

In Apartheid times, when black workers poured through these terminals, Reverend Theo Kotze saw Mowbray not merely as a peripheral suburb or a transport hub, but also as the center of something that could emerge in the zone between a failing old order and a much needed new order, then still painfully distant but simmering. He saw it as a place of connection that potentially could work across the forced separation that marked Apartheid, a challenge to its spawning alienation. This, then, is where Kotze opened the regional office of the Christian Institute of South Africa (CI).

The Institute had been founded by concerned Christians to nurture the power of faith against the rule of Apartheid, using the most humble of tools of congregate resistance and emergence: Bible study, lunch served to all whatever their "color" or faith, truth-telling meetings, and highly practical ministries to help those displaced from their homes or needing medical care—a place to connect across the barriers when very few such places existed.[1] Those goals required that Kotze leave his relatively peaceful white congregation on the other side of the city in the balmy suburb of Sea Point with its wind-protected beaches. Mowbray, Kotze recognized, and not Sea Point or the inner city center where the Institute was initially located, helped keep the city humming with the largely black labor force upon which it was built. It was where things could break open and break through.

Boundary leadership is the practice of leadership in the boundary zone, the space in between settled zones of authority, where relationships are more fluid, dynamic, and itinerant. Sometimes this kind of leadership is felt to be positive, but frequently disquieting. As we will explore, the paradigm of religious health assets finds its way into transformational practice mostly where people imaginatively exert their influence in malleable social spaces, histories, and hopes. The multiple interplay of the ideas we have introduced are mental tools to bring out that dense complexity into view, tools that require boundary leaders.

The idea of a "boundary leader" has its own limitations. Both words draw the mind toward fixed, clear lines of authority or place. Yet everything we argue implies a richer, more dynamic approach with a language appropriate to the turbulent complexity and vitality of life. When we speak of boundaries, then, we will use the language of turbulence to underscore the complex motion between the layers and on the boundaries between things, and we shall think of boundary leaders as people exerting their influence on turbulent human systems. We would also wish for a better word than "leader" to describe those who help move human systems toward health. Social phenomena are influenced by individuals, but these individuals are almost always defined by the wider movement that expresses and carries their life.

Earlier we explored how the idea of tangible and intangible religious health assets prompts a different, potent way of seeing community in relation to proximate and distal patterns of health for individuals, families, and social networks.[2] Those assets weave together and constantly change in ways that are difficult for formal structures to see, map, follow, and control. Nevertheless, they are still at work, whether the formal structures and their positional leaders see them or not, and they have effect at social scale even when that effect is hard to monitor. Boundary leaders are attracted to the broken, and broken-open, spaces in between formal structure and "legible" functioning. More than just being in between boundaries, and more than seeing the complex and turbulent reality of boundary zones, they consciously, intentionally seek to engage and influence the social networks alive in them. Boundary leadership, we will suggest, is thus critical for how leaders work with religious health assets in seeking the health of the public.

The people disembarking from the trains in Mowbray moved across boundaries that were cultural, economic, racial, and political. The patterns that shaped their health could be described in the language of status (low), determinants (pathological), and patterns (grossly disparate). The story of the CI is relevant to the health of the public in its direct confrontation of the fundamental social determinants of community health, and in its role as an explicitly religious health asset designed to heal an ill body politic. It was a beautiful expression of what we have come to call a "web of transformation," reflecting the *social* embodiment of boundary leadership. The CI modeled a social form and a pattern of leadership that are expressions of the leading causes of life, and of religious health assets where people of faith engage the social determinants of health.

Celebrating exceptional leaders and extraordinary institutions is not our intent here, therefore. More important is the pattern of how they emerge from within a weave of social life that finds a way to thrive even amid the constraints and pathologies of a particular order. At the heart of the idea of boundary leadership lies a way of seeing the boundaries where things converge for ill or for good, and the zones between things that appear disconnected but are not. It describes the practices and journeys of those humans who influence social networks and institutions across their boundaries and boundary zones and, in the process, form new social wholes that are healed. They also hope for social well-being of the kind predicted by public health or provoked by basic religious aspirations but never achieved, a commitment to the "not yet" that drives the creative human imagination to transform "what is" into "what should be." The world—as understood by boundary leaders such as Kotze, or another to whom we will turn, Dr. Martin Luther King, Jr.—is not only broken, but also breaking open, in ways that allow for intrinsic wholeness to emerge—on streets as gritty as the suburbs of Cape Town or downtown Memphis.

LEGIBILITY AND ILLEGIBILITY, LITERAL AND PARTICIPATORY KNOWLEDGE

James Scott has explored the curious failure of many modern states to improve the human condition despite power and resources that would seem to predict success.[3] The basic problem rests in the self-limiting capacity of large-scale systems. They must record, filter, classify, and control millions of details, and yet they fail to read the complex, often contradictory and shifting ways of human beings and natural life. States see only partially, yet they act as if they view the whole; and thus, their schemes fail.

The emergence of state forestry in Germany, a useful example described by Scott,[4] radically impinged on people's ways of living with and in a forest in favor of the instrumental rationality that governs the production of wood. The limited goals of a forestry industry further grossly oversimplified the social and ecological life forests contain, ultimately in self-defeating ways, so that new schemes had to be created to overcome the problems the old ones had created. The same tools that make some of that complexity visible, through counting, documenting, organizing, and controlling arrangements and activities, inherently hides the rest of its complexity, thus making it illegible.

How the state sees reality is thus powerful in one way but powerless in another because it cannot account for much of what is actually going on. That which is not noticed can produce pathologies, as became obvious in the effect of forestry science on the loss of resources for food, fuel, shelter, and recreation by peasants who depended upon them, and in the ecological blowback from the trend to monoculture with its destruction of critical habitats, interdependent vitalities, and water reticulation and retention systems. Just because a state cannot see something does not mean it is not there or it is inconsequential.

Wendell Berry, writing from his Kentucky farm, describes the opposite way of seeing as "the empathetic mind," which fears the oversimplification that strips key vitalities from living phenomena, especially those that involve long-term relationships between particular local physical and social ecologies.[5] Berry argues that even those aspects of human ecologies that are formally religious— the standard traditions and their orthodoxies—contain far more richly layered nuances than is accounted for by their ordained managers. Religious leaders thus also frequently lose their capacity to read the complex characteristics of human ecologies when they rigidly defend fixed articulations of their tradition. Academics, too, Berry argues, can be dangerous when their mental tools for abstraction remove them from accountability to lived reality. The empathetic mind fears the collapsing of messy, living complexity into elegant abstraction.[6] An empathetic mind is thus one major characteristic of boundary leadership. It stands against simpleness (naiveté, innocence, lack of penetration), though not against simplicity (intelligibility, clarification). It includes the specifically religious, faithful, or spiritual openness to what physicist David Bohm calls "the unlimited."[7]

Bohm also argues that human intelligence or wisdom is served by two kinds of discourse or knowledge: literal and participatory.[8] Literal knowledge serves technical challenges of the kind that states (or other bureaucracies) find useful for managing forests, automobile inspection, or emergency departments of hospitals. Participatory knowledge learns and knows by participating in the phenomenon of interest. It has an interest in "knowing" that has no immediate utility, and expects and responds with reverence rather than fear to the vital complexity of social and physical ecologies, aware of what it does not fully understand. This nonanxious humility frees one to move toward actions that go beyond functional or instrumental rationality, to see what might not otherwise be seen, and to hope for things that might not otherwise be hoped, precisely because one recognizes that our profoundly limited minds must engage living phenomena that are not themselves so limited.[9]

Boundary leadership embraces such participatory knowledge, and boundary leaders thus read beyond simplified and constrained legibility. They live in the spaces in social wholes that are not congruent with (and thus transgress) the lines of control, ownership, naming, and accountability that states, as well as organizations that think like states, prefer. They are not, like states or religious institutions, intent on defining and policing boundaries. When they do think literally (what should we do about this?), they do so in ways that reflect their participation in a whole that envelops them and through which they find sustenance. This accounts for what, in iconic boundary leaders such as Kotze or King, often appears as courage but is actually more like a habit.

Consider Era Chandrasekaran, a former insurance sales representative in India who has set loose a swarm of disconcertingly hopeful projects, including *Udhavum Ullangal* (Tamil for "Helping Hearts"). Helping Hearts provides skilled intervention for men whose lives are marked by mental illness. However, they are actually drawn into a wholly new social ecology in which medical care is only one dimension of healing.[10] The men, volunteers, and medical professionals (working outside their "normal" place of formal service) participate in a life that welcomes all of them into a new way of being in the world, a "new normal." Volunteers are trained to administer appropriate psychiatric pharmaceuticals correctly and to monitor and record each man's response so that the physician who visits each month can optimally adjust the medication. Efforts are made to reach out to the families of the men, from which they are frequently severed because of their unpredictable behavior and the fearful stigmatization attached to untreated mental illness. Very practically, the men also work to beautify the community by planting trees on the city streets, a therapy for the men, who have a chance to do something visibly constructive for others, and therapy for the community, which receives a chance to appreciate and thank them.

Where the traditional way of life for these men was filled with fear, stigma, exclusion, and disgrace, the new normal sees human beings capable of contributing to the health and well-being of the whole community. The first step toward that new normal is the vision, even in broad outlines, of the possibility of something new emerging in the boundary zones that otherwise block imagination and separate people.

In Service of the Whole

Customarily, we describe something like Helping Hearts through its founder, as a story of personal virtue and charisma. Chandrasekaran tells the opposite story, of a world in which almost everyone wants to help others and everyone is capable of doing so. Helping for him is normal, not extraordinary. He does not wait for a few heroes; he expects thousands to create the spaces in which millions can live. This means transgressing all sorts of boundaries—Chandrasekaran and most volunteers, for example, are Hindu, but the medical staff are from the Christian Medical College of Vellore—in service of the whole. The same could be said about King, another iconic boundary leader, whose way of leading, not his uniqueness, is what needs emulation.

A Christian, a Baptist, and educated in a seminary associated with Walter Rauschenbusch and the social gospel movement, King was never contained by those identifiers or boundaries. King was drawn to the one place in Memphis where all its humans connect with raw physicality—trash collection, a root public health function. In 1968, the waste from homes of every economic, racial, and political description was carried from backyards in open steel tubs on the heads of Black men to open trucks that would take the trash to dump into open pits a few miles outside of town. Civil life depended on this function being performed effectively, but the men who actually performed this common good were themselves denied human decency or fairness. Exposed to gross filth with hardly any protection from the elements and without enforced health standards regarding the kind of waste carried, they were also almost entirely without health care or security against intimidation, and paid at such low wages that they were virtually a subhuman class of servants.

King called them sanitation workers, wanting to express that their labor had dignity and deserved respect.[11] The health of the workers and, quite directly, the health of the polis that required their work rested on righting deeply broken relationships that cracked along racial and class lines. King aimed the weight of his celebrity, intelligence, and presence at this fractured boundary, and helped to break it open so that something new could grow through.

Kotze of South Africa and King in the United States shared a personal relationship with a less well-known boundary leader, the Reverend Clarence Jordan, who spent his life leading a small, odd, radical but influential experimental farm in Americus called Koinonia, deep in the heart of Georgia clay.[12] Jordan's farm was a religious health asset. He intended its life to be an attestation of faith against racism, itself a health liability, and it paid careful attention to what we now call the social determinants of health, introducing ecologically sensitive farming and affordable housing, from which, under Millard and Linda Fuller, arose Habitat for Humanity.

King, Kotze, Chandrasekaran, and Jordan understood themselves to be religious actors, engaging deadly social brokenness while moving toward an emergent wholeness that did not yet exist, but that could be imagined and brought into being. All four found their lives on the boundaries between things broken and breaking that needed to be healed, where what was right needed to emerge. They crossed, transgressed, and transformed otherwise moribund or deadly boundaries.

Boundary leadership is foundational to the emergence of the health of the public, because it engages with social wholes that are sufficiently inclusive to be relevant to the fundamental determinants of health. It is also consistent with the deepest intellectual perspectives of public health, seeing less like a state than do most public health agencies, usually extensions of states. Such agencies keep data about matters that are relatively easy to count, and they read the health-related risk factors that are relatively easy to describe. Increasingly, they do so in language that privileges individual rational choice-making actors ("consumers"), rather than persons who are members of a complex social ecology, a public whose health as a whole is decisive.

Boundary leaders serve the emergence of healthier publics as they read and participate in social wholes, including aspects that are proximate to health (such as access to medical care or food) and distal (such as the intractable racism engaged with such tenacious humility by Koinonia Farm). If Bohm emphasizes the polar distance between literal and participatory thinking, and Scott that between legible and illegible thinking, then boundary leaders live like spiders in a web of relationships suspended in creative tension between those two ways of thinking and being. In apprehending the relation between the literal and the participatory, the legible and the illegible, they acquire a vital, critical edge in understanding the social whole, out of which they act. In Berry's language, their empathetic mind is their power. With it, they are able to confront crisis and imagine new possibilities for engagement, finding a way where others cannot.

Iconic boundary leaders are usually understood within the frame of the movement they have led and the specific reality they fought: Apartheid for Kotze, American racism for King and Jordan, caste and mental illness for Chandrasekaran. Yet clearly, none enclosed their own lives inside such simple lines. The eclectic nature of their learning and intentionally extended collaborative relationships indicates the complexity at the heart of their identity. King and Kotze, though they never met, both maintained active correspondence with Jordan. That is not a surprise. It is what one should expect to find happening in a larger whole.

Boundary leaders thus not only create social capital relevant to their own movements but also tend to nurture it widely, beyond their own most obvious purposes, because they sense the deep links between apparently diverse activities that make up the social whole. When Jordan's farm faced failure because of a near-total local economic boycott, King used the social capital resting in the networks of Dexter Avenue Baptist Church to market their produce a hundred miles away. When associates of Kotze needed sanctuary from the attention of the Apartheid state, Jordan gave them a place to rest and regain strength. All three knew that their particular struggles expressed a deeper, broader emergence of life.

THE BOUNDARY LEADERSHIP CYCLE

The idea of boundary leaders originally emerged from the work of the Interfaith Health Program at The Carter Center in dialogue with the Public Health Leadership Institute meeting at The Fetzer Institute in the spring of 2001. That conversation produced a "Call to Colleagues" in the domains of both public health and religious leadership, recognizing that they were parts of a larger social whole that needed to be brought together.[13] The group named as its primary goal:

> *Justice*—a word implying peace, wholeness, virtue and well being, not only of individuals, but of communities and the social connectedness from which we each can find meaning, hope, and sustenance. Together we recognize the concern for individuals and families that need immediate aid and healing. However, our primary focus is on the wholeness of people as they live and develop complex relationships in the wholeness of community.

The Call expressed an expansive vision emerging from the fruitful boundary zone between religion and public health, shared by leaders from within both horizons, based on what were seen as a rediscovery of "the heart of meaning and service out of which our vocations developed long ago." Moreover, it suggested new possibilities "for advancing the health and wholeness of our communities, [and] amplifying the possibilities of deep collaboration with others."[14]

That same year the Centers for Disease Control and Prevention (CDC), charged with leading public health efforts for the US government, approached the Interfaith Health Program, wanting to support an educational program to recruit and train leaders able to lead toward the vision of the Call to Colleagues. In 2002, the Institute of Public Health and Faith Collaborations created for this purpose initiated what it eventually called a Boundary Leadership model,[15] using a team-based educational logic based on a circle of seven mutually interacting values identified by Brad Gray and Mimi Kiser, as shown in figure 7.1.[16]

Above all, the cycle models the conviction that boundary leaders generally are not "natural," that is, born such; they emerge by being transformed through a relationship they may not have expected to be transformational at all.

Kotze of the CI is an exemplar of boundary leadership, and he certainly had gifts of communication, but he was transformed into being that leader by the movement in which he took part. Unable to become the architect he had hoped

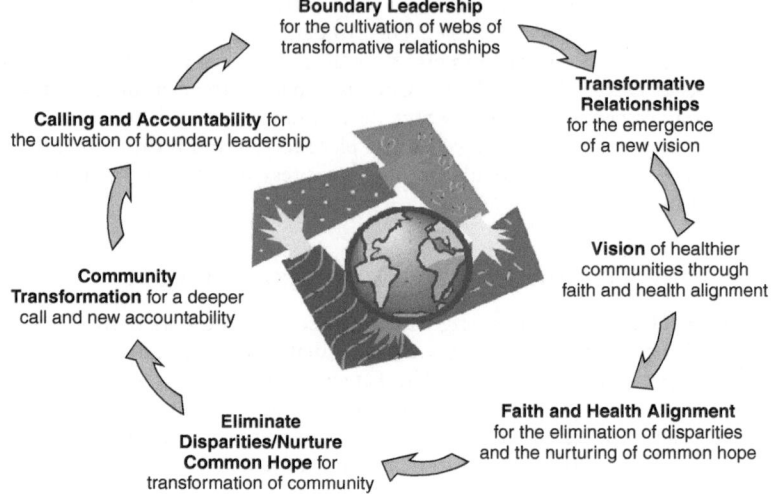

Figure 7.1   Boundary leadership cycle.

to be, he ended up as an official on the gold mines of the Witwatersrand until he was led to become a Methodist pastor. In that role, he encountered international Methodists who, in the postwar era, believed a renewal of the church was vital, envisaging a "church without walls." The idea spawned others,[17] but in his time and in South Africa, Kotze immediately recognized that in his church and society the walls between black and white were rigidly entrenched. A church without walls would take those boundaries down. Exactly that is what Kotze, crucially supported by some others, did quite literally to the fence that guarded the lawn of his Sea Point church, intended to keep out the black servants of whites, for whom there was no park and little place to rest.[18] Dr. Beyers Naudé, founder and national director of the CI, noticed this kind of leadership, and invited Kotze to open a regional office in Cape Town. And so that movement carried him too.

Similarly, King is an icon of boundary leadership transformed into being that leader by the simple, innocuous steps of being recruited by other pastors to head a committee. When he became chair of the Montgomery Improvement Association, it was partly because he was seen by his congregation, by his community, and by himself as a stabilizing, moderate, nonprovocative person who would not add divisive energy to a volatile situation. The initial goals as articulated by King were remarkably and explicitly modest, not even subversive of the underlying segregation legislation, so nobody expected the bus boycott to last more than a few days.

King led the process, but he was transformed by the movement he found in the tumultuous boundary zones of race, class, politics, and faith, where others too were evoking and making legible a new vision of American society. King was drawn from literal leadership (nominal and formal) to participatory leadership (deeply engaged with others) through a movement not limited to bus riding but distinguished by its participation in "the unlimited" (Bohm again), as mediated through the extraordinarily powerful imagery, language, rituals, and resilient practices of the Black church.

This view on boundary leadership matches other models of leadership for community transformation on the side of public health, ones tuned to the underlying social, economic, political, and culture determinants of health and drivers of ill-health.[19] Such leadership has to involve far more than the managerial and technical competencies of the kind that typically fill up the curricula for public health officials, or many other public professionals for that matter. The key CDC-supported publication on "Competency Development in Public Health Leadership" includes the competencies of transorganizational linking, team building, motivation, and political engagement.[20] This model, in turn, influenced the framing mission of the Center for Community Transformation of the Chicago Theological Seminary (CTS), whose faculty added a branch of competencies relating to spiritual life. They include some that Bohm would regard as participatory ("being fully present to the human spiritual reality without fear" and "being about one's own journey of faith and service"), and some more classically literal ("appreciate the literature and practices of faith traditions in the context of current crisis" and "develop rituals of passage, growth and lament, memory and encouragement").[21]

The cycle of values shown above represents a realization that boundary leaders at their best are unpredictable in their journey, impact, and success. They intuitively, often quite intentionally, cultivate webs of transformative relationships, which tend to favor the emergence of a new vision while seeking to align existing or emerging strengths (such as religious health assets) that nurture common hopes. Boundary leaders are thus central for transformation of community. If this is so, then agencies and institutions that live on the interface of religion and public health need to cultivate boundary leadership as an essential element in tackling the huge challenges they face.

Nobody that helped design the model of a cycle of values imagined that reality follows such a simple path. Like all models, it is a simplification of actuality. However, whatever the actual shape of the journey across the lived topography and chronology of any life, the model makes clear that the path of transformation of the self and of social wholes moves in ways that are only partly predictable. It projects and embraces not just actuality, but possibility. This way of understanding the contributions, challenges, and motivations of leadership is consistent with what both faith and public health leaders now understand to be necessary in the contested emergence of the health of the people in relation to social wholes.

CHARACTERISTICS OF BOUNDARY LEADERSHIP

The pattern of life of boundary leaders typically includes certain felt strengths and weaknesses shaped by their insertion between literal and participatory ways of being, and between legible and illegible ways of thought. Whereas no particular personality type seems linked to capacities for boundary leadership, over time a similar array of felt strengths and weaknesses develops that go with the role, usually reflecting the holistic and systemic contributions boundary leaders make for the health of communities or social systems.

Embracing Complexity of Persons and Systems

Boundary leaders see their apparent weaknesses and strengths as such because they are empathetic persons attentive to their own lives in relation to the lives of others, aware of the complexity this introduces into any situation. They live in such complexity without reducing reality to any one aspect of it, and that in itself requires certain strengths and exposes personal weaknesses. That boundary leaders are often religious or deeply spiritual is hence not surprising. Openness to complexity without being overwhelmed means, in Bohm's sense, to live in dialogic relationships that are open to the unlimited. Substantial dissonance, tension, turmoil, and even transformation at a personal level, is thus not an uncommon experience in boundary leadership.[22]

It is typical of many kinds of leaders, even in traditional positional roles that stay within particular boundaries, to experience times of doubt and surprise at their capacity to assume the expectations placed upon them. This is not what marks a boundary leader. Boundary leaders face the same challenges as others in this respect, but they add something crucial that is intrinsic to their peculiar way of reading reality (not like a state or bureaucracy) and to their membership of a body of people alive in the emergence of a new social whole. They do not merely excel or succeed in changing a challenged organization, but see beyond any particular organization or movement to grasp a larger whole, legible and illegible, bounded and unbounded, including, critically, that which lies in the interstices between boundaries (where a great many people find themselves, and where health is at great risk).

This theory of boundary leadership begins not with global icons, but from observing the pattern of lives of those who do the work of community organizing in the mundane venues of neighborhood-level congregational programs and public health efforts.[23] Here, mostly outside the walls of clinics or other important buildings, it is easier to see and experience the broken, breaking, and emergent nature of social life. Here people who lend their lives to the social efforts of health improvement often find that they themselves are "illegible" to the formal structures that may employ them, doing more complicated work than is accounted for by "deliverables" couched in the language of "measureable outcomes." The formal structure is likely to ask for the number of children immunized but not about those human dynamics and webs of trust needed for one real mother to make the string of choices that result in her child being touched by a nurse who can apply the needle. The boundary leader—the one who makes that pattern of healthy relationships happen repeatedly—is largely illegible to those who only count needles.

Living with Misunderstanding

Boundary leaders are thus often misunderstood by their organizational structure or profession. They commonly feel marginalized, invisible, undervalued, or even endangered professionally. The way they work and where they undertake their work simply bursts the bounds of standard role and job expectations. So their accountability and even allegiance to their institution is likely to be suspect, precisely when they ignore boundaries or succeed in crossing them, as they do what they see as necessary. Their institutions, by contrast, tend to set boundaries and to police them, creating lines of command and accountability defined in terms of those boundaries.

Boundary leaders thus have complex professional journeys with complicated career histories that may appear suspect to those on more traditional paths. They may even be regarded as misfits or recalcitrant rebels. In one sense, they are rebels, as understood by Albert Camus who, though aware of its destructive potential, saw in rebellion—properly understood as action that transcends the stasis of the actual in advocating for new possibility—the decisive dynamic of a hopeful civilization.[24]

Clarence Jordan, an agriculturist holding a PhD in New Testament Greek, thus found himself standing in a worn red clay field in South Georgia trying to plant pecan trees. He did so as an expression of his particular reading of his religious texts about a new order of life trying to break into the lived social reality. It is unsurprising that his journey is hard for others to understand. So it is with public health epidemiologists, experienced at investigating toxic outbreaks, who find themselves in a dialogue with seminary presidents. However, those who see the need for such a dialogue have entered into the world inhabited by boundary leader personalities.

Creating Bridges and Keeping Them Open

Boundary leaders, then, are partly engaged in developing *bridging* social capital as part of their core work. Religion is commonly associated with bonding social capital because of its role in forming and holding the perimeter around a religious community. However, religion as expressed in the life of boundary leaders, through their participation in the "unlimited," provides the energy to move across boundaries and build bridges for others to cross as well.[25] Thus they frequently have very broad networks of relatively thin relationships, which may come at the cost of depth, not unlike rural pastors who play a crucial role in holding widely scattered people together, and they often lack safe, deep, and personal relationships. What boundary leaders invest in building and holding open bridges also comes at a personal cost of felt vulnerability and marginalization. They go against the established grain (of congregations, communities, organizations, societies, and academic disciplines) and frequently face a multiplicity of unfulfilled or delayed hopes. However, this too, ironically, exemplifies a systemic strength, for those hopes contain seeds of possibility waiting for a season in which they might sprout. They may not sprout, but only those hopes nurtured in broken ground make it possible.

Generating new bridging capital is also an expression of the systemic role of boundary leaders in the social whole. Boundary leaders frequently express a confidence grounded in their wide networks. Because of their complex personal journeys, they read and speak multiple languages of community and see emergent social wholes invisible to those with more fixed lenses and literal minds. By necessity of their vulnerability, they know a lot about organizational behavior and understand how to avoid its dangers. They tend to be resilient and flexible. They are frequently described by themselves and others as imaginative: they not only see what has happened before, what is happening now, and what has not yet happened, but also, they see differently. They tend to integrate these dimensions of the real rather than disaggregate them.

Engendering Webs of Transformation

The social structure in which boundary leaders move and work is a web of transformation. Their common pattern is to move in networks that are functional bridging assets for the tasks of organizing, communicating, learning, and engaging in social change. Similarly, they are drawn to networks in which participatory social knowledge is alive to the unlimited, transformational energy that creates powerful and unpredictable bonding social capital. Often boundary leaders say that they feel more powerful bonds with the odd assortment of people they find in their boundary networks, as was typical of the CI lunches in Mowbray, than they do with their formal colleagues in their credentialed identity. Such unorthodox social bonds formed in the boundary zones are magnets that hold together what would otherwise be unlikely groups of people, but whose conjoining produces powerful energies and actions, and experiences of a surprising social whole that is itself a sign of what might be possible at larger scale.

Similarly, boundary leaders help systems gain many efficiencies through aligning and connecting assets that already exist but are, for many reasons, otherwise inaccessible or invisible. A simple example involves a family whose father, after developing eleven bedsores in a poorly run nursing home, was admitted to Methodist Extended Care facility in Memphis. This purely medical intervention was greatly strengthened by the relationship between the Faith and Health office of the hospital and the patient's pastor, an experienced chaplain whose congregation was well organized into care teams. The pastor and the care teams (without cost to hospital or patient) provided important support to patient and family in helpful, tangible ways (walking the dog while the family were with their father) and important nontangible ways (lowering the energy of fear, mediating anger at the poor care provided earlier, and thus making good decisions going forward more likely).

Boundary leadership, concretized here in the form of a paid "navigator," enabled existing religious and other health assets to come into alignment to the benefit of the patient, and it fulfilled the mission of all the relevant and interested parties. It is important to note in this example that we are not describing a means of outsourcing an institution's legitimate responsibilities, for the hospital does not shirk the material costs involved. Moreover, were it simply to abrogate its responsibilities and cast them onto its network of community-based collaborators, it would not work; nor would the hospital's basic problem—how to deliver health care efficiently, effectively, and sustainably in the long run—be solved. The alignment we are describing is not first a social contract but a human necessity, all the more so where health systems and health policies are in crisis.

Boundary leaders also play transformative functions that help the social system gain new intelligence by aligning what is already known in one part of the system with what is known in another. Research indicates that 70 percent of patients in any emergency room in Memphis claim to have been in a house of worship within thirty days prior to admission.[26] Most clergy might be surprised to learn this. However, even if only half are telling the truth, it suggests that it might be important for the hospital to understand what the congregation knows about health, what motivates and animates their health-seeking choices and behavior, and what kind of providers they turn to under what circumstances.

Nevertheless, congregations usually have very little organized knowledge about how formal health facilities operate or what their standards of admission or payment are. However, both organizations are interested in and relevant to the health of its members/patients. Boundary leaders will help one system learn from the other and gain new synergistic intelligence by building a web of trusted relationships across the boundary zones that keep them apart.

In exactly this way and for these reasons the Congregational Health Network (CHN) covenant between congregations and the hospital system was drafted by Memphis Methodist Le Bonheur Healthcare (MLH), largely by pastors who shared their intellectual assets so that the hospital could design the relationship to reflect what the pastors knew about the life of their members and neighbors, and not just what the hospital knew about disease.[27] The design, nurture, and implementation of this program exemplify boundary leadership at work.

Holding the Negative Valence

Much that is found in and outside boundary zones is broken, the debris of destructive processes, scattered fragments of life, or the asymmetrical play of power. Fears and negativity may thus dominate such spaces, the effect of perceived (and sometimes real) threats to one's existence. Unrealistic or distorted expectations may then be directed like a lightning rod toward someone in authority or power. This is a phenomenon familiar to therapists working in the one-on-one relationship of counselor and client, and it has parallels at social scale, especially where conflict or uncertainty reign. Here, boundary leaders play a similar role in the social dynamics of community, practicing what psychologists and psychotherapists often colloquially refer to as "holding the negative valence."[28]

In psychiatry, holding the negative valence is how a good therapist keeps people with borderline personality disorders centered—stalkers, self-mutilators, obsessives, and people who put one foot on a pedestal or in the gutter—while not being pulled into the negative effects or bent thought patterns emanating from that person. Typically, a patient engaging in negative valence "attacks" a therapist or other authority figure, irrationally erupting out of their own perceptual and cognitive distortions. The therapist's job is to remain objective, not fight back, and to hold the negative valence steady, not escalating it, until the patient learns to develop his or her own internal sense of stability.[29]

Boundary leaders frequently find themselves in the middle of negative valence partly because they evoke fears from those whose stability—personal, ideational, or organizational—is threatened. However, because they see the social whole as generally positive, they hold the negative valence until the balancing positive become visible to others. This is of course no easy task, but it is characteristic.

Boundary leaders such as Kotze, King, Jordan, and Chandrasekaran, however, do far more than hold the negative valence. By avoiding swimming in negative racism and the competitive violence common in the broken zones within which they moved, they actively sought to turn it around. They used their personal powers of expression and positional leadership to evoke a participatory interpretation of the emergent social possibility. In short, against the negative valence, boundary leaders also hold open a positive valence until it can be seen and experienced by others, initially at small, then at larger scales, pulling together scattered and broken parts toward a stable center of a new, emerging whole. People who do not want that new whole are often threatened by this positive valence, of course. Nevertheless, the point remains.

Like therapists, boundary leaders are not always appreciated by those in whose interests they act. This is especially so if a boundary leader's larger view of reality transcends parochial community claims, inviting it beyond an accustomed comfort zone, and exposing it to risks it may not welcome. Why not strengthen the walls against risk, rather than moving toward it? Kotze's growing critique of the international economic system that for long made Apartheid durable is one example, and it lost him many affluent supporters. King's move from Dexter Avenue Baptist Church to the streets and alongside sanitation workers, the white poor, and the Vietnamese, disturbed the sense of identity of some of his community, exposing him to additional vulnerabilities and stresses.

Unlike therapists, few boundary leaders are trained to hold the negative valence, so they often experience the resistance as personal vulnerability even as they discover new strengths. Trained or not, however, they characteristically attempt that task, drawn by the contrasting positive valences necessary and vital to the way life creates new social wholes. The movement that claims them thus transforms them at the same time.

Social Embodiment

The characteristics of boundary leaders we have outlined can be understood in relation to any social situation and found among people in countries and institutions on every continent. Within any particular field of activity, and across congruent fields and geographical locations, boundary leaders are also surprisingly often aware of each other. The webs of transformation they inhabit, usually persisting as flexible and resilient social forms, frequently impact on each other because of their common search to embody the social whole.

Indeed, how boundary leaders socially embed themselves in our contemporary context is as important as any characteristics they might share. In our view, some forms of contemporary embodiment are particularly important to the shared passions and commitments of religious and public health leaders. To describe them, we draw some relevant insights from the history of one of the boundary institutions we have referred to in discussing the characteristics of boundary leadership.

The CI's web of relationships extended far beyond its structure. Not only was it led by boundary leaders, but also it was a boundary institution, working in the boundary zones. In this context, it embodied four basic social commitments that may be generalized for other contexts in our time.[30] The first was to reinvent and reconstitute the "political proper,"[31] which refers to the communicative action necessary for public discourse in service of the life of a people in a particular society. This is a vital counter to the instrumental, purposive rationality that governs the system imperatives of the marketplace and state bureaucracies. A healthy polis is the aim of such discourse, though it often is overridden by the intrusions of an instrumental rationality that systematically distorts or manipulates public discourse in the interests of a particular part of the whole. However, the whole requires a mutually accountable discourse, extended in principle to all. That requires that all have the capacities to enter into that discourse voluntarily, free of unreasonable constraint—exactly not the situation under the constraints imposed by the Apartheid state.

The second commitment of the CI was explicitly to confront the public lie of segregation, black inferiority, and African ignorance that so comforted the white rulers of South Africa. This is not unlike the way in which Memphis sanitation workers had to confront the social lie of white racism by claiming, "I am a man."[32] The public lie is all too often with us, and worryingly, it has gained greater political respectability in many places in recent times. In the context of health, it includes the subtle suggestion that one's health is entirely one's own doing, one's ill-health entirely the result of one's own choices and actions, erasing in the process the social determinants of health. Boundary leadership will confront the public lie, at every level, and from any source.

The CI's third commitment, aware of the broader social and economic forces undergirding Apartheid, was to challenge the logic of the global political economy. From a systemic point of view, boundary leadership, its social webs, and its occasional boundary institutions are relevant to proximate threats to the health of the public, just as they are to the proximate affects of racism. The Institute for Public Health and Faith Collaborations, for example, was funded by the CDC in part because of its concern to eliminate racialized disparities in health. Indeed, most of the teams that attended the Institute meetings were drawn from existing community projects bearing the names of the diseases they were organized to address: human immunodeficiency virus (HIV), diabetes, obesity, mental illnesses, hunger, and cardiovascular diseases. These teams tended to see and organize around literal knowledge using standard ways of gathering health data, and demand legible organizational accountability that overlooked the illegible processes so critical to the more radical and hopeful potential of their labor. More broadly, as we discuss in the next chapter, threats to the health of the public are deeply rooted in the pathologies of our current global political economy. Taking those seriously also represents a basic task for boundary leadership in our time.

Finally, the CI sought to engage the pathogenic religious (in this case, Christian) ideology supporting Apartheid, from within that same tradition, critically interpreting its normative texts, just as the early leaders of the civil rights movement in the United States did in their response to racism. It was a simultaneous application of a hermeneutics of suspicion and a hermeneutics of reconstruction or innovation, which is easy to be missed by those unfamiliar with religious dynamics. However, it is a key ingredient for boundary leaders in building their applied social intelligence and evoking a mature faith from religious leaders.

Congruent with those four loci of social embodiment—reinventing and reconstituting the public proper, exposing the public lie, challenging the instrumental logic of the political economy, and critically interpreting normative traditions for positive transformation—we may add three others that carry the deep social intelligence of boundary leaders. They include the capacity to listen to others, especially those whose voice is normally diminished by coercive power and authority; ways of acting in solidarity with others for the interests of the whole; and ways of living that are healing for the persons who encounter each other in that process.[33]

Such capacities to embrace social and human complexity express precisely what we have been describing as the participatory knowing and being that marks boundary leadership. Boundary leaders act in social webs that express a commitment to justice with a compassion for persons. Boundary institutions structure their life and activity, drawing vitality from opening spaces for the voices and experiences of those who are excluded by society and marginalized by the dominant powers of the state and the market. Boundary institutions, exemplified by *Udhavum Ullangal*, the CI, and Koinonia Farm, move between people who would normally not meet each other, addressing those who suffer with hope and confronting those who cause suffering with the face of the one who suffers.[34] And finally, boundary institutions are comprehensive in their reach and complex in their response. In this sense, sophisticated rather than naïve, they are capable of working out of and into many roles rather than being locked into one.

They are thus social embodiments of boundary leadership, beyond individual action, however potent such individual action may be. Boundary leadership is transformative, always arising out of some social stirring that finds and nurtures the life in one human connecting to others. This reflects the logic of the leading causes of life, which assumes that life, emerging out of but going beyond existing orders of life and thus subversive of any stasis, will always make way for new, more complex forms of life.

RELEVANCE TO THE FIELD:
WHAT IT LOOKS LIKE IN PLACE

What, then, is the relevance of boundary leadership to a health care system? Let us consider the formal health system in Memphis as an example. As elsewhere, Memphis struggles financially to support its public hospital, the Regional Medical Center at Memphis (The Med), 30 percent of whose patients are unable to pay anything, with most of the rest covered by subsidized government programs such as Medicaid and Medicare that pay significantly lower than break-even rates. Occasionally public discussion focuses on whether the hospital would be better placed under the umbrella of one of the private systems, such as the faith-based MLH. However, since the facility has been underfunded for many years, whoever owns it will need to replace it soon.

Hospital buildings are very expensive: a rule of thumb in 2010 is that it costs roughly $1million per room/bed. By comparison, adult community programs costs about half a million. If a 100-bed hospital, fully built and equipped, costs roughly $100 million, a 400-bed facility around $400 million, one must give serious thought to what the public really needs. Do the people of Memphis need 300 beds? Why not 242? What analysis justifies the capital for what size facility? What is the health logic most relevant to understanding the journey and conditions of the patients that will eventually fill up those beds? What practices, in medical and human terms, will serve them best? Does the practice of boundary leadership have anything to offer to such profoundly concrete social and political deployments of financial assets?

In Memphis' public hospital, about a quarter of the beds are used for "classical" hospital needs: casualties of trauma, violence and emergencies such as heart attacks, and a small number of active psychiatric illness cases. Most of the remaining beds are filled with people with four other, clearly identified conditions. First, and most difficult, are the large numbers of frail elderly with conditions that cannot be managed by their existing home support network that, reflective of long-standing patterns of race and poverty, is often scattered and shattered by the difficult social conditions of Memphis and the Delta. Their situation is often exacerbated by the lack of other institutions equipped to care for long-term elderly of diminished capacity, especially those with little or no insurance. Not surprisingly, then, old people tend to linger as long as possible in the hospital, inappropriately.

Second, large numbers of people suffer from late-stage complications of chronic conditions that, painfully obviously, could be managed effectively outside the hospital, but they are not, so they easily become more complex. This too is exacerbated by the nasty interweave of poverty and race that means there are fewer, less intensive, clinical care options outside the hospital. People before retirement age, especially men, are very poorly covered by disease management programs and frequently lose employment along with their health, arriving in the hospital like old people though they are not.

Third, many beds are filled with sick, fragile, or underweight babies and their unhealthy mothers. It takes little sophisticated analysis to establish the links between poverty, race, and gender here, and many millions of dollars could have been better spent on prevention than on providing the facilities needed to respond after the fact.

Finally, to all of this one may add that a large part of the demand for the outsized emergency room facilities (accounting for well over $100 million of projected capital need) is best understood as undiagnosed, poorly managed mental health issues that reflect the predictable damage of life stresses associated with race, gender, and poverty in a fragile economy filled with many insecure low wage jobs. These stresses show up as violence and self-destructive choices of many kinds. Truly unanticipated "accidents" are a minority.

These four kinds of patient—the frail elderly, people living with late-stage chronic complications, fragile babies and mothers, and those dealing with the mental and emotional issues of life traumas—fill up the hospitals, a reflection of the disparities in Memphis that are responsible for a large portion of suffering treated in ways that are unnecessarily burdensome, highly costly, and painfully inappropriate.

A tertiary hospital is a very blunt instrument to deal with this. Even a superficial review of the literature relevant to those four conditions makes it obvious that a large body of best practices exist that make hospitalization at a late stage totally unnecessary. Abundant models of community, neighborhood, and even home-based care exist that cost far less in capital and staff than a large hospital, many of the best practices being combined with professional medical care. Once one starts to look at this array of health needs differently, it becomes abundantly clear that many of the conditions could be served by common infrastructure.

Any boundary leader would recognize the need and the opportunity. The key is to see the social whole on which such common social infrastructure might rest and find its own life, as part of the care of people for whom a hospital is inappropriate and too institutional. It would be a core competence of boundary leadership in this context to create systems of health that result in more health, not just more hospital rooms. However, it would require thinking beyond the vision, say, of a new public hospital, to focus on the social infrastructure for far more appropriate and effective programs at community and neighborhood levels.

Such is the mundane but critical work of boundary leaders. In the context of MLH and its seven hospitals, it has led to the creation of the CHN, which embodies the humble but revolutionary work of bringing hundreds of diverse congregations (heading toward four hundred at the time of writing) into alignment with each other around a common covenant appropriate to the vision of creating a healthier Memphis community.[35] Things that are impossible even to imagine without a critical scale of action and a web of trust are easy to implement once the boundary institutions function. Where once broken neighborhoods sent a constant flow of impossibly complex health issues into expensive institutions that could not begin to respond, either with the compassion or science that the twenty-first century should make easy, now it is possible to see very different action and science with both proximate and distal implications. A few, skilled boundary leaders can make it possible for elders, those living with diabetes and HIV, pregnant moms, and those traumatized by mental stress, to experience a very different journey.

If a good modern hospital staffed to deal with the car crashes, violence, burns, and truly sophisticated medical problems is always necessary, the community will nevertheless be far healthier when boundary leadership has seen, named, and called into alignment the full health assets in a different and more scientifically grounded way.

BOUNDARY LEADERS AS KEYSTONE SPECIES IN THE TURBULENCE OF LIFE

Of course, the story in Memphis is not likely to evolve exactly as we might hope. The theory of boundary leadership includes an expectation that one can and does fall short of one's own expectations. We might say that it includes its own failure in its theory of success. However, no effort fails entirely or completely, allowing some of its emerging social and intellectual capital to be reconstituted and incorporated into the next step of the journey. Boundary leaders participate in the emergence of social wholes and know that no one step of that journey is definitive. Life moves, and even if bound to a particular local expression, remains uncontained by it. Life in every sense is contingent, passing, dependent, and in service to others, and to this boundary leadership surrenders itself, finding sustaining meaning in doing so. It is driven by hope, in other words.

Boundary leaders think in terms of social wholes that function more like ecologies than concrete and steel buildings or electronic instruments. They are somewhat akin to what biologists call "keystone species," upon which the ecology of other species depends.[36] The wolves in Yellowstone Park are keystones in that ecology, just like salmon in rivers of the Northwest. Remove them and the ecology generally declines. Keystone species thrive only when they live in a way that serves the life of the whole. So boundary leaders thrive only when their social ecology flourishes, in the sense of continuing to unfold and emerge toward its intrinsic possibility.

Systematically incorporating complexity into one's thinking and imaginative construction of possibilities for transformative action is thus a crucial, determining feature of boundary leaders. In this way, they go against the grain, at least where those who seek to reduce or simplify the complexity of life in order to study, manage, or control it dominate the day, pressing their agendas upon the science and practices relevant to the health of the public and drawing the bulk of resources to their cause.

Equally crucial and determining in boundary leadership is the attention it gives to what happens in the boundary zones. Focusing leadership around the boundaries rather than in the center is a great advance, not unlike the impact of following Antonovsky's attention on salutogenesis away from pathology. We specifically therefore do not mean by a boundary leader a person who, in seeking power and influence or acting self-interest, moves across or over boundaries for their own ends. Boundary leadership turns attention away from the centers of power to the edges, transforms the imagination about the nature of what happens on the edges, and breaks open spaces to create opportunity to nurture the new for the sake of the whole.

Just as salutogenesis can turn into a static analysis of factors and measures, so too can boundary leadership drift back toward old ideas about lines of demarcation while using new language. Boundary language is intended to reflect images of the shifting, chaotic, often unpredictable zones along tidal estuaries or forest edges, not the demarcations of political maps and organizational charts. A "traditional" leader, by contrast, hears "boundary" and generally only sees sharp lines between this, and that. Perhaps, then, we need an appreciation for the turbulence that is common at the edge of any changing environment, between fluids (as in a river) or between a gas and solid (as a wing moves through the air); or, perhaps, between groups of people?[37]

Turbulent systems are difficult to describe precisely, much less predict. Research on such systems not only illuminates their extraordinary complexity, but it also provides innovative engineers tools for using turbulence without anxiety. It offers a rich language for describing liquid boundaries, where two fluids reacting with each other and moving smoothly and slowly in adequate space are described as "laminar." One can imagine as laminar a group of people adapting well and smoothly to their changing circumstance with plenty of space, time, and resources. Indeed, as suggested by fluid dynamics, creating turbulence in small amounts can be the key to controlling the unpredictable and inefficient outbreak of larger turbulence later.[38]

Working with turbulence rather than unrealistically aspiring to eliminate it is a key insight for boundary leaders in dealing with the complex reality we call the public and its health. The social implications of the metaphor point to the role of boundary leaders in steering systems toward the logic of life, with an appreciative eye for the complex intricate whorls, eddies, and flow of energy in the boundary layer of what we might call a river of life.

Memphis has learned many lessons from its great Mississippi river, including the unpredictability of its massive forces of change. As John Barry describes the river, "It roils. It follows no set course. Its waters and currents are not uniform. Rather, it moves south in layers and whorls, like an uncoiling rope made up of a multitude of discrete fibers, each one following an independent and unpredictable path, each one separately and together snapping like a whip."[39] King was a master of the whorls at the boundaries of black, white, rich, and poor. Boundary leaders generally, drawn to the human boundary layers of social groups in motion, similarly appreciate the rich and intricate flow of ideas, energy, resources, meaning, and agency—let us say, life—in turbulent spaces.

From the center, the boundaries look like places for civil negotiation— the use of power, finance, or even violence—where something is lost or won. Boundary leaders are comfortable with the unpredictable liveliness of the layers and zones beyond the illusional, controlling power of elites. Too complex for negotiation or instrumental, linear control, and far too alive to be smooth and predictable, the boundary layers are where leadership delights in the whorls and eddies of living systems.

Why is this so important? Simply because those who hope for the health of the public need a way of understanding the complex flows of change that encourage both humility and hopefulness at the boundaries between what is and what could be. The traditional language of public health is simply not robust or bold enough to describe the turbulence of human systems. Similarly, most existing models for its leadership are inadequate to influence those complex flows. Boundary leadership, undergirded by a nonanxious view of social turbulence, may be more suited to the relevant social realities.

8

THE CHALLENGE OF SYSTEMS

The paradigm we have outlined for understanding religion and the health of the public rests partly on the credibility of each component idea, and partly on how those components *as a whole* serve the work of better reflection and action. Here we reflect on one last critical component, the link between the health of the public on one hand, and polity and economy on the other. This link seems obvious, as farming is to weather and climate. However, no aspect is as challenging or contested, and we tread warily in this respect. Faith, health, politics, and economics: each is an aspect of human life that might be designed to rule the others, each has appeared to do so in different times and places, and each is complex beyond measure.

In recent years, there has been enough reliable data about a range of health and social indicators of well-being, gathered across and within enough nations, to allow for a systematic comparison of patterns and relationships between the factors. One of the finest attempts to see those patterns in their impact on large-scale health outcomes is Wilkinson and Picket's *The Spirit Level*, which explores the extraordinary way in which equality between the citizens of a state correlates closely across a very wide range of indicators. They demonstrate that once a people has gained a basic level of safe food, clean water, sanitation, housing, and primary health care, additional financial gain does not have much effect on well-being or happiness.[1] Characteristics of social relationships—trust, cohesion, and participation—are better correlated with improved health outcomes. Equity, meaning more than raw economic equality and simple political participation, is the best predictor of social-scale health.[2] "Modern societies," they say, therefore, "will depend increasingly on being creative, adaptable, inventive, well-informed and flexible communities, able to respond generously to each other and to needs wherever they arise."[3]

These are qualities of living social bodies that resonate closely with several concepts introduced in this volume, including the leading causes of life and boundary leadership. Their understanding of how inequity "gets under the skin" is also very similar to the way we describe the self and health seeking, although they do not include spiritual or religious aspects.[4] What they see—and what we are also trying to bring to focus—is society functioning as a whole system, only partly captured in the separate languages of economics, politics, sociology, or health.

Some will notice that we have not focused directly on themes fundamental to the way in which social ordering or disorder happens, such as gendered or racialized patterns of exclusion or diminution, many of which also challenge religious traditions. This is by choice, not a lack of awareness. While such patterns are an irrevocable part of the mix, gender analysis, for example, being both a fundamental touchstone of how poverty and inequality play themselves out and a key source of the kind of theory of human capabilities offered by Martha Nussbaum upon which we depend,[5] they are not our focus here. Our aims are more modest here, primarily addressing the implications for health and health systems of two particular dimensions of any political economy, power, and knowledge,[6] in relation to what it means to be a citizen rather than a "patient" or a "consumer of health," how pathologies of power affect this, and what it might mean to meet the challenge of systems—political and economic, private and public—that seem an irrevocable part of the life of any health or religious practitioner, leader or academic. Power and knowledge are golden threads that weave their way across all the critical fault lines, including gender, race, and socioeconomic status, providing penetrating entry points into the entire range of issues with which polity and economy are concerned. The reader will find them mirrored in all our key concepts, beginning with the importance of making visible the contribution at community level of religious health assets (RHAs).

If economy and polity is the concert hall, the stage upon which our concepts must play, then religion and health are the spotlights by which they come into focus. If faith, health, politics, and economy are the instruments in a jazz ensemble, we listen not for careful orchestration but for how each accompanies or disrupts the other—noting that not all jazz is good, while some is shockingly bad.

SETTING THE STAGE

An autobiographical narrative sets the stage. We were part of the pilot research team from the African Religious Health Assets Programme (ARHAP) that first systematically mapped and assessed RHAs for the World Health Organization (WHO) in the famous Copperbelt region of Zambia. By the 1990s, endemic malaria had been eradicated from the Copperbelt, a major victory at the time. However, times changed, and the human immunodeficiency virus (HIV) had arrived. So had the season of the Structural Adjustment Programs (SAPs) that enforced dramatic changes in funding and policy for all governmental services, including health. The Copperbelt's two major towns, Kitwe and Ndola, though reasonably stable economically until then, experienced a sustained downturn after privatization kicked in at the beginning of the 1990s.

When we arrived with other ARHAP researchers in Ndola in 2006 to conduct a pilot study on RHAs, malaria was again endemic, killing mainly young children. We visited the impressive Ndola General Hospital, and while waiting in the parking lot for a senior physician, our host, we observed the activity around us. There was little activity, and the parking lot was almost empty. Beyond the lot, however, a gate opened into a compound from which pickups regularly exited, passengers already in the back joined by others waiting outside, all chanting and praying as they drove away. Puzzled, we wondered what we were seeing.

When the physician finally arrived, he explained that the internal road we were looking at led to the mortuary. The people on the trucks, family and friends, were there to fetch the body of a deceased person before proceeding to a burial ground somewhere. The constant stream was because HIV infected people were dying in significant numbers, arriving too late for treatment or possibly already dead. While it did have a maternity ward, the hospital processed death more than it delivered life.

A second surprise awaited us—the main building. In the large reception area, only two people waited, there was no one attending. In the wards above, we saw mostly empty beds. It was all a result of user fees, our host explained, which was a conditionality of international loans at the time. In Zambia roughly two-thirds of the population lives on less than US 1$per day, and inequality is high,[7] so even low user fees force households to decide between traveling to the hospital and feeding a baby. Usually, the baby wins.

Outside again, our host indicated a separate door into the main building. Here people moved in and out regularly. It was the entrance for the privately insured patients who could pay fees—corporate employees, government officials, expatriates, and tourists—and who received full, high-quality care in a walled-off section of the same floors we had seen empty otherwise. The divide between the health of the rich and the poor was set, literally, in stone.

The previous evening we had been in a poor, subeconomic Ndola "compound," sitting on a back pew in a local Pentecostal Sunday worship service. It was as rudimentary a church as one could get, with gaping split pine walls roughly wired together, patchy plastic sheet roofing flapping in the wind, crude benches, and a dirt floor. One incongruity stood out: an impressive set of high-tech electronic musical instruments fronted the low stage on which stood a lectern. The place thrived, rocked by song, praise, and preaching as vibrant as the hospital reception area was lifeless. Many of those present, mostly younger, were likely unemployed,[8] and almost a quarter HIV infected, with a life expectancy of a paltry forty years.[9] Unsurprisingly, the religious messages were of hope and assurance, punctuated by amens, hallelujahs, and ululations. Furthermore, woven into them were words about bodily care, protected relationships, compassion, and the need to express one's own agency against the threat of death or the devil.

Little of this would directly change the general epidemiological profile or aggregate health outcomes of those present, yet one might expect their resilience to grow and their quality of life to improve, partly because of a reenergized sense of coherence and of connections to others in the congregation supporting them. We expected that Charismatic Pentecostals would pay scant attention to the political and economic realities of their lives, but we were soon disabused. SAPs, the pastor and others claimed, had negatively affected the health of the congregation, with ongoing effects long after the specific policies had changed.

They were acutely aware, they said, of how their religious lifeworld and their health were inseparably bound to the functioning of other systems.

ON CITIZENS IN SOCIAL SYSTEMS

SAPs are no longer the policy of the World Bank or International Monetary Fund (IMF)—Poverty Reduction Strategy Papers (PRSPs) are[10]—but the particular policy is not the point. At stake is the way in which people locally are often still significantly limited in their choices by the choices and actions of others at a distance over whom they have no control. These are people who reflect interests often not consonant with or even inimical to theirs. This reality persists even in the face of "consultations" with stakeholders or "participatory" processes specified in policy documents.[11] Deeply affecting those other interests are system imperatives that carry with them a logic and rationality that has no necessary link to the communicative logic and lifeworld interests of local people.

It is not a matter of "bad people"—though bad people all too often do make good use of their opportunities in this regard—but of skewed rationalities, of what Habermas calls systematic distortions in the social fabric introduced by the penetration into lifeworlds, including the sphere of the public, of the instrumental logic of markets and bureaucracies that now tend to shape a world system. To counter these distortions, a link between economy and polity has to be constructed so that citizens rather than the imperatives of the systems meant to serve them are prior. That requires strengthening the meaning of citizenship where it is strong and, where weak, fighting for the conditions, the processes, and the institutions that enable it. To be a citizen in a healthy political economy means to be a person, in multilevel relationships with other persons, who has access to and the use of the full range of capabilities that define what it means to be human.[12]

In our collaborative research to understand RHAs, we have been repeatedly confronted with how strongly their nature, scale, and potential are determined by historical, political, and economic dynamics directly relevant to health. Paying attention to religion and the health of the public has meant dealing with the question of how that public is constructed, damaged, or voided—the question of citizenship, its value, the norms attached to it, and the rights that accompany it. This is a loaded question, especially in Africa where, during colonization, only a privileged few, principally European settlers and colonizers, had citizenship status and rights. Indigenous populations were, in the classical sense of feudal Europe, subjects of the elite and generally excluded from citizenship rights.[13]

Unsurprisingly, the struggle for citizenship has been a mark of post–World War II. It has included the struggle for full citizenship by women among others—by no means assured even in Europe or North America. It remains a central concern for public health, because citizenship in its fullness means equitable access to the goods and services of health for all as a basic right, while that right often remains unsecured, as seen, for example, in the inequitable burden of ill-health borne in many contexts by women.[14] Citizenship is also the necessary counter to the erosion of the public sphere by the systemic imperatives of markets and state bureaucracies.

For all these reasons, citizenship should be a central plank in any health care reform that aims to meet the goals of health for all in a healthy political economy. Health care organizations, however, tend to think not of citizens but of patients, organized by their disease and means of payment. Herein lies a profound challenge: is the human being, called a patient, an object receiving targeted technical interventions aimed at one of their troubled organ systems, a "consumer" of services rather than a citizen?

An RHA approach requires an awareness of the extent to which people are able to act as citizens, to have a say in determining which health interventions are best, how they should occur, and what changes might shift the social determinants of their health. A health citizen describes a role quite different than a health consumer. Health citizenship is thwarted or undermined by skewed or asymmetrically distributed power, producing inequities and disparities that undermine the health of the public.

"PATHOLOGIES OF POWER"

If health is a very good indicator of the skewed nature of social realities, the failings of global public health, Farmer argues, are related to what he calls "pathologies of power."[15] Epidemiological data is unequivocal in its depiction of the inordinately high burden of disease and ill-health among the relatively poor. The data represents a human drama of enormous proportions, largely unseen by those who are *not* poor, and marked by deep violence to the bodies and lives of a great many people, especially women who face what in South Africa and elsewhere has been called the "triple oppression" of being female, poor, and black.[16] The asymmetry of power, Amartya Sen thus notes, "can indeed generate a kind of quiet brutality."[17]

The picture is particularly bleak in some parts of Africa that lack financial resources, managerial and professional capacities, scientific personnel, facilities, and infrastructure to deal with illnesses that are mostly preventable and controllable. Failure of governance might be part of this, especially where available resources are misapplied, or reappropriated for the security of the elites, while one cannot ignore the murky world of illegal trade in narcotics, arms, human trafficking, and body parts.[18] The reach of nation-states is also more limited, perhaps declining,[19] and transnational realities increasingly define the economic terrain within which they must act.[20]

Many health systems are either collapsing or in trouble,[21] and financing them is a major conundrum, increasingly a basic concern of public health.[22] Here a market model of competition governs the dominant approach, but whatever their strengths, market rationalities reflect an inherently limited way of determining what to do. As Habermas notes, the market is essentially "deaf to information that is not expressed in the language of price,"[23] and whereas nothing is particularly fair or just about wastefulness and inefficiency, while grounds exist for arguing that markets are better mechanisms than, say, government bureaucracies, for dealing with waste and inefficiency, the limits remain. Partly because of serious distortions created by deep-seated asymmetries in power, markets fundamentally fail to meet the assumptions of perfect competition and equal access upon which their promise of justice depends. Thus, far from solving crucial problems of access and distribution, Habermas argues, "Real markets reproduce, and exacerbate, existing relative advantages of businesses, households, and individuals *ex ante*."[24]

The resulting inequalities are a key indicator of the health of the public,[25] they evoke the question of human rights,[26] and they challenge public health whose central role, Gilson believes, "is to manage the processes through which the meaning of the health system to society, and so its contribution to broader societal value, is established."[27] Again, we face the issues of citizenship and the common good. Neither can be established without dealing with the sources, conditions, and potentialities that govern the ability of citizens to enter with effect into the public sphere, while protecting that space from being undermined by the systemic interests of power and money.

The idea of RHAs should be understood within this frame. Paying attention to the health assets that people hold also highlights how they might exercise their agency. Equally, it means questioning the increasingly obvious deficits of a utilitarian view of economy in which people are simply "consumers" or "stakeholders" and not, first and foremost, citizens and persons. It also means, therefore, challenging reductionist rationalities that eliminate anything resembling religious faith or the religious mind from view, thereby discarding significant wellsprings of moral action and intention, especially those that trace histories of struggle for freedom, justice, and the good of all.

One example of such reductionism can be seen in the unfortunate saga of primary health care (PHC). Its formalization in the WHO's Alma-Ata Declaration, a propitious moment in the history of public health, was motivated by a recognition that high-tech, expert-driven, and facility-oriented medicine had limited impact on poorer or more disadvantaged populations who bear the greatest burden of ill-health. Reviewing its subsequent history, we quickly discover that the original impulse of PHC—to give local communities some responsibility for planning and implementing their own health services backed by state resources—was quickly undermined.[28] Other imperatives were at work.

Leaving aside those who simply appropriated resources meant for others to themselves, these imperatives included fiscal constraints on states that prevented a fully implemented system of PHC, and practical constraints in training and retaining PHC workers in local areas. Soon a reduced concept of "selective primary health care" emerged, effectively removing infrastructural support for community-based health workers and transferring responsibility back to state organs and aid agencies, both thoroughly undermining the integrative principles of PHC.[29] States and other agencies simply took "the decision making power and control central to PHC away from the communities and delivered it to foreign consultants with technical expertise in these specific areas," favoring instead more easily controllable "vertical, definable, time-limited programs."[30]

In 1993, the World Bank Report, *Investing in Health*,[31] had the effect of further eroding local control. Whereas it recognized that the economy had to be organized in a way directly relevant to health of the public, its view of health sector reform largely remained within the dominant economic philosophy of the time to herald "an emphasis on using the private sector to deliver healthcare services while reducing or removing government services. User payments, cost recovery, private health insurance, and public–private partnerships became the focus for delivery of healthcare services."[32] The notion of a common good that shaped the origins of public health had largely given way to the instrumental priorities of efficiency. Efficiency, however, is surely not *the* public good where gross disparities mean that large portions of the citizenry are effectively excluded from economic life altogether. The tail (efficiency) wags the dog, perhaps is detached from the dog, or used by some to punish the dog for being poorly fed.

Twenty years later, despite changes to offset the negative effects of such policy interventions, the crisis in public health appears to have deepened, as we have repeatedly noted. Moreover, though 150 years of science has produced a vast range of medical and pharmacological tools to extend the promise of health, the mundane nature of appropriate interventions remains strikingly similar to those prevailing at the dawn of the public health movement: mobilizing communal, social, and material assets to protect or improve water, food, housing, education, and the essentials of disease prevention, including immunization. While the fundamental determinants of health remain superficially addressed or unaddressed, the scientific engine races ahead, propelled largely by commercial rather than public motives, disrupting and challenging the economics of health care delivery systems everywhere. Simultaneously, state institutions fail many citizens living on the margins or outside of the money economy. Experts gathering in Memphis or Cape Town in the name of public health will therefore drive through neighborhoods whose health is most obviously limited not by the failure of medical technology, but by issues of political economy.

CHALLENGING SYSTEMS

On the one hand, systemic imperatives are part and parcel of our lives, and dealing with them is a challenge for anyone who wishes to alter or change them for the better; on the other, pathological configurations of systemic forces also need to be challenged. This dual responsibility is the lot of daily life for public health and religious leaders engaged with the world. Diseases and conditions common to the citizens at the center, rather than on the periphery, of political and economic attention attract the bulk of funding, time, and creative attention of those that produce knowledge and technologies. Diseases of temperate and urban environments have a panoply of pills, whereas people in tropical and rural places are often left to their prayers. Health sciences and technologies thus inescapably reflect political economic realities, raising again the question of what it means to be human beings as citizens of a public. The tools of medical science do not invent themselves. They are subject to the system imperatives of markets or state agencies, deeply influenced by money and power, and embroiled in a logic shaped by instrumental rather than communicative purposes.

Of course, they are subject to system imperatives. One cannot evade such systemic imperatives in modern, large-scale societies, and they have their place. Yet, when system imperatives of markets or bureaucracies override or "colonize" (Habermas) the lifeworlds of people, running rampant, they damage the health of people and of the public. Attempting to ameliorate their effects on the determinants of health by, say, volunteering time and money for worthy organizations may be positive but it is insufficient, perhaps even misleading, if the priorities are not reversed.

We do not think that systems are god-given. One can challenge the way they work and the priority they are given. However powerful and enduring their impact, they are the making of, and subject to, human choices and actions. If one wants a communicative (human) rather than an instrumental (nonhuman) rationality to prevail—the thrust of all the concepts we have introduced—then another imperative for health is necessary, based on a fundamental moral view of human beings as ends in themselves rather than as a means to some other end. Thus, within a health system, one would clearly distinguish between kinds of knowledge relevant to the instrumental purposes of science or governance, and those relevant to citizenship and communicative ends, with the former always subject to the latter. Hospital administrators, medical personnel, public health advocates, and even religious leaders—indeed, anyone who works in and with one or another system, no matter at what level—all face this perennial tension between instrumental purposes and communicative action, which often confounds the highest aims of public health or the most holistic visions of religious faiths.

No administrator of a health care facility wishes for his or her reception rooms to empty, or for their back doors to be filled with wailing mourners like those we saw leaving the gates of Ndola hospital. If the hard, painful edges of the global political economy were visibly present at Ndola, they are quite as real in Memphis, where leaders of a faith-governed hospital must calculate how to provide care for an increasing number of those without funds while trying to keep up with expensive new technologies seen as necessary by physicians and academic partners, and face demands to increase quality as measured and mandated by government regulators.

Arguably one of the organizations with the most agency in the region, the leaders of Methodist Le Bonheur Healthcare (MLH) nonetheless work in the context of a limiting political economy. Adopting novel community alignment strategies, they must still consider a future filled with constraints intrinsic to the systems in which they operate. These include multiple layers and facets of government affecting every aspect of their work and of the lives of their patients and their neighborhoods, a panoply of corporate partners and technology providers with their own interests, and dozens of health care professionals each with their own aspirations. All function within particular systemic imperatives that favor—often demand—a particular way of seeing, acting, and relating. Local choices are shaped by a global matrix. Many of the hospital's physicians are from

India, Lebanon, and Bangladesh, while Memphis is the hub of FedEx, a major Canadian National Railroad terminal, and the Mississippi river highway that carries grain destined for many places around the world.

Still, within the health care facility itself a conceptual cocoon pressured by system imperatives tends to make some choices more chooseable and others entirely unthinkable. Health care in the United States is commonly viewed less as a right or common good than a commodity, and though health care services are highly regulated by many different public entities and bound by multiple guilds, all of which shapes costs and accessibility, a critical question is which provider is most efficient or competitive. Some providers are owned by shareholders and are expected to pay taxes on their profits, whereas others are accountable to provide community benefit in lieu of taxes. All compete with each other to attract patients, physicians, employees, and capital.

Within this framework, Porter and Teisberg insist that the inefficiencies that cause health care services to be so expensive and thus inaccessible result either from insufficient competition between providers or from competition over the wrong things measured in the wrong way.[33] They advocate economic rewards that will force providers to compete based on treatments for medical conditions rather than based on discrete interventions.[34] Though sharply focused on the US political economy, they extrapolate their views globally, suggesting that state monopolies over health care elsewhere should be broken up too to allow for competition for gains in prevention and long-term care, or for alliances with providers in the United States and Europe that offer lower-cost surgical services.[35]

A rather different approach, emphasizing the Institute of Medicine's (IOM) "quality of care" model, comes from Boston's Institute for Healthcare Improvement (IHI), which seeks multisectoral collaboration to advance the "triple aims" of lowering cost, advancing quality, and improving "population" health.[36] The IHI, moving from the institutional health care environment into the far more complex arena of local community life, and believing in the power of measuring objective outcomes, focuses on the challenges faced by governmental players dealing with "socially complex patients" from fractured communities.[37] Its approach, somewhat in the direction we propose, includes new forms of collaborative action between health care organizations and community health assets. Highlighting the "role of strong partnerships between health care and community organizations," it pays attention to the health-seeker's assets, including family support, church groups, community ties, and relationships with other social service providers.[38]

Porter and Eisberg, and the IHI, are concerned with particular process improvements in the existing systems. They teach us something about how systems work, and there is no lack of improvements required to be made—hospitals even struggle to get their physicians to wash their hands, for instance. However, neither fully addresses the tension between instrumental and communicative action within health systems in the context of asymmetries of power and knowledge. We are interested in how organizational decisions in Ndola, Memphis, or anywhere accord with broader social goals, within which administrative and technological capacities should be located, that have to do with a vision of the human and social conditions that favor the health of the public as a whole.

Knowledge and its technologies here are important. They are needed by health system decision-makers to determine how to allocate resources, material and human. A host of scholars, think tanks, and others invest huge resources in the development of knowledge and its technologies. However, most implementation is instrumental, designed for greater medical, managerial, and financial efficiencies, rather than for the human persons that the system is meant to serve. The issue is thus not whether knowledge and information is valuable but, rather, what value one prioritizes.

PURPOSES OF KNOWLEDGE

There are many ways of organizing and using the ever-increasing arrays of knowledge about the health of the public. Internally a health care system hopes for better quality and efficiency in treating patients. Thus many organizations, including MLH, now invest hundreds of millions of dollars in electronic medical records, a revolutionary improvement over the clutter of paper previously used to manage the journey of a patient in the medical environment to one that makes legible almost every aspect of that journey in close to real time. The electronic view is designed to strengthen the capacities of the providers of care. Yet, it only indirectly serves the powers of the patients and their families, and illuminates only a small portion of their health journey, largely restricted to encounters within the hospital.

Other tools, not necessarily linked, illuminate the treatment journey between providers of medical care to enable medical services rendered at one center to be visible to providers at another, including competitors. This information exchange is designed to keep track of expensive duplication of services, so that the patient receives only what is medically appropriate for their presenting condition. Some tools are emerging that would help the community by mapping a broader range of health delivery services from social agencies. This would restrict recipients from getting more than is considered appropriate by the providers, who otherwise have little way of knowing when someone else has already given some medical service. Producing more transparency and less "waste" or duplication, it presumably spreads resources further, though at the same time it increases the power of providers, not a neutral effect.

Those who run or serve systems, we have said, tend to view matters using an appropriate instrumental logic, fine in its place. However, recalling Scott's analysis, those in the system often find it very hard to see beyond its imperatives. Public health institutions, like state bureaucracies, are drawn to what he calls "simplifications," measures, and methods that make social reality manageable, legible. Market-based corporations do the same. All then struggle to comprehend the complexity of the lives of communities or individual people, which are reduced to "interested, utilitarian facts...nearly always written...documentary facts,...typically static facts,...also aggregate facts, [and] therefore...standardized facts."[39] The facts, not the voices or the stories, are most easily digested into uniform policies and standardized practices.

Large systems thus tend to produce policies and implement practices based on "planning for abstract citizens."[40] The consequent weaknesses in grasping the lifeworlds of real citizens are exacerbated if the state or the market has no deep interest in those who live at a distance from the centers of power or wealth, or where civil society is weak or nonexistent. Thus, Scott believes, we need to make space "for the indispensable role of practical knowledge, informal processes, and improvisation in the face of unpredictability," which requires an emphasis on "process, complexity, and open-endedness."[41] Such practical knowledge, *métis* in Greek philosophy, is something ordinary people usually possess but to which systems are often oblivious. The tension between expert knowledge and local or indigenous knowledge, or what we would call instrumental versus communicative knowledge, Scott suggests, is thus "not simply theoretical but also political."[42]

Knowledge, however, is being produced at an unprecedented rate. With innovations like software company SAP's HANA in-memory database technology, petabytes (quadrillions) of data can easily be searched in short periods of time economically, a new capability that fundamentally changes the scope and diversity of quickly accessible information.[43] Ultimately, though, quantity or speed is not the issue, for knowledge might even be dangerous to some when it makes it easier for privileged powers to extend their dominion and remove the hiding places of those that remain resistant to such powers. It is not equally safe for all to be visible on all maps, and visibility is not an automatic desire, as Scott shows in his studies on resistance to domination,[44] while a persuasive presence in the public arena is not guaranteed merely by an ability to communicate.

Considerations of knowledge in relation to power, its asymmetries, and its systemic distortions were at the forefront of ARHAP's development and use of its set of tools for assessing and mapping RHAs. The tool-set, originally called PIRHANA ("Participatory Inquiry into Religious Health Assets, Networks and Agency"), rests on several relevant, interrelated theoretical frameworks: Paulo Freire's pedagogy of "dialogical action" that highlights the agency of the poor or the marginalized; Asset Based Community Development theory, supported by a Sustainable Livelihoods Framework, that focuses on the "portfolio of possible assets" poor households have from which they can draw, and on their "vulnerability context"[45]; the Appreciative Inquiry approach to community transformation that pays attention to the "energy for change" in people's experience of past successes and current aspirations[46]; social capital theory to understand RHA networks and ties[47]; and, action methodologies such as Participatory Rural Appraisal to define a range of exercises that enable community members to express their concerns and share their wisdom about their lives, while giving them ownership of that information and an ability to act upon it. More recently, the tool-set and approach has been further adapted for building partnerships between providers and local communities.

Despite this formidable array of integrated ideas, it is clear to us and others in ARHAP that the tool-set can (and will) be easily turned to instrumental rather than communicative purposes. No method, tool, or instrument can obviate the question of how it is used and for what purposes. The purposes of knowledge, and the conceptual frame or "data model" used to assemble it, are therefore critical. This moves us quite sharply from what is *capable* of being known, to what one *wants* to know that is relevant to the health of the public. Our answer to the question of what ends govern the creation or use of knowledge will determine whether our "data model" is restricted to managing the relationships among citizens, marked as they are by patterns of difference, privilege, and partition, or extended to enhance the communicative action that will enable and maintain the greater health of the public and its citizens.

Every provider of health services, public and private, religious or not, faces such issues. Some will operate out of an integrated and expanded view of their community, others will not. That, in turn, may produce asymmetries of power between providers themselves. While *all* providers may appear to their "consumers" to be powerful, those that accept a disproportionate share of poor people may be financially weaker in relation to others who manage to avoid the poor. Yet, one that cares for the poor may create political currency that results in economic gains through policy or pricing advantages.

We are thus dealing with a *political* economy, not a pure financial market. In this regard, we place the concepts that are central to our paradigm of religion and the health of the public in the long tradition that views politics and economics as two sides of the same coin, a tradition echoed within the field of health in the life and voice of Rudolf Virchow. A physician and social reformer, Virchow is still revered nearly two hundred years after his birth for two streams of science that are now seen as distant from each other, cellular pathology and his analysis of what we now call the social determinants of health—poverty and its comorbidities: bad housing, lack of sanitation, clean water, and food.

Virchow believed that "Medical science is in its innermost core and being a social science," and that politics is best understood as "medicine in the largest sense."[48] His insistence on experimental medical science established the intellectual credibility of the field and gave it a methodology for continuous, rigorous development. His understanding of the social determinants of health remain part of the public health field, visible today in the "Spirit of 1848" caucus in the American Public Health Association, even if it is still a distinctively minority voice nearly lost amid the dominant focus on simpler constructs of disease transmission and the instruments of intervention. He saw that society could choose health for itself, not just for particular individuals. We think that is still true despite the ever-increasing complexity of the systems that open up or constrain that choice.

REIMAGINING THE HEALTH OF THE PUBLIC

If medicine is at heart a social science and politics is medicine writ large, then it is also true that the deepest roots of religious imagining aim at a fulfilled life in a healed and whole society and world. None is separable from economy and politics, a conceptual whole despite the functional separation of economic agents and political leaders, who are better understood as a double helix continually shaping each other in an indivisible dance. Their combined effect on the health of the public is shared for good, ill, or something in between, as is their effect on the language, imagination, and the forms of faith. Any individual actor with a particular role in, say, a religious institution or health facility, will be constrained by the systemic imperatives at work in that context and their particular social environment. Every actor will be faced with systemic distortions that inhibit the goal of health for all in a healthy political economy.

It might make a technically minded administrator's eyes glaze, but any durably effective leader simply must take account of the systemic and structural forces that impact on public health and health systems. Africa, for example, was shaped by historic traumas and material legacies of the slave trade, colonization, and wealth extraction all of which shaped the more recent reality of trade marginalization and frequent failures of governance. This indicates that health cannot be viewed merely as a commodity or service to consumers, or as a matter of better knowledge and science. The fractures and malignancies that result from the use of power or money are neither merely coincidental nor simply effects of the ambiguous complexities of social life. They certainly have direct consequences on the health of the public.

Religious leaders who are close to their communities, such as the Pentecostalist pastor in Ndola, know this. Similarly, public health practitioners and theorists are aware that the model of political economy that strips the commons and reduces life to its monetary value contradicts the basic instincts of their field. Whether they believe such developments are a result of a conscious intentionality, or of unintended collateral damage issuing from the unbridled pursuit of economic gain (which Scambler calls "disorganized capitalism"),[49] many public health practitioners wish for another direction.

A recent report of the National Association of County and City Health Officials in the United States, for example, states that "The so-called disparities in health status that we find among population groups are unjust and inequitable because they result from preventable, avoidable conditions and policies" which, in turn, arise from "systematic, avoidable, disadvantages [that] are interconnected, cumulative, intergenerational, and associated with lower capacity for full participation in society."[50] As Farmer shows,[51] such disparities are not particular to the United States but global in reach. Equity, as a key measure of health, has thus gained recent attention. The Regional Network for Equity in Health in Southern Africa (EQUINET) defines equity as (1) "addressing differences in health status that are unnecessary, avoidable and unfair," (2) "directing more resources for health to those with greater health need," and (3) "having the power to influence decisions over how resources for health are shared and allocated."[52] Similarly, the World Development Report, whatever its weaknesses, suggests that reconfigurations of public health investment should aim at systemic interventions benefitting the most vulnerable.[53] As Fabienne Peter (quoting Robertson) indicates, "this is not so much a new public health as a return to the historical commitments of public health to social justice."[54]

Adopting the language of equity brings into view the asymmetries of power and wealth of the global political economy, but it may not alter them. As EQUINET's Steering Committee, clearly disturbed by a cooption of language, notes:[55]

> "Poverty alleviation" and "equity" are terms that are also appearing in the language of international finance institutions, international agencies and donors. The *language* is being incorporated but do we all mean the same thing? The 2000 World Health Report, for example, identifies countries such as India as having *unfair* health financing systems because the rich are paying more as a share of their income, for their health than the poor.

Simply measuring and describing avoidable inequalities in health, or focusing on health status and health sector inputs with a view to vertical equity (preferentially allocating resources to those whose health status is worse) is unlikely to change much for two reasons.[56] First, as long as such analyses focus narrowly on health and fail to address the systemic maldistribution of resources that feeds poverty and impacts negatively on the health of populations, the deep structural impediments to "health for all" will remain untouched. Second, if such analyses are cast primarily in the language of inputs and outcomes while ignoring the agency of those people for whom health is intended, effectively turning them into a passive recipients of care, then the communicative action necessary to altering their conditions will be undercut. Thus, we wish to speak of health of citizens rather than recipients, consumers, or even patients.

If good public health practice encourages people and communities to take part in decisions about their own health, is supportive of people's initiatives, and advocates international support to countries that move in this direction, why is it so hard to give effect to a commensurate vision of public health? Consider one example, that of the 2000 World Development Report. It was preceded by a series of participatory "Consultations with the Poor" conducted by local organizations, drawing in more than sixty thousand poor women and men in sixty countries.[57] What did that impressive number of poor people say? Their responses, we are told, reflected "an overwhelming feeling of powerlessness on their part, mostly negative experiences with governments, and a generally poor quality of health and social care services. While those interviewed generally appreciated the work of non-governmental organizations (NGO)...they had mixed feelings about them, preferring the dependability of their own local networks."[58]

The report then recommends recognizing the realities of poor people and investing directly in their organizational capacities, which is a start. However, how will one invest in their organizational capacities if they distrust their governments and are hardly enthusiastic about NGOs or other external agents? Who will find, identify, and invest in the local networks that people find more dependable, and with what criteria? What if doing so damages them, either because of the tension, distrust, and enmity money tends to breed among people struggling for resources, or because hostile agents of government prefer not to have well organized communities confronting them about questionable activities or gains? In short, what will change the structural and systemic conditions of poverty, alienation, and marginalization so clearly articulated by the Consultations with the Poor?

One cannot simply listen to people or record what they say, clearly, but must pay attention to their freedom and dignity, again introducing the question of justice (or its absence) in health. The practice of public health rests on a moral vision and not just a science or technology, and one significant criterion in determining whether or not a health system is just is whether it pays attention to what *all health citizens* find generative or life-giving, or what *they* experience as a threat or diminution—a critical indicator of respect for their knowledge and their capacity to survive or thrive.

In health, as elsewhere, this implies a need to mediate "between the necessary leadership or polity from 'above' (*techné*) and the experience and wisdom (*métis*) of those who are 'below,' taking into account the asymmetries of power that this equation represents."[59] We are very close here to a basic religious insight, namely, the idea of mutual reciprocity or, more commonly, of "doing unto others as you would have done unto you,"[60] which can also be summed up in Paul Ricoeur's profoundly simple aphorism that a healthy society depends on establishing and maintaining ways of "living well with and for others in just institutions."[61]

Living well with and for others is the practical project that justice enables and that injustice undermines. None of the three important terms dealt with earlier, "reciprocity," "quality of life," or "decent care,"[62] can be reduced to individual healthy behavior. Separated from conceptions of justice, such notions are likely to betray the very thing they seek. Further, if we accept that trust is a vital element of any practice of reciprocity, quality, and decency, then without a sense of justice as a basis for trust among those who are the intended recipients of health interventions, nothing fundamental is likely to change.

Everything we claim here suggests that a purely formal view of justice—as expressed in a contract, governed by procedural rules, managed by thousands of legal experts, and focused ultimately only on "what?" and "why?"—is, if necessary, insufficient. It should, in principle and practice, be subsumed under a view of justice predicated upon reciprocity in relationships with others, governed not merely by procedural rules proscribed by formal law, but by discursive rules responsive to the question, "who?"

The "who" here is human: first, by virtue of the imaginative capacity to act, and second, by virtue of the experience of suffering. In Ricoeur's words: "With the decrease of the power of *acting*, experienced as a decrease of the effort of *existing*, the reign of suffering, properly speaking, commences."[63] The two things stand in direct correlation to each other and should change how we think about public health interventions. The most obvious but radical implication would be to redirect efforts, resources, money, and institutional priorities toward enhancing the power of acting. It is precisely on these grounds that we work with the ideas of assets and agency, and the notion of the leading causes of life.

CHANGING STANDARDS OF ACCOUNTABILITY

It takes no great insight to discern that one's life experience affects the way one sees and thinks. It is simply true that those whose lives have led them to be at the central levers of power and money will generally think of public health in ways not informed by the experience of other citizens who are the "least." It is not just that one's life experience is privileged, but one lives in streams of knowledge that are also privileged, that tend to pose, disseminate, and favor questions tuned to the privileged. One lives in a privileged ecology of knowledge. We draw an analogy with Alice O'Connor's analysis of the historical construction of what she calls "poverty knowledge."[64]

Central to her arguments is that a basic change in the way we think is necessary for dealing effectively with poverty (health, in our case). O'Connor argues that the existing body of knowledge on poverty (in the United States, at least) is itself the problem. It conceives of poverty primarily in terms of "individual failings rather than structural inequality," or "cultural and skill 'deficits' rather than the unequal distribution of power and wealth" and, thus, instead of inquiring into the political economy of the late twentieth century, it is "about the characteristics and behaviour and...the welfare status of the poor."[65]

Why this bias, asks O'Connor? First, poverty knowledge is shaped heavily by the "enormous influence" of foundations and government agencies over research agendas and funding, partly determining what will count as "policy-relevant"; second, it is fuelled by a widespread disjunction between relevant disciplines, a separation of "academic" from "applied" policy research; and finally, a disconnect between social scientists and those they research.[66] "Authoritative poverty knowledge," as O'Connor calls it, thus does little to alter the conditions of poverty so assiduously and thoroughly studied. The credentialing of such knowledge controls and replicates it as new generations of students are taught what counts and what not, faculty learn what will earn or jeopardize promotion or tenure, scholars discover what will be accepted or rejected by their guilds and journals, and all learn what will or will not get a grant.

These socially constructed and historically conditioned patterns are hard to overcome. In Kuhn's paradigm theory language, the exemplars of a particular science determine which puzzles are worth considering, set the way in which puzzles are framed, provide the lexicon for describing them, define the training of the next generation, and provide the standards by which solutions are judged.[67] They shape a way of seeing.[68] Thus Bophal, reviewing numerous standard epidemiological textbooks, shows that though there is diversity in concepts, content, and approach, "Most exemplars [are] related to etiologic research rather than public health practice," resulting in an "increasing inability of epidemiology to solve socially based public health problems."[69]

This analysis raises one fundamental question: To what does one hold oneself accountable? The norms and values of good scientific practice provide one standard of accountability, which is well policed. Powerful mechanisms ensure that its accountability is met, or its lack exposed. There are consequences to not meeting these standards. However, is that enough to advance the health of the public? Following O'Connor's argument,[70] the single most important challenge is to make health a legitimate *public* policy concern, placing issues such as health-seeking behavior or quality of care in the context of inequality.

Making public health genuinely part of the public domain will, in our time, mean recovering and reinventing "the public" as a determining point of reference for health care. In turn, it means putting into its proper place—open to public scrutiny and accountability—what is usually described as private enterprise in health, but in fact is more like one component of a large interlocking community of powerful decision-makers accountable primarily to each other.

One option, already hinted at in our discussion of *métis* as crucial knowledge born from local experience, is to develop ways of being receptive to the expressed will of the relevant population, enacted where it matters most to them. As Habermas suggests, "The political public sphere can fulfill its function of perceiving and thematizing encompassing social problems only insofar as it develops out of the communication taking place among *those who are potentially affected*."[71] The work of such communication comes close to the meaning of "decent care,"[72] but it would also help us discern and respond better to the impact systemic deficiencies have upon those for whom care is meant.

9

RELIGION AND THE HEALTH OF THE
PUBLIC: DEEP ACCOUNTABILITY

"For the hardest problems, the problems that would not give way without long looks into the universe's bowels, physicists reserved words like *deep*."
James Gleick, *Chaos: Making a New Science*[1]

Better theory enables better practice, or it is not worth the bother. If a theory does not help those in positions of influence to guide efforts and alignments relevant to the health of their community, it is little better than intellectual entertainment, a distraction. Good theory helps people in positions of influence, many of whom might not think of themselves as "leaders," to achieve deep accountability for how they use their influence and live their lives. They seek accountability that is deep-rooted in an understanding of the complexity of life and in respect for its forms, aware of the turbulence it contains, sensitive to the variety of levels and scales at which human relationships matter, and worthy of the weight their decisions must support over time. We have defined health as comprehensive well-being, and linked it to freedom via Amartya Sen's theory of development, and to justice by calling on Paul Ricoeur's analysis of ethics as rooted in an understanding of the self as constituted by another. Deep accountability for health takes account of all three dimensions of human life.

Accountability per se, however important, is not enough. The standard language of accountability pervades discourse around health policy. Recent US reforms, for example, include a move toward "accountable care organizations," simply meaning that somebody be held accountable for the various paid providers who offer services for an episode of treatment. Deep accountability would hold a more rigorous standard by including all of those involved in the journey of health, understood in light of the earlier chapters of this book.

Deep accountability, in a time when public health faces many crises and the sphere of the public itself has been variously undermined, challenges many people. The health of the public, for instance, is affected by choices made by influential people, especially in states and markets, who seldom look beyond the interests of their own institution or specific field of activity. Transdisciplinarity, often extolled in the academy and crucial to any understanding of complexity, is mostly marginalized, leaving boundary-guarding disciplinary guilds relatively unscathed and boundary-crossing thinkers comparatively isolated. In public health, people largely continue thinking within institutional confinements. Religious or faith leaders equally prefer the comfort of their familiar domains of language and logic, seldom feeling the need for wider accountability. Moreover, few are sufficiently aware of what people in local communities, however meager their resources, do about their own health.

The ecology of contemporary social life is marked by ever-expanding hybrid organizational forms, emerging and mutating faster than typologies can name them. Thousands of new nongovernmental organizations explode into being like beneficent viruses, playing roles previously thought to need a government or, perhaps, a religious structure. Their work engages many determinants of health, with proximate and distal effects, using tangible and intangible means, at individual and social levels. If those in public organizations tend to think and act like states, and those in religious structures think and act like guardians of a bounded world, then those in the new hybrids regularly invent their logic as they go.

Alignment in the resulting cacophony is accidental at best, and even common accountability is rare, especially for distal health improvements that require choices sustained over time. Obvious reasons for bad alignment include differing interests and incentives, the fragmented plethora of professional guilds that influence decisions about policy and practice, and the machinations of power and money. Leaders, especially those carrying titles that imply a capacity to deliver a social good—"director of public health" or "archbishop," say—face complexities that affect the health and well-being of entire publics. Their leadership burden is heavy, awkward, and slippery. If their theory of leadership is simply contained within their institutional identities—religious, secular, or public—neither director nor archbishop will be able to be accountable for the health of the whole public. This holds especially true if they adopt a practice of dominion and control to secure their structural center of power, establishing boundary patrols that, ipso facto, tend to negate any realistic accountability for a complex, turbulent social reality.

It may seem naïve to suggest that better theory would make a difference; however, we think it does. Better theory helps leaders to live their lives accountable to a foundation deep enough to rest their life choices on. Living in a world of turbulent human systems, where should they lend their energy, imagination, presence, and capacity for risk, informed by what hope? Current theories of complexity make clear that linear, reductionist approaches to complex problems are not very effective. They are better suited to standard or "legitimate problems," amenable to any skilled scientist using available techniques after appropriate contemplation and calculation.[2]

Complex problems—as are most matters connected to the health of the public—require some capacity to deal with unpredictability and nonlinearity, including both the positive and negative sides of life. The challenge is conceptual, as neuroscientist, psychiatrist, and MacArthur "Genius Award" Fellow Arnold Mandell saw in critiquing the dependency of psychiatry on psychopharmacology, which generally fails to produce cures. Traditional approaches, he argued, are far too linear and reductionist: "The underlying paradigm remains: one gene→one peptide→one enzyme→one neurotransmitter→one receptor→one animal behaviour→one clinical syndrome→one drug→one clinical rating scale. It dominates almost all research and treatment...."[3] And it is inadequate to life.

If the complex problem is one in which unpredictability ("noise," standard science might say) and nonlinearity (or noncausal events) are definitive, how does one approach it? In the science of complexity the answer, concerning natural or social phenomena, lies in recognizing that certain patterns always repeat themselves at particular scales, with a definable relationship between those patterns that can be understood and leveraged. Edward N. Lorenz, an iconic figure in complexity theory, studying three-dimensional dynamical systems in meteorology, found not just unpredictability, but also fractal patterns, "suggestions of structure amid seemingly random behaviour."[4] Erwin Schrödinger, quantum physicist, saw half a century ago that life has the "astonishing gift of concentrating a 'stream of order' on itself and thus escaping the decay into atomic chaos."[5] Complexity, it turns out, is about generative patterns of order and of life. Properly understood, complexity is the friend of accountable leadership, precisely because life is not supposed to sit still.

This is what we point toward in using the term "deep," and to speak of it as fractal is an accurate way of describing the patterns of complexity that repeat themselves at different levels always in new ways. It is also a rather precise way of describing what this book is about. Ideas like religious health assets (RHAs), leading causes of life, healthworlds, congregational strengths, and boundary leadership are descriptions of particular patterns we believe to be relevant, in different ways at every scale, to describing the complexities of health and its relation to religion. Not at all arbitrary, these patterns variously repeat themselves in multiple contexts and over time, they are significant for understanding health interventions and goals, and they open up significant areas of inquiry that are largely undeveloped and poorly understood.

If that is what we mean by "deep," what of "accountability?" Accountability can be viewed in several ways. In its simplest form, it values counting. Better theory makes possible better counting in the sense of tracking and measuring more appropriate, useful, relevant things over more illuminating periods of time. One could count the number of pills an individual person, the "patient," receives from their physician, and one could measure their cost. Better would be to count all the pills the person receives from all health providers they might encounter, make sure the combined effect of all those pills is optimal, and count the cost of the whole in relation to the conditions the pills are supposed to improve.

Better still would be to know if the person-as-patient understands their situation and the purpose of the pills sufficiently to enable them to begin to act as a person-with-agency in their own health. Even further, to arrive at an accurate understanding of what influences their health—and thus would guide appropriate action—one would include all those involved in the health of that person. That most of those factors are obviously beyond the professional competency or interest of specialized providers acutely sharpens the need to broaden accountability to align those who make up the ecology of care around that one human being.

The best theory thus allows all involved to be accountable for their individual contribution to the full effect of their combined efforts. That full effect is best understood not in the light of a theory of disease, but in the context of a living person in a social system that is itself alive. *Bophelo* allows for such better theory, in Lesotho however limited its resources to sustain good practice, as in countries awash with technical, professional, and material resources who might equally fail in practice.

The conceptual foundations we have sketched provide one framing set of ideas, a transformational ensemble, for establishing deeper accountability on both sides of the interface between religion and the health of the public. Whatever particular words we use to express them, the ideas are more general, resting on potent insights and a rich array of empirical and theoretical studies drawn from a wide range of congruent disciplines. A decade ago, Chatters spoke of the very limited "extent to which the research and practice communities endorse the proposition that religious involvement is significant for individual and population health."[6] Acutely aware of this, we believe that the grounds for seriously rethinking this interface are powerful, and much clearer now than before.

The picture is clearest when one explores the narratives of people who seek their and their community's health in the face of challenges that should defeat them. Here the real meaning of RHAs, leading causes of life, strengths of people who congregate, and boundary leadership emerges in the face of sometimes helpful, sometimes unhelpful, and sometimes downright hostile forces of polity and economy. Barely visible in the data that makes up the work of epidemiologists and informs public health decisions, here we see measures of deep accountability—for the deepest accountability is to generative life.

DEEP ACCOUNTABILITY IN HEALTH ORGANIZATIONS

Our call for better theory comes at a time when it is increasingly obvious that great opportunities exist for integrated work, for blending many kinds of organizations, networks, associations, and institutions that fill the organizational ecology of our planet. Specific collaborations aimed at particular diseases— some well-known and long feared, such as drug resistant TB, polio, and malaria, and others long neglected and unknown in the developed world—have attracted unprecedented resources from coalitions that blend public and private funds. Other initiatives, focusing on developing key technologies such as vaccines unlikely to interest the market, have emerged with demonstrable success at large scale. Fiduciary and governance models are as complex and varied as the underlying conditions and linking opportunities. Leaders are thus constantly hearing about collaboration and being offered toolkits filled with instruments and forms to bring order to the chaos of opportunity.

One example of this heightened priority is *Real Collaboration*, by authors long at home in leadership roles of global health initiatives linked to The Carter Center, the Centers for Disease Control and Prevention (CDC), and the Gates Foundation.[7] They describe a new landscape marked by higher expectations and fragmented organizational architecture that makes collaboration vitally important but also difficult to achieve. Leaders of partnerships now have the opportunity to seek funding from more sources, working harder to connect with ministers and staff in countries with new governmental structures, staying abreast of many others likely to be working in the field of activity, being alert to changes in official policy, and all the time working harder at the human relationships within and around the partnership.

It is important to note that the driving energy here is not a new sense of the problems but the opposite—a new sense of the real opportunities within reach of resources, science, and connectivity. Yet, the actual tools remain instrumental, not dynamic, evidencing a trust in order rather than generativity, in structured management of resources rather than animate networks of humans finding life in and through turbulence. Their book's toolkit offers list after list of roles and concrete tasks to be filled in and checked off, artificially assigning order.[8] The tools and processes are Newtonian, because the theory underneath the tools offers leaders nothing more. Moreover, it is remarkable that a book on collaboration, so filled with noble purpose in the great tradition of global public health, fails to mention the role of faith in any fashion, avoiding its problems and blinding the new global partnerships to its assets. It is thus likely to promote the same instrumental projects and activities of the past, with pretty much the same incremental results and missed opportunities. It projects into the future the same self-inflicted blindness public health has shown toward its past, adopting an oversimplified history that does not fully account for its own successes, and robs leaders of the full vision of what is possible to achieve with a fuller menu of dynamic assets.

There is more to which leaders can be accountable. The answer is not just to add another category into the toolkit about religion, extending the instrumentalizing process to partnerships with faith leaders and their networks, institutions, or assets. Better accountability means paying attention to the full generative flow of life that leaders should be expected to appreciate, nurture, encourage, protect, and tend. It requires a blended intelligence: one that integrates a wide variety of information—community wisdom, clinical data streams, academic research, and the best practice knowledge from local and international partners—to enable better practices.[9] Leaders should be accountable (first, to themselves) for such blended intelligence. Furthermore, from our point of view, the newly successful global collaborations are better explained by a theory of blended intelligence, which is another way of describing the kind of interface between religion and the health of the public we have unpacked, not unlike the history of iconic public health landmarks that we have described in relation to the RHAs that helped enable them.

Increasingly, innovative thinkers in health care are formulating such accountability frameworks for improving care at system level, centered on the needs of the patient (in their lexicon) or the person (in the broader, community-based and nonhospitalcentric focus). For example, the Institute of Medicine's (IOM) focus on quality care attempts to break out of the linear traps described by Mandell with a call to elevate care to its highest level by attending to the key dimensions of STEEEP: safe, timely, effective, efficient, equitable, and patient-centered.[10] While not as comprehensive as one could hope in seeing the whole system of care outside the walls of the hospital and clinics, the simple recognition from this powerful guild that community and social determinants may play a pivotal role in accessing and delivering quality care, focused on the patient/person journey, signals a huge shift in benchmarking a more complex and multifaceted view of health.

Our own approach to deeper accountability emphasizes this nonlinear view of care further and calls particular attention to assets for health beyond formal facilities. Its usefulness can be seen in something as simple as observing one life's journey of health. Let us give a concrete example of this.

Clearly visible from Gunderson's office, Senior Vice President for Faith and Health at Methodist Le Bonheur Healthcare (MLH) in Memphis, stands an eight-story public housing unit. Here one woman has found her life for more than eight decades. Barely lower-middle class, high school uncompleted, marrying, birthing, and outliving her husband, she watched her children move north to Chicago. Carried on the currents of minimal public assistance, eventually she approached the ending of her days, close to a religious hospital that has a growing record of her ever more complex medical conditions. Increasingly frequently, she was readmitted into the hospital for reasons that could be addressed or even prevented by nonclinical care giving: taking medication off schedule, slipping and falling while bathing, and unable to care for a wound on her foot without assistance.

A member for many years of a small Baptist congregation, the women in her prayer group visited her, sometimes even the pastor, all quite overmatched by the practical barriers that the medical care system presents to one with so little means. However, this particular hospital has begun to follow a different theory, one that locates it as one component in a large complex of religious assets that share the care for this one woman. With eyes that see not just like a state, a medical provider, or a hospital facility, but also like the RHA it is, it has perceived the possibility of constructing webs of human trust across and between forms and structures that health care facilities usually cannot see at all. This involved many detailed changes in the internal ways and means of the hospital, though none involved any substantive change in clinical treatment. The key is a web of trust, of which the hospital is only one part.

The hospital had to work for that trust, which cannot be taken for granted at all. Moreover, it had to be institutionally concretized, beyond marketing slogans and great science. At root, it is embodied in the relationship between a paid "navigator," Jean, who is able to follow the thread of trust into the woman's apartment, mediated by the pastor who cares for the woman and trusts Jean. Jean connects what was disconnected and invisible. She makes permeable and communicative (Habermas) those institutional spaces that were opaque and circumscribed. She invites into the shared work of hospitality those who were not just unwelcome, but also invisible. Once the embodied web extends into that life, many things previously invisible, unimaginable, or remote become much easier. If this sounds magical, it is entirely natural, in the sense that the new, more inclusive order reflects the nature of life, its capacity for new connections, deeper coherence, relevant agency, generativity, and hope. A leader who knows that and does not work with that natural flow of life should be held accountable, in the same way they would be for withholding evidence-based treatment.

A hospital normally can only do things it can pay somebody to do. However, with new eyes, it now sees a way to have an employee, Jean, spend her time aligning and animating other human assets and networks the hospital does and should not pay. This care-giving "team" comprising the pastor, the women of the prayer group, and the informal network of residents in the town block, loosely but effectively aligned yet working as a social whole, does a very remarkable thing. It creates a web of care that can help her with bathing, general wound dressing, taking medication on schedule and correctly, and getting her to the hospital when she needs to be there, not too late to help. Her continuum of care is rooted in a web of trust that overtly includes and provides critical support for the medical facility

She is one of hundreds of similar patients moving across social webs that influence their journeys in remarkably tangible ways, measurable by the hospital: patients like her, coming across the slender filaments of embodied trust, cost about 25 percent less, saving the payers about $8,500 per visit, and not because they were denied anything they needed, but because they came at a time in their condition when they needed less costly treatment. Moreover, they tend to come back to hospital about 20 percent less often, and even show half the mortality, both outcomes apparently affected by the presence of relevant social supports.[11] Such indicators are what the hospital sees in the end, but they are the result of things, invisible and uncontrollable by such systems. In a very practical way, an older woman, appropriately afraid of strangers, can now safely admit into her apartment visiting nurses who are trusted because someone she already trusts (her pastor) extends the web of trust to include them. Her web of trust now includes people with very tangible relevance to her healing process.

The invisible but highly relevant social assets of the patient's reality change what the hospital cannot change—the journey of health that begins outside its doors—and they affect the hard outcomes of the journey. A new standard of quality, and a different view of collaboration, starts to come into view as this peripheral vision sharpens. What if every patient came at the right time? What if they all came accompanied by a trusted and competent friend? What if they were not afraid and thus prepared to receive treatment?

If all one can see are professional guilds aligned by payment systems accountable to the low standard of legal liability, it is not possible to imagine accomplishing what only a social whole can do. A relevant theory of alignment and collaboration should turn on enough light to see the whole community. The turbulence is then no longer purely threatening but is a condition navigable by leaders building systems appropriate to their fluid environment, ones that enable enough caring people to share the opportunity to enhance the life of the whole. Memphis is an ironic scandal, precisely because it is a small city filled with obvious health assets made distant by equally obvious social and political failures. It would seem clear that connecting things should not be so difficult. They are there to see, if one knows what to look at: a task not of imagining a distant future, but of seeing the images right down the street. The assets are there, and they are good for health, both individual and public.

Deep Accountability in Religious Leaders

Recently one of us, together with staff from the *Masangane* HIV and AIDS program, the comprehensive, integrated faith-based initiative to which we have referred before that had arisen from the regional Moravian Church to help deal with the pandemic, visited the public hospital in Mount Fletcher in the Eastern Cape, South Africa, one of four sites for antiretroviral treatment (ART) in the region. The ART unit is fully staffed and equipped, ready to treat thousands of people living in homesteads spread out across wide-flung hills whose immune systems are crashing. We had brought a patient, a thirty-five-year-old woman critically ill from AIDS-related complications, who had finally agreed to acknowledge her situation. We travelled in the pickup belonging to Masangane. We left behind another woman, so emaciated and weak that we could not move her into the pickup. A fully equipped ambulance was necessary, but none was at hand then or for the next couple of days (she eventually died).

For the many households in this area public transport is seriously limited, private vehicles rare or too expensive to hire, and vehicular access difficult. Lying just below the majestic mountains of Lesotho, the land is worn, the *dongas* or erosion gullies deep. Jobs are hard to come by, and a hundred years of forced labor migration movement to the gold mines and factories of the Witwatersrand is definitive. Home, family, community, and land have all been disrupted in the process, traditions undone and reinvented.

This is a reality not peculiar to Apartheid, nor restricted to the African continent. Like many people in rural or marginalized communities worldwide, people from here must look for jobs elsewhere than their home place. On the outskirts of the distant cities, they settle temporarily in tin shacks or under plastic sheets, alienated or undone, but at least within possible reach of work or resources. Perhaps they send remittances back home. They frequently do return, to care for a sick loved one, participate in a family ritual, attend a funeral, or simply to die where their ancestors are buried. Furthermore, in Africa, they most often conceive of the health and well-being of individuals and communities through religious narratives, symbols, and rituals, distinctly social in their patterns. Meanwhile, people left behind in the rural areas, mostly women, have begun to die from AIDS, leaving more children orphaned, left to the care of whoever is available. Caregivers themselves—grandmothers especially—either battle to cope, or become sick and die themselves.

Among those increasingly distressed by the devastating effects of AIDS are religious leaders, often despairing and searching for a response. The Reverend Mgcoyi, a leading Moravian pastor in the region, anguished by the visible pain, motivated by the hope his faith proclaimed, was certain that preaching, praying, and visiting the ill and the bereaved was simply not enough. Gathering a small team around him, he began Masangane. In Xhosa it means, "let us embrace," directly attacking the problematic religious and cultural stigmatization of those with HIV and AIDS, folding them into a congregation and community instead of casting them out.[12] Masangane workers, themselves beneficiaries of the program and openly HIV positive, had brought this woman to the hospital in Mount Fletcher. Without them, she would never have reached an ART site where she could get help.

For all practical purposes, with no transport at its disposal, the ART unit had no way of reaching people in its area, and people frequently had great difficulty getting to the hospital. Bringing this woman in met a massive need. Finding people in time also mattered. This means knowing the local communities well enough, not only being regularly present to them, but also accompanying people in their journey of health before and after any hospital or clinic visit, mentoring, encouraging, monitoring, supporting, and drawing them into relationship with others to help sustain the lifelong treatment that is likely. Such responsibilities cannot be borne by formal health facilities like a hospital.

Despite the daunting challenge, limited resources, and a handful of person-nel (much of it voluntary), Masangane has done a remarkable job for almost ten years now. Reverend Mgcoyi was intelligent enough to know that his position, used properly, could work toward breaking stigma, and that religion could be a health asset. He offered one priceless asset: trustworthy authority. Religious (or traditional) authority can serve unhealthy ends in support of questionable ideas; but equally, it can serve health. This was, after all, a time when South Africa's notorious minister of health repeatedly spoke of ARTs as poison, undermining their use and piling confusion upon confusion among the populace. Mcgoyi had immediate and trusted access to communities through the congregations embedded in them, themselves representing locally rooted, long-standing, and durable religious traditions of care and compassion. A boundary leader, he understood the importance of a web of trusted relationships.

Masangane is more than a single pastor or team, but works through a web of relationships that extend from its members in the community, to local doc-tors, initially to Médicins Sans Frontières (who provided its first trained nurse), later to the local state hospitals, to a German church worker resident in South Africa able to act as intermediary to international funders and supporters, and to partners in those bodies themselves. Also alongside Masangane are community-based orphan care groups initiated by local people, often from faith convictions or a traditional African religious sense of responsibility for the community. These webs of trust describe the multilayered nature of accountability, and no layer is less important that the other. As a whole, they represent a vital, complex, but quite understandable pattern of elements that describe a health system adequate to the challenges, much of it resting in RHAs.

While such assets are all too often misaligned with, and unrecognized or unsupported by the formal health system, perhaps even regarded with suspicion and hostility, religious leaders do have a responsibility for changing that situation. Strategically, given the scale and scope of RHAs, if only 10 to 20 percent of the religious bodies in any particular community were to be engaged in aligned and accountable practices working for the health of the public, potent resources would be unleashed toward the comprehensive well-being of all.

Deep Accountability in the Social Whole

No conscientious accounting for the health of individuals is possible if one excludes the social, environmental, and economic conditions that impact on community or population-scale health. It cannot be done simply by aggregating individuals, as if that describes the social. Yet Margaret Thatcher's view that there is no such thing as society, only individuals,[13] permeates much policy and practice. It plays itself out theoretically and practically in the instrumental and mathematical reasoning that dominates much policy and decision making, in the current widespread adoption of rational choice theories of human behavior,[14] and, in the context of public health, in an emphasis on the quality of life defined all too often in terms of individual choices about what foods to eat, exercise to take, and the like.

Margaret Radin, seeking a new vision of the common good,[15] shows that the same ethos that governs the commodification of health has intensified in every other aspect of human life, including religion, to our detriment. We share Radin's view, consciously arguing for the primacy of the social that, following Ricoeur among others, is grounded in the nature of human being. Personal choices are certainly real, and they do carry responsibility. However, unless they are wholly trivial, they are affected by and have effects upon others. Even individual choice is thus social.

Consider avian flu, AIDS, smoking, obesity, violence, suicide, or depression. The specific etiologies of these phenomena may be quite different, but all are social in various ways. Avian flu becomes a threat in the context of commercial chicken production; HIV is made more likely in the context of fractured family structures and gender asymmetry; smoking reflects a pathological social formation using cynical tools of mass persuasion aimed at the young; obesity appears as an aggregation of bad food choices by individuals only by disguising the complexity of causes that are social and economic. Similarly, violence is patterned, gendered, and located in gross disparities that makes a social framework of understanding primary; suicide (in the United States) is biased toward older white men; and most depression is best understood through the social dynamics of a person's life in relation to socially formed expectations and fears that affect emotional fitness for the journey of life.

Each of these phenomena is social *before* it is personal; each is personal in the context of a social reality. Furthermore, each offers opportunities for seeing the role of faith—also social, in essence—in understanding how the patterns of pathology rather than generative life gain momentum. Rather than asking largely functional questions—what does faith *say* about smoking or condoms, for example?—it is more useful to ask how faith in practice is potentially transformative (or complicit) in the social patterning that creates the phenomena. In that regard, though we have at several points indicated our profound personal and theoretical awareness of the pathologies of religion or faith, we have nevertheless privileged the search for transformative understandings, practices, and models of comprehending faith and religion. That there are theoretical, practical, and strategic grounds for doing so, we show in this work as we have searched for a more productive view of the interface between religion and public health. We want a stronger basis for mutual accountability between thinkers and actors on both sides of that interface, which may exist not only between different people, but also within the same person, perhaps even as a kind of experiential and methodological split personality.

Here we turn, too, to the idea that health is not merely a state of being, but a journey that integrates our social and personal lives. We are in motion from the day we move down the birth canal. We move always, and the cumulative moves are a journey, though never apart from the journeys of others. Even when it appears lonely, we move in social fields of reality that attract, repel, influence, and speed us along, just as our journey influences that of others in ways we may only dimly perceive. Persons, neighbors, societies, and global traditions and cultures are in motion, not necessarily predictably. Indeed, the idea of globalization can be understood in terms of growing mobility and movement, of people, ideas, information, goods, and services, with mixed consequences. The choices for good and bad we or others make about our journey are important because they shape our well-being.

This too is a way of looking at social accountability, now as something more than a calculus of rights and responsibilities according only to the needs or demands of the moment. To see health as a journey adds to body, place, and space the ingredient of time, with important implications for health practices and health institutions, including for the way its leaders behave. Hospitals, congregations, and social service agencies have reason to work together because their members, patients, and clients are the same human beings, at various points in their life span going to, through, and beyond different doorways along the way.

This is not a trivial observation. Institutions that care about the people have good reason to look up and down the journey those people are on, even if only to ensure a smooth, efficient passage along the way. The institutional reality of a health care facility is changed if its self-image shifts from seeing itself as a fixed a point of service, to that of a landmark on a longer path toward health. Anything done in a hospital or a clinic is only a part of a larger continuum of care, and this needs to be accounted for institutionally. The key questions will then be: (1) How does this (or that) medical intervention fit into the journey? (2) To what does it need to be linked? and (3) How do we enable that link?

Accountability then shifts from a focus on the autonomous quality of the event of service in one place, to an optimal alignment with other institutions, upstream and downstream, in the different places that a person occupies in space and time. Advancing the quality of life for the whole—individuals, their families, those who serve them, and the communities that hold them—over a life span, becomes the most fundamental point of health care. Not the same as controlling disease, or keeping someone alive with the use of advanced technologies, it concerns how one experiences the longer journey. While medical facilities and health systems need to be available for some of that journey, most of it occurs elsewhere. The key question then becomes: What advances the quality of life over the long haul, sustainably? With this as a critical indicator of what a medical system can offer, or better, of whether or not what it can offer is adequately conceived, we arrive at a different norm of accountability.

A similar point could be made about religion, often a key factor in a person's journey. Better religion is not about stasis, but about informing a life journey in ways that enhance the well-being of persons and the societies within which they exist. Religious bodies that care for sick individuals or work for public well-being may occupy different buildings, speak different languages, or compete with each other for cash, attention, and political support, as with any human institution and, like much other work in the world of health, fail to see the whole to which they are accountable. People who run soup kitchens, for example, rarely spend much time working on mental health policy, although they are sure to observe that many of their clients suffer from at least one chronic mental health condition.

The paradigm we seek must hold in creative tension the moral and intellectual forces that spin away from each other. What kind of religion and what kind of science makes that more likely? What kind of paradigm will undergird those common passions and enable them to find their way toward the choices that lead to life? Those have been guiding questions for what we here term deep accountability. It is the kind of accountability that seeks exemplars, to use Thomas Kuhn's term, capable of illuminating both complexity and the limits to any one route to grasping that complexity. It is accountability that ties targeted, narrowly disciplined but vital health interventions in one aspect of human life to other congruent aspects of life, and ultimately to the totality of life together. It requires building new standards of accountability capable of matching such goals, and ways of measuring or making legible what such standards mean.

This is because life, and not simply death, is at stake. Therefore, we need boundary leaders, people alive to the possibilities of lending their influence and energies to life at community scale in complex combinations of skills, disciplines, and interests. Moving across divides of language, guild, position, and discipline they see health in a larger conceptual whole, embodied in a more vital social whole. They can imagine not just healing past and present wounds, but nurturing the conditions in which social life, tumbled and turned by positive turbulence, might expand.

Given a theory to guide them, they may even imagine transformation and, testing that imagination against the times, find it not delusional to be accountable deeply for what matters most, generating the life that comes next.

NOTES

1 SEEING DIFFERENTLY: CHANGING THE PARADIGM OF THE HEALTH OF THE PUBLIC

1. Personal communication, June 13, 2011.
2. Molly Caldwe Crosby, *The American Plague: The Untold Story of Yellow Fever, the Epidemic That Shaped Our History* (New York: Berkley Books, 2007).
3. See African Religious Health Assets Programme, "Appreciating Assets: The Contribution of Religion to Universal Access in Africa" (Cape Town: ARHAP, Report for the World Health Organization, 2006). Also available at www.arhap. uct.ac.za.
4. See Southern Africa AIDS Training Programme & the International HIV/AIDS Alliance, *CBO/NGO Support: The Role and Value of NGO Based CBO/NGO Support Providers in the Response to HIV/AIDS in Southern and Eastern Africa: A Case study of CHEP*, The SHARE Series (Harare: SAT/International HIV/AIDS Alliance, 2004).
5. On the vital role of grassroots intermediary organizations, see Thomas F. Carroll, *Intermediary NGOs: The Supporting Link in Grassroots Development*, Library of Management for Development (West Hartford, CT: Kumarian Press, 1992); James R. Cochrane, "Trustworthy Intermediaries: Role of Religious Agents on the Boundaries of Public Health," in *When Religion and Health Align: Mobilising Religious Health Assets for Transformation*, ed. James R. Cochrane, Barbara Schmid, and Teresa Cutts (Pietermaritzburg: Cluster Publications, 2011), 150–63.
6. Paul Germond and Sepetla Molapo, "In Search of *Bophelo* in a Time of AIDS: Seeking a Coherence of Economies of Health and Economies of Salvation," *Journal of Theology for Southern Africa* 126 (2006), 27–47.
7. See chapter 8.
8. Robert Skidelsky, "The Remedist: Why John Maynard Keynes is the Man of the Year," *The New York Times Magazine*, December 14, 2008, 21–22.
9. Jim Yong Kim et al., eds., *Dying for Growth: Global Inequality and the Health of the Poor* (Monroe, ME: Common Courage Press, 2000), 23.
10. Said Amir Arjomand, "Religion and the Diversity of Normative Orders," in *The Political Dimensions of Religion*, ed. Said Amir Arjomand (New York: State University of New York Press, 1993), 45–68.
11. Richard Hofrichter, ed. *Health and Social Justice: Politics, Ideology, and Inequity in the Distribution of Disease* (San Francisco: Jossey-Bass [John Wiley & Sons], 2003).
12. B. J. Turnock, *Public Health: What It Is and How It Works*. 2nd ed. (Gaithersburg, MD: Aspen Publications, 2001).
13. George Rosen, *A History of Public Health* (Baltimore, MD: Johns Hopkins University Press, 1999), 18–19.

14. Lucy Gilson, "In Defence and Pursuit of Equity," *Social Science and Medicine* 47, no. 12 (1998): 1891–96.
15. Laurie Garrett, *Betrayal of Trust: The Collapse of Global Public Health* (New York: Hyperion, 2000), 585.
16. The term comes from Klaus Nürnberger, *Prosperity, Poverty and Pollution: Managing the Approaching Crisis* (London: Zed Books, 1999).
17. Elaine Cameron, Jonathan Mathers, and Jayne Parry, "'Health and Well-Being': Questioning the Use of Health Concepts in Public Health Policy and Practice," *Critical Public Health* 18, no. 2 (2008): 225–32; see also Sandra Carlisle and Phil Hanlon, "'Well-Being' as a Focus for Public Health? A Critique and Defence," *Critical Public Health* 18, no. 3 (2008): 263–70.
18. See, for example, Gabriel A. Almond, R. Scott Appleby, and Emmanuel Sivan, *Strong Religion: The Rise of Fundamentalism Around the World* (Chicago: University of Chicago Press, 2003); Peter L. Berger, "Reflections on the Sociology of Religion Today: The 2000 Paul Hanly Furfey Lecture," *Sociology of Religion* 62, no. 4 (2001): 443–54; José Casanova, *Public Religions in the Modern World* (Chicago: University of Chicago Press, 1994); Roland Robertson and JoAnn Chirico, "Humanity, Globalization and Worldwide Religious Resurgence," in *The globalization reader*, ed. Frank Lechner and John Boli (Oxford, UK: Blackwell Publishers, 2000), 93–98.
19. Harold G. Koenig, Michael E. McCullough, and David B. Larson, *Handbook of Religion and Health* (Oxford: Oxford University Press, 2001).

2   THE HEALTH OF THE PUBLIC AND THE RELIGIOUS MIND: CONNECTIONS AND DISCONNECTIONS

1. David R. Kinsley, *Health, Healing and Religion: A Cross Cultural Perspective* (Upper Saddle River, NJ: Prentice Hall, 1995).
2. Personal information, discussion with Pope Shenouda III of the Coptic Church, which still uses the pharaonic tongue in its liturgy; its key title for Jesus Christ is *Sine*, the Healer.
3. The French Annales school coined the historical concept of the *longue durée* prioritizing "long-term" historical structures and mentalities over events, and emphasizing a history from below; see Fernand Braudel, *On History*, trans. Sarah Matthews (Chicago: University of Chicago Press, 1980); Lucien Febvre, *A New Kind of History and Other Essays*, trans. Peter Burke and K. Folca (New York: Harper & Row (Harper Torchbooks), 1973).
4. S. W. B. Newsom, "Pioneers in Infection Control: John Snow, Henry Whitehead, the Broad Street Pump, and the Beginnings of Geographical Epidemiology," *Journal of Hospital Infection* 64, no. 6 (2006): 210–21.
5. John Duffy, *The Sanitarians: A History of American Public Health* (Urbana, IL; Chicago: University of Illinois Press, 1992).
6. Robert D. Morris, *The Blue Death: Disease, Disaster, and the Water We Drink* (New York: Harper Collins, 2007).
7. Dorothy Porter, *Health, Civilization and the State: A History of Public Health from Ancient to Modern Times* (New York: Routledge, 1994).
8. Ibid., 81–87; George Rosen, *A History of Public Health* (Baltimore, MD: Johns Hopkins University Press, 1999), 263–66.
9. *Lancet*, June 23, 1855, cited in Steven Johnson, *The Ghost Map: The Story of London's Most Terrifying Epidemic—and How It Changed Science, Cities, and the Modern World* (New York: Riverhead Books (Penguin), 2006), 186.
10. Ibid., 74.

11. Newsom, "Pioneers in Infection Control."
12. Johnson, *The Ghost Map*. 18.
13. Or perhaps eighty-nine, as reported by S. P. W. Chave, "Henry Whitehead and Cholera in Broad Street," *Medical History* 2, no. 2 (1958): 92.
14. Newsom, "Pioneers in Infection Control," 213–14.
15. Johnson, *The Ghost Map*. 194.
16. Chave, "Henry Whitehead," 95.
17. Johnson, *The Ghost Map*. 171.
18. Ibid., 175–77.
19. Chave, "Henry Whitehead," 96–97; Johnson, *The Ghost Map*. 178–80.
20. Henry Whitehead, "Report on the Cholera Outbreak in the Parish of St. James, Westminster, During the Autumn of 1854," http://johnsnow.matrix.msu.edu /work, accessed August 10, 2009, (1855), 132.
21. Johnson, *The Ghost Map*. 195–96.
22. Ibid., 202.
23. UCLA, "Whitehead," University of California Los Angeles, School of Public Health, http://www.ph.ucla.edu/epi/Snow/whitehead.html, accessed October 1, 2009.
24. Duffy, *The Sanitarians*. 157.
25. Rosen, *A History of Public Health*. 23–24.
26. Vivian Nutton, "The Medical Meeting Place," in *Ancient Medicine in Its Socio-Cultural Context, Volume 1*, ed. Ph. J. van der Eijk, H. F. J. Horstmanshoff, and P. H. Schrijvers, The Wellcome Institute Series in the History of Medicine (Amsterdam; Atlanta, GA: Rodopi, 1995).
27. Bronwen L. Wickkiser, *Asklepios, Medicine, and the Politics of Healing in Fifth-Century Greece: Between Craft and Cult* (Baltimore, MD: Johns Hopkins University Press, 2008).
28. Ravi P. Rannan-Eliya and Nishan De Mel, "Resource Mobilization in Sri Lanka's Health Sector," Institute of Policy Studies, Harvard School of Public Health & Health Policy Programme, http://www.hsph.harvard.edu/ihsg/publications/pdf /No-42.pdf, accessed April 21, 2010.
29. Porter, *Health, Civilization and the State*. 22.
30. Peter van Minnen, "Medical Care in Late Antiquity," in *Ancient Medicine in Its Socio-Cultural Context, Volume 1*, ed. Ph. J. van der Eijk, H. F. J. Horstmanshoff, and P. H. Schrijvers, The Wellcome Institute Series in the History of Medicine (Amsterdam; Atlanta, GA: Rodopi, 1995), 154. See also Jole Agrimi and Chiara Crisciani, "Charity and Aid in Medieval Christian Civilization," in *Western Medical Thought from Antiquity to the Middle Ages*, ed. Mirko D. Grmek (Cambridge, MA; London: Harvard University Press, 1998), 182.
31. Peregrine Horden, "The Earliest Hospitals in Byzantium, Western Europe, and Islam," *Journal of Interdisciplinary History* xxxv, no. 3 (2005): 376.
32. van Minnen, "Medical Care in Late Antiquity," 159.
33. See Rosen, *A History of Public Health*. 22–24.
34. See James C. McGilvray, *The Quest for Health and Wholeness* (Tübingen: German Institute for Medical Mission, 1981), 2–3.
35. Christoffer H. Grundmann, *Sent to Heal!: Emergence and Development of Medical Missions* (Lanham, MD: University Press of America, 2005).
36. See, for example, the chapter on missions in James R. Cochrane, *Servants of Power: The Role of English-Speaking Churches, 1903–1930* (Johannesburg: Ravan Press, 1987). Albert Schweitzer represents a classic example of the ambiguities in medical mission approaches: clearly holding a patriarchal view on Africans, he also felt a deep responsibility to atone for what he describes as the unbearable injustice and cruelty done to African people by European colonizers. See Albert Schweitzer, *Zwischen Wasser und Urwald: Erlebnisse und Beobachtungen*

eines Arztes in Urwalde Äquatorialafrikas (München: Verlag C. H. Beck, 1963), 147–48.

37. See Andrew M. Eason, "'All Things to All People to Save Some': Salvation Army Missionary Work Among the Zulus of Victorian Natal," *Journal of Southern African Studies* 35, no. 1 (2009): 8.

38. For a brief summary of some of these factors, see Christoffer H. Grundmann, "Mission and Healing in Historical Perspective," *International Bulletin of Missionary Research* 32, no. 4 (2008): 187.

39. For example, see Ivan Illich, *Medical Nemesis: The Expropriation of Health* (Toronto: Bantam, 1979).

40. This story, in its larger context of the history of Christian medical mission in the 1960s and 1970s, comes from McGilvray, *The Quest.* 32–41.

41. Ibid., 33.

42. Ibid.

43. Ibid., 34.

44. Several of these associations and their partners are today gathered in the Africa Christian Health Association Platform; see www.africachap.org.

45. *Deutsches Institut für ärtzliche Mission;* see http://www.difaem.de/.

46. The following discussion rests heavily on the account by McGilvray, *The Quest.* 9–22.

47. Ibid., 27.

48. Ibid., xv.

49. Gillian Paterson, "The CMC story, 1968–1998," *Contact* 161/162 (1998): 3–52.

50. John H. Bryant, *Health and the Developing World* (Ithaca, NY: Cornell University Press, 1970).

51. McGilvray, *The Quest,* 42–54.

52. James C. McGilvray, "The Church and Health: Reflections and Possibilities," *Contact* 81 (October 1984): 7.

53. Peter Bellamy, "The Significance of Bob Lambourne's Writing Today," *Contact* 81 (1984): 12–15.

54. Robert A. Lambourne, "Secular and Christian Models of Health and Salvation," *Contact* 1 (1970): 2.

55. Ibid., 3.

56. Ibid., 4.

57. Bryant, *Health and the Developing World.*

58. John H. Bryant, "Five Challenges to the Churches in Health Work," *Contact* 42 (1977): 1.

59. J. H. Bryant and David Jenkins, "Moral Issues and Health Care," *Contact* 4 (July 1971): 11.

60. John H. Bryant, "Five Challenges to the Churches," 1.

61. McGilvray, *The Quest.* 46.

62. Ibid., 49, 51.

63. Ibid., 52.

64. See Marcos Cueto, "The Origins of Primary Health Care and Selective Primary Health Care," *American Journal of Public Health* 94, no. 11 (2004): 1865. While groundbreaking at the time, this approach did not survive well: "The percentage of villages with a cooperative medical system fell from 90% in the 1960s to 5% by 1985. .... [The] Collapse of the cooperative medical system and change in the role of barefoot doctors resulted in a huge decline in primary health-care coverage in rural areas," according to Daqing Zhang and Paul U. Unschuld, "China's Barefoot Doctor: Past, Present, and Future," *The Lancet* 372, no. 9653 (2008): 1865–67. More recent reforms have tried to reverse this situation; see Guy Carrin et al., "The Reform of the Rural Cooperative Medical System in the People's Republic

of China: Interim Experience in 14 Pilot Counties," *Social Science & Medicine* 48, no. 7 (1999): 961–67.

65. For a more detailed description, see McGilvray, *The Quest*. 55–69.
66. Ibid., 70.
67. World Health Organization, *Health by the People* (Geneva: World Health Organization, 1975).
68. Ibid., "Declaration of Alma-Ata," from the *International Conference on Primary Health Care* (Alma-Ata, USSR: World Health Organization, 1978).
69. See, for example, Raymond Aron, *Progress and Disillusion: The Dialectics of Modern Society*, The Britannica Perspectives (New York: New American Library, 1968); Robert Nisbet, *History of the Idea of Progress* (New York: Basic, 1980).
70. Michael D. Bordo, Alan M. Taylor, and Jeffrey G. Williamson, eds., *Globalization in Historical Perspective* (Chicago: University of Chicago Press, 2003).
71. William H. Foege, J. D. Millar, and D. A. Henderson, "Smallpox Eradication in West and Central Africa," *Bulletin of the World Health Organization* 52, no. 2 (1975): 209.
72. William H. Foege, "Keynote Speech, the Thomas Francis Jr. Medal in Global Public Health," University of Michigan, www.polio.umich.edu/program/foege.html, accessed October 26, 2010. See also a recent comparison of smallpox and polio vaccination campaigns in India, by S. Bhattacharya and R. Dasgupta, "A Tale of Two Global Health Programs: Smallpox Eradication's Lessons for the Antipolio Campaign in India," *American Journal of Public Health* 99, no. 7 (2009): 1176–84.
73. "Herd immunity" was the standard approach of the time, which Foege and his colleagues discarded to initiate their surveillance-containment model; see, William H. Foege, "Smallpox Eradication: William Foege Oral History—Interviewed by Victoria Harden," Centers for Disease Control and Prevention, http://www .globalhealthchronicles.org/smallpox/record/view/pid/emory:15jvg, accessed October 26, 2010. That this model was key to their success is challenged by Edward H. Kaplan and Lawrence M. Wein, "Smallpox Eradication in West and Central Africa: Surveillance-Containment or Herd Immunity?" *Epidemiology* 14, no. 1 (2003): 90–92. And, in response, it is vehemently defended by Svetlana S. Marennikova, "Commentary: Perspectives on Smallpox Eradication," *Epidemiology* 14, no. 1 (2003): 93.
74. Much of the following narrative is drawn from Billy Woodward, Joel Shurkin, and Debra Gordon, *Scientists Greater Than Einstein: The Biggest Lifesavers of the Twentieth Century* (Fresno, CA: Linden Publishing, 2009).
75. Foege, "Smallpox Eradication."
76. Foege, Millar, and Henderson, "Smallpox Eradication in West and Central Africa," 216.
77. William H. Foege, Donald Millar, and J. Michael Lane, "Selective Epidemiologic Control in Smallpox Eradication," *American Journal of Epidemiology* 94, no. 4 (1971): 311.
78. Data from Foege, Millar, and Henderson, "Smallpox Eradication in West and Central Africa," 215.
79. Ibid., 209.
80. Foege, Millar, and Lane, "Selective Epidemiologic Control in Smallpox Eradication," 312.
81. Foege, "Smallpox Eradication."
82. Jean Roy, "Smallpox Eradication: Jean Roy Oral History—Interviewed by Victoria Harden," Centers for Disease Control and Prevention, http://www .globalhealthchronicles.org/smallpox/record/view/pid/emory:15n9k, July 13, 2006, accessed January 24, 2010, 15–17.
83. Cueto, "The Origins of Primary Health Care," 1864–74.

84. World Bank, *World Development Report 1993: Investing in Health* (New York: Oxford University Press, 1993).
85. John J. Hall and Richard Taylor, "Health for All Beyond 2000: The Demise of the Alma-Ata Declaration and Primary Health Care in Developing Countries," *Medical Journal of Australia* 178 (2003): 20.
86. Paul Farmer, *Pathologies of Power: Health, Human Rights and the New War on the Poor* (Berkeley, CA: University of California Press, 2003); Laurie Garrett, *Betrayal of Trust: The Collapse of Global Public Health* (New York: Hyperion, 2000); Jim Yong Kim et al., eds., *Dying for Growth: Global Inequality and the Health of the Poor* (Monroe, ME: Common Courage Press, 2000).
87. Lucy Gilson et al., "Challenging Inequity through Health Systems," (Geneva: WHO Commission on the Social Determinants of Health, 2007); Richard Hofrichter, ed., *Health and Social Justice: Politics, Ideology, and Inequity in the Distribution of Disease* (San Francisco: Jossey-Bass [John Wiley & Sons], 2003); Nancy Krieger, "Why Epidemiologists Cannot Afford to Ignore Poverty," *Epidemiology* 18 (2007): 658–63.
88. World Health Organization, *The World Health Report 2008: Primary Health Care—Now More than Ever* (Geneva: World Health Organization, 2008).
89. World Health Organization, *Building from Common Foundations: The World Health Organization and Faith-Based Organizations in Primary Healthcare* (Geneva: World Health Organization, 2008).
90. Robert W. Amler and H. Bruce Dull, eds., *Closing the Gap: The Burden of Unnecessary Illness* (New York: Oxford University Press, 1987), vii, Preface.
91. Jimmy Carter, "Foreword," in Ibid., 1.
92. James P. Wind, "One Congregation's Experience," *Second Opinion*, March 13, 1990, 87.
93. Gary R. Gunderson, "The Task Ahead," in *Faith and Health* (Atlanta, GA: Interfaith Health Program, The Carter Center, 1994), 1.
94. Miriam Kiser, Deborah L. Jones, and Gary R. Gunderson, "Faith and Health: Leadership Aligning Assets to Transform Communities," *International Review of Mission* 95, no. 376/377 (2006): 50.
95. Thomas A. Droege, "Congregations as Communities of Health and Healing," *Interpretation* 69, no. 2 (1995): 118.
96. Kiser, Jones, and Gunderson, "Faith and Health," 57.
97. Ibid., 52.
98. For one account of ARHAP, see James R. Cochrane, "A Model of Integral Development: Assessing and Working with Religious Health Assets," in *Religion and Development: Ways of Transforming the World*, ed. Gerrie ter Haar (London; New York: Hurst & Co; Columbia University Press, 2011).
99. African Religious Health Assets Programme, "Appreciating Assets: The Contribution of Religion to Universal Access in Africa" (Cape Town: ARHAP, Report for the World Health Organization, 2006).
100. See Joshua Cooper Ramo, *The Age of the Unthinkable: Why the New World Disorder Constantly Surprises Us and What We Can Do about It* (New York: Little, Brown and Company, 2009).

3   Religious Health Assets: What Religion Brings to Health of the Public

1. See the Resident's Association report, ratified by Drs. H. Weber and J. O'Riain: "This is to advise you that even the groundwater seeping from the earth below IY is so badly polluted with the bacteria associated with human faeces that direct contact with the water could prove fatal." Hout Bay Resident's Association, "Poisoned

Earth," *Hout and About* http://www.houtbay.org.za/Newsletters/200809_
HoutAbout.htm, accessed October 22, 2011.
2. This discussion draws on Jan Froestad, "Health, Democracy and Governance in
South Africa: Two Case Studies," unpublished paper (Bergen: University of Bergen,
2002); and James R. Cochrane, "Religion in the Health of Migrant Communities:
Cultural Assets or Medical Deficits?" *Journal of Ethnic and Migration Studies* 32,
no. 4 (2006): 715–36.
3. Paul Farmer, *Infections and Inequalities: The Modern Plagues* (Berkeley, CA; Los
Angeles: University of California, 1999).
4. Jan Froestad, "Environmental Health Problems in Hout Bay: The Challenge of
Generalising Trust in South Africa," *Journal of Southern African Studies* 31, no. 2
(2005): 342.
5. Ibid., 350–51.
6. Ibid., 343–47.
7. Ibid.
8. Department of Health, "Restructuring the National Health System for Universal
Primary Health Care," (Pretoria: Government of South Africa, 1996).
9. Froestad, "Environmental Health Problems," 344.
10. Department of Health, "A Policy for the Development of a District Health System
for South Africa," (Pretoria: Government of South Africa, 1996), 25.
11. James C. Scott, *Domination and the Arts of Resistance: Hidden Transcripts* (New
Haven, CT: Yale University Press, 1991).
12. Froestad, "Health, Community and Governance," 10.
13. Jan Froestad, "The Incapacitating Impact of Distrust: Observations from the
Health Sector," in *Trust in Public Institutions in South Africa*, ed. Steinar Askvik
and Nelleke Baak (Aldershot, UK: Ashgate Publishing, 2005), 167; citing Piotr
Sztompka, *Trust: A Sociological Theory* (Cambridge, UK: Cambridge University
Press, 1999).
14. Froestad, "Environmental Health Problems," 335.
15. Ibid., 336.
16. Claus Offe, "How Can We Trust Our Fellow Citizens?" in *Democracy and Trust*,
ed. Mark E. Warren (Cambridge, UK: Cambridge University Press, 1999).
17. Froestad, "Environmental Health Problems," 335–36.
18. Offe, "How Can We Trust Our Fellow Citizens?" 48.
19. Ibid., 52.
20. Lucy Gilson, "Trust and the Development of Health Care as a Social Institution,"
Social Science & Medicine 56 (2003): 1453.
21. By self-referential politics, we mean here that kind of discourse, oriented toward
coordinated action and in principle open to all, where citizens may state their
validity claims and have them tested in argument, properly free of the instrumental demands of business or bureaucracy, state or market; see Jürgen Habermas,
The Postnational Constellation: Political Essays (Cambridge, UK: Polity Press,
2001).
22. On "legibility," see chapter 8; also James C. Scott, *Seeing Like a State: How Certain
Schemes to Improve the Human Condition Have Failed* (New Haven, CT; London:
Yale University Press, 1998).
23. John P. Kretzmann and John L. McKnight, *Building Communities from the Inside
Out: A Path toward Finding and Mobilizing a Community's Assets* (Chicago: ACTA
Publications, 1993).
24. Acceptability, by those for whom any intervention is meant, is here crucial to
sustainability.
25. Kretzmann and McKnight, *Building Communities from the Inside Out.* 9.
26. For a particularly relevant discussion in the context of religion and health, see Steve
de Gruchy, "Of Agency, Assets and Appreciation: Seeking Some Commonalities

between Theology and Development," *Journal of Theology for Southern Africa* 117 (2003): 20–39.

27. Scott, *Domination and the Arts of Resistance*.

28. David Bohm, *On Dialogue* (London; New York: Routledge, 1996).

29. de Gruchy, "Of Agency, Assets and Appreciation."

30. Charles Elliot, *Locating the Energy for Change: An Introduction to Appreciative Inquiry* (Winnipeg: International Institute for Sustainable Development, 1999), 43.

31. The tool-set is known as PIRHANA—Participatory Inquiry into Religious Health Assets, Networks and Agency; see www.arhap.uct.ac.za.

32. Lewis Carroll, *Through the Looking Glass and What Alice Found There* (New York: Random House, 1946).

33. Paul Ricoeur, *The Rule of Metaphor: Multi-Disciplinary Studies of the Creation of Meaning in Language*, trans. Robert Czerny, Kathleen McLaughlin, and John Costello (Toronto: University of Toronto Press, 1977).

34. Notable in this regard is the highly popular work by Richard Dawkins, though his analysis shows little of the intellectual attention to counterfactual information one would expect from someone who explicitly appeals to rigorous science; see Richard Dawkins, *The God Delusion* (Boston: Houghton Mifflin, 2006).

35. Ellen L. Idler, "Religious Involvement and the Health of the Elderly: Some Hypotheses and an Initial Test," *Social Forces* 66, no. 1 (1987): 226–38; Ellen L. Idler, "Religion and Aging," in *Handbook of Aging and the Social Sciences*, ed. Robert H. Binstock and Linda K. George (San Diego: Elsevier, 2006).

36. See Cochrane, "Religion in the Health of Migrant Communities," originally presented in 2003.

37. Nancy Krieger, "Proximal, Distal, and the Politics of Causation: What's Level Got to Do with It?" *American Journal of Public Health* 98 (2008): 227, 223. She argues that biomedical interventions generally focus on proximal factors, or "downstream" health interventions, to the exclusion of distal or "upstream" issues. A social determinants approach does the opposite. However, both rest on a reductionist causal logic. "The basic point," she notes, "is that societal patterns of disease represent the biological consequences of the ways of living and working differentially afforded to the social groups produced by each society's economy and political priorities."

38. A potent illustration of this widely recognized dynamic may be found, in the context of how art is produced, in John Berger, *Ways of Seeing* (Harmondsworth, Middlesex, UK: Penguin, 1972).

39. Paul Farmer, for example, has explicitly acknowledged his debt as a clinician to the religious notion of the "preferential option for the poor"; see Paul Farmer, *Pathologies of Power: Health, Human Rights and the New War on the Poor* (Berkeley, CA: University of California Press, 2003).

40. Geoff Foster, "Study of the Response by Faith-Based Organizations to Orphans and Vulnerable Children: Preliminary Summary Report," (Nairobi: World Conference of Religions for Peace; United Nations Children Fund—UNICEF, 2003).

41. See, for example, the important study by Steffen Fleßa, *Gesundheitsreformen in Entwicklungsländern: Eine kritische Analyse aus Sicht der kirchlichen Entwicklungshilfe* (Frankfurt am Main: Verlag Otto Lembeck, 2002).

42. Christoph Benn, "The Influence of Cultural and Religious Frameworks on the Future Course of the HIV/AIDS Pandemic," *Journal of Theology for Southern Africa* 113 (2002): 3–18.

43. Liz Thomas et al., "'Let Us Embrace': Role and Significance of an Integrated Faith-Based Initiative for HIV and Aids: Masangane Case Study" (Cape Town: African Religious Health Assets Programme, University of Cape Town, 2006).

44. African Religious Health Assets Programme, "Appreciating Assets: The Contribution of Religion to Universal Access in Africa" (Cape Town: ARHAP, Report for the World Health Organization, 2006).

45. What one means by compassion and love is a key question, and the researchers involved spent much time exploring that in terms of affective and material dimensions of health. Our interest here is primarily to indicate the importance of perceptions for behavior and action; see, for example, Benn, "The Influence of Cultural and Religious Frameworks"; George Lakoff and with Mark Johnson, *Philosophy in the Flesh: The Embodied Mind and Its Challenge to Western Thought* (New York: Basic Books, 1999); George Lakoff and - Mark Johnson, *Metaphors We Live By*, 2nd ed. (Chicago: University of Chicago Press, 2003 (1980)); Ricoeur, *The Rule of Metaphor*; R. Jones, "Cognitive Frames and Cultural Responses to Aids Education" (paper presented at the 12th International Conference on AIDS, Geneva, 1998).

46. E. Murphy and R. Dingwall, *Qualitative Methods and Health Policy Research* (New York: Aldine de Gruyter, 2003).

47. See also de Gruchy, "Of Agency, Assets and Appreciation."

48. Susan P. Shapiro, "Agency Theory," *Annual Review of Sociology* 31 (2005): 263–84.

49. Ibid., 268.

50. Paul Ricoeur, *Oneself as Another* (Chicago: University of Chicago Press, 1992), 320. Emphasis ours.

51. David Korten, *Getting to the 21st Century: Voluntary Action and the Global Agenda* (West Hartford, CT: Kumarian Press, 1990).

52. Two efforts at assessing assets that make this link explicit are Kelvin Jasek-Rysdahl, "Applying Sen's Capabilities Framework to Neighborhoods: Using Local Asset Maps to Deepen Our Understanding of Well-Being," *Review of Social Economy* LIX, no. 3 (2001): 313–29; Nicol E. Turner and Randal D. Pinkett, "An Asset-Based Approach to Community Building and Community Technology" (paper presented at the Shaping the Network Society: The Future of the Public Sphere in Cyberspace, Directions and Implications of Advanced Computing, Seattle, WA, May 20–23 2000).

53. Martha C. Nussbaum, "Adaptive Preferences and Women's Options," *Economics and Philosophy* 17, no. 5 (2001): 67–88.

54. These capabilities relate to: life, bodily health, bodily integrity, senses, imagination and thought, emotions, practical reason, affiliation (recognition and dignity), other species, play, and control over one's environment (political and material); see Martha C. Nussbaum, "Human Capabilities, Female Human Beings," in *Women, Culture and Development: A Study of Human Capabilities*, ed. Martha C. Nussbaum and Jonathan Glover (Oxford, UK: Clarendon Press, 1995): 61–104; Martha C. Nussbaum, *Women and Human Development: The Capabilities Approach* (Cambridge, UK: Cambridge University Press, 2000).

55. See T. M. Scanlon, "Value, Desire and Quality of Life," in *The Quality of Life*, ed. Martha C. Nussbaum and Amartya Sen (New York: Clarendon Press, 1993), 201–07.

56. Steve de Gruchy et al., "Participatory Inquiry on the Interface between Religion and Health: What Does It Achieve, and What Not?" in *When Religion and Health Align: Mobilizing Religious Health Assets for Transformation*, ed. James R. Cochrane, Barbara Schmid, and Teresa Cutts (Pietermaritzburg: Cluster Publications, 2011), 43–61.

57. Institute of Medicine, "The Future of Public Health," (Washington, DC: National Academy Press, 1988).

58. Barbara L. Norton et al., "Community Capacity: Concept, Theories, and Methods," in *Emerging Theories in Health Promotion Practice and Research: Strategies for Improving Public Health*, ed. Ralph J. DiClemente, Richard A. Crosby, and Michelle C. Kegler (San Francisco: Jossey-Bass [John Wiley & Sons], 2002), 195.

59. Ibid.

60. Felix-Burdine & Associates, "Model of Community Capacity for Health Improvement," (Allentown, PA: Report for the Robert Wood Johnson Foundation, 2000).
61. R. J. Chaskin et al., *Building Community Capacity* (New York: Aldine de Gruyter, 2001). Cited in Norton et al., "Community Capacity: Concept, Theories, and Methods," 204–05.
62. This notion comes from the sustainable livelihoods framework (SLF), though its theorists generally (contrary ARHAP's position), see religion as a negative factor; see de Gruchy, "Of Agency, Assets and Appreciation."
63. Laurence R. Iannaccone and Jonathan Klick, "Spiritual Capital: An Introduction and Literature Review" (Cambridge, MA: Paper Presented in the Spiritual Capital Planning Meeting, 2003).
64. Laurence R. Iannaccone, "Religious Practice: A Human Capital Approach," *Journal for the Scientific Study of Religion* 29, no. 3 (1990): 297–314; Rodney Stark and Roger Finke, *Acts of Faith: Explaining the Human Side of Religion* (Berkeley, CA: University of California Press, 2000).
65. Bradford Verter, "Spiritual Capital: Theorizing Religion with Bourdieu against Bourdieu," *Sociological Theory* 21, no. 2 (2003): 152.
66. Peter L. Berger and Robert W. Hefner, "Spiritual Capital in Comparative Perspective," Institute for the Study of Economic Culture, http://www.spiritualcapitalresearch-program.com/pdf/Berger.pdf, accessed June 6, 2011.
67. Robert D. Woodberry, "Researching Spiritual Capital: Promises and Pitfalls," Spiritual Capital Planning Meeting, http://www.spiritualcapitalresearchprogram.com/pdf/woodberry.pdf, accessed February 10, 2010.
68. Ibid.
69. Viktor E. Frankl, *Man's Search for Meaning*, Revised & Updated ed. (New York: Washington Square Press, 1997 [1946]).
70. Krieger, "Proximal, Distal, and the Politics of Causation," 221.
71. Ronald S. Burt, "Social Holes Versus Network Closure as Social Capital," in *Social Capital: Theory and Research*, ed. Nan Lin, Karen Cook, and Ronald S. Burt, Sociology and Economics: Controversy and Integration (New York: Aldine de Gruyter, 2001).
72. Linking capital is an extension of the idea of bridging capital, defined as "norms of respect and networks of trusting relationships between people who are interacting across explicit, formal or institutionalized power or authority gradients in society"; see Simon Szreter and Michael Woolcock, "Health by Association? Social Capital, Social Theory, and the Political Economy of Public Health," *International Journal of Epidemiology* 33 (2004): 655.
73. For a fuller and nicely nuanced discussion, see Sarah Ferlander, "The Importance of Different Forms of Social Capital for Health," *Acta Sociologica* 50, no. 2 (2007): 115–28.
74. Thomas et al., "Let Us Embrace."
75. George Davey Smith and John Lynch, "Commentary: Social Capital, Social Epidemiology and Disease Aetiology," *International Journal of Epidemiology* 33 (2004): 691–700.
76. Simon Szreter and Michael Woolcock, "Rejoinder: Crafting Rigorous and Relevant Social Theory for Public Health Policy," *International Journal of Epidemiology* 33 (2004): 700–04. Preceding the emergence of social capital theory in the society-and-health movement, some theorists spoke of "relational position" as an important social determinant of health; see S. M. Miller, "Thinking Strategically About Society and Health," in *Society and Health*, ed. Benjamin C. Amick III, et al. (New York & Oxford: Oxford University Press, 1995), 342–58.

77. For a profound study of such intermediary organizations, see Thomas F. Carroll, *Intermediary NGOs: The Supporting Link in Grassroots Development*, Library of Management for Development (West Hartford, CT: Kumarian Press, 1992).
78. See chapter 8, "Boundary Leadership."
79. Nancy Tatom Ammerman, with et al., *Congregation and Community* (New Brunswick, NJ: Rutgers University Press, 1997), 349.
80. The dangers of exclusion—a potential threat to the well-being of others—are well expressed by Jacques Derrida, "Faith and Knowledge: The Two Sources of 'Religion' at the Limits of Reason Alone," in *Religion*, ed. Jacques Derrida and Gianni Vattimo, Cultural Memory in the Present (Cambridge, UK: Polity Press, 1998), 1–78.
81. For a philosophical grounding to this distinction, particularly in the idea of a three-fold difference in *mimesis* between a prefigured, a configured, and a reconfigured narrative construction of world, see Paul Ricoeur, *Time and Narrative, Volume 3*, trans. Kathleen McLaughlin and David Pellauer (Chicago: University of Chicago Press, 1988).
82. See Murphy and Dingwall, *Qualitative Methods*.
83. Following Immanuel Kant, we are committed to a view of reason (or *Vernunft*, the German word carrying the nuance of "the sense of things") in which the orders of reality are ultimately comprehensive and unified, even if our representations of that reality cannot be other than partial and limited.
84. Scott, *Seeing Like a State*. Scott's study begins with the application of state rationality to the science of forestry in Germany, and shows how ambiguous its results were, yielding some value but unwittingly losing other value.

4   LEADING CAUSES OF LIFE: PATHOLOGY IN ITS PLACE

1. Marshall Kreuter et al., "Understanding Wicked Problems: A Key to Advancing Environmental Health Promotion," *Health Education & Behavior* 31, no. 4 (2004): 441–54.
2. Jonas Salk, *The Survival of the Wisest* (New York: Harper & Row, 1973).
3. See Heather Wood Ion, "Creating an Epidemic of Health" (Presentation, the Epidemic of Health Meeting, Center of Excellence in Faith and Health, Methodist Le Bonheur Healthcare, Memphis, TN, 2011); also, Bill Moyers, *A World of Ideas II* (New York: Doubleday, 1990), 238–39.
4. Thomas L. Friedman, "Global Weirding Is Here," *New York Times*, February 17, 2010.
5. Nov. 5, 2003.
6. The term is derived from the Latin *salus* (health) and the Greek *genesis* (origin), and describes an approach focusing on factors that support human health and well-being, rather than on factors that cause disease.
7. Aaron Antonovsky, *Unraveling the Mystery of Health: How People Manage Stress and Stay Well* (San Francisco: Jossey-Bass Publishers, 1987), preface xi.
8. Aaron Antonovsky, *Health, Stress and Coping* (San Francisco: Jossey-Bass Publishers, 1979), 123.
9. Antonovsky, *Unraveling the Mystery of Health*. 19.
10. Monica Eriksson and Bengt Lindström, "Validity of Antonovsky's Sense of Coherence Scale: A Systematic Review," *Journal of Epidemiology and Community Health* 59 (2005): 460.
11. See chapter 2.

12. Thomas A. Droege, "Congregations as Communities of Health and Healing," *Interpretation* 69, no. 2 (1995): 117–29.
13. Personal communication with author Gunderson, Lake Burton, fall of 1992.
14. Author's (Gunderson) personal records; see also William H. Foege, Robert W. Amler, and C. C. White. "Closing the Gap. Report of the Carter Center Health Policy Consultation," *Journal of the American Medical Association* 13, no. 254 (10) (1985): 1355–58.
15. Ibid.
16. Antonovsky, *Unraveling the Mystery of Health.* 12–14.
17. Monica Eriksson and Bengt Lindström, "A Salutogenic Interpretation of the Ottawa Charter," *Health Promotion International* 23, no. 2 (2008): 198.
18. Bengt Lindström and Monica Eriksson, "Contextualizing Salutogenesis and Antonovsky in Public Health Development," *Health Promotion International* 21, no. 3 (2006): 239.
19. Such language of life allows one to take into account other epistemologies of health, as seen in such ideas as *seriti* (energy, Sesotho) in relation to *bophelo* (comprehensive well-being), or *Qi* (energy, Chinese) in relation to *yangsheng* (life); see, for example, Judith Farquhar and Zhang Qicheng, *Ten Thousand Things: Nurturing Life in Contemporary Beijing* (New York: Zone Books, 2012); Judith Farquhar and Zhang Qicheng, "Biopolitical Beijing: Pleasure, Sovereignty, and Self-Cultivation in China's Capital," *Cultural Anthropology* 20, no. 3 (2005): 303–27; Giorgio Agamben, *Homo Sacer: Sovereign Power and Bare Life* (Stanford, CA: Stanford University Press, 1998).
20. Gary R. Gunderson and Larry Pray, *Leading Causes of Life* (Memphis, TN: The Center of Excellence in Faith and Health, Methodist Le Bonheur Healthcare, 2006).
21. Corey L. M. Keyes, "Complete Mental Health: An Agenda for the 21st Century," in *Flourishing: Positive Psychology and the Life Well-Lived*, ed. Corey L. M. Keyes and Jonathan Haidt (Washington DC: American Psychological Association, 2003): 293–312; Martin E. P. Seligman, *Learned Optimism: How to Change Your Mind and Your Life* (New York: Knopf; Penguin Books, 1991, 1998); Martin E. P. Seligman, *Flourish: A Visionary New Understanding of Happiness and Well-Being* (New York: Free Press, 2011).
22. Corey L. M. Keyes, "The Mental Health Continuum: From Languishing to Flourishing in Life," *Journal of Health and Social Behavior* 43 (2002): 207–22.
23. The original adaptation was done by Gunderson.
24. Kenneth I. Pargament, *The Psychology of Religion and Coping: Theory, Research, Practice* (New York: The Guilford Press, 2001).
25. Such as the Stop Asthma program in Atlanta, Georgia, which approaches the lives of its participants as a whole in understanding and responding to their condition; personal communication, Joyce Essien, MD, February 22, 2010.
26. Antonovsky, *Unraveling the Mystery of Health.* 164.
27. Ibid., 165.
28. Ibid., 170.
29. Ibid.
30. Tom Munnecke, "Ensembles and Transformations," (San Diego, CA: Report for the Science Applications International Corporation, 2000).
31. Precisely this view of causation grounds Einsteinian science against Newtonian physics, even if it remains hard to grasp for the lay person who experiences both space and time as substantial, whereas they are representational constructions of the human mind, as the theory of relativity insists. Heisenberg's principle of indeterminacy, and quantum mechanics in general, further erode any idea that we can grasp as essences or substances in themselves.

32. One could name the causes of life differently, but this would change little if, as we argue, the phenomena we claim as causal are relatively adequately grasped in our model.

33. Viktor E. Frankl, *The Doctor and the Soul, from Psychotherapy to Logotherapy*, trans. Richard Winston and Clara Winston (New York: Bantam, 1971).

34. Viktor E. Frankl, *Man's Search for Meaning*, revised & updated ed. (New York: Washington Square Press, 1997 [1946]), Harold Kushner, foreword, ix.

35. Gordon Allport, "Preface," in ibid., 11.

36. James Pennebaker, *Opening Up: The Healing Power of Expressing Emotions* (New York: Guilford Press, 1997).

37. Stewart Wolf and John S. Bruhn, *The Power of Clan: The Influence of Human Relationships to Reduce Heart Disease* (New Brunswick, NJ: Transaction, 1993).

38. Paul Germond and Sepetla Molapo, "In Search of *Bophelo* in a Time of AIDS: Seeking a Coherence of Economies of Health and Economies of Salvation," *Journal of Theology for Southern Africa* 126 (2006): 27–47; see also Paul Germond and James R. Cochrane, "Healthworlds: Conceptualizing Landscapes of Health and Healing," *Sociology* 44, no. 2 (2010): 307–24.

39. Frans de Waal, *The Age of Empathy: Nature's Lessons for a Kinder Society* (New York: Harmony Books, 2009).

40. E. Eger et al., "Familiarity Enhances Invariance of Face Representations in Human Ventral Visual Cortex: Fmri Evidence," *Neuroimage* 26, no. 4 (2005): 1128–39.

41. Gregory L. Fricchionne, "Separation, Attachment and Altruistic Love: The Evolutionary Basis for Medical Caring," in *Altruism and Altruistic Love*, ed. Stephen G. Post and Lynn G. Underwood. (Oxford, UK: Oxford University Press, 2002), 346–61.

42. Pierre Bourdieu, *The Logic of Practice* (Cambridge, UK: Polity Press, 1990); James S. Coleman, *Foundations of Social Theory* (Cambridge, MA: Harvard University Press, 1990); Nan Lin, Karen Cook, and Ronald S. Burt, *Social Capital: Theory and Research* (New York: Aldine de Gruyter, 2001); Corwin Smidt, ed. *Religion as Social Capital: Producing the Common Good* (Waco, TX: Baylor University Press, 2003).

43. Sarah Ferlander, "The Importance of Different Forms of Social Capital for Health," *Acta Sociologica* 50, no. 2 (2007): 115–28; Jonathan Lomas, "Social Capital and Health: Implications for Public Health and Epidemiology," *Social Science and Medicine* 47, no. 9 (1998): 1181–88; Catherine Scott and Anne Hofmeyer, "Networks and Social Capital: A Relational Approach to Primary Healthcare Reform," *Health Research Policy and Systems* 5, no. 9 (2007): 1–27; Marshall W. Kreuter, Nicole A. Lezin, Laura Young, and Adam N. Koplan, "Social Capital: Evaluation Implications for Community Health Promotion," in *Evaluation in Health Promotion: Principles and Perspectives*, ed. Irving Rootman, Michael Goodstadt, Brian Hyndman, David V. McQueen, Louise Potvin, Jane Springett, and Ziglio Erio (Copenhagen: World Health Organization Regional Publications, European Series, No. 92, 2001), 439–62.

44. Zygmunt Bauman, *Globalization: The Human Consequences* (Cambridge, UK: Polity Press, 1998).

45. See chapter 3.

46. Albert Bandura, "Self Efficacy Mechanism in Human Agency," *American Psychologist* 37, no. 2 (1982): 122–47.

47. John L. McKnight, *The Careless Society: Community and Its Counterfeits* (New York: Basic Books, 1996).

48. Geoff Foster, "Study of the Response by Faith-Based Organizations to Orphans and Vulnerable Children: Preliminary Summary Report," (Nairobi: World Conference of Religions for Peace; United Nations Children Fund—UNICEF, 2003).

49. Gabriel Marcel, *Homo Viator: Introduction to a Metaphysics of Hope*, trans. Martha Crauford (New York: Harper and Row (imprint: Harper Torchbooks/Cathedral Library), 1962).

50. He was also the major influence in Jürgen Moltmann's famous theological formulations of hope; see Jürgen Moltmann, *Theology of Hope: On the Ground and the Implications of a Christian Eschatology* (New York: Harper and Row, 1967).

51. Ernst Bloch, *The Principle of Hope*, trans. Neville Plaice, Stephen Plaice, and Paul Knight, Vol. 2 (Cambridge, MA: MIT Press, 1986).

52. Ernst Bloch, *The Utopian Function of Art and Literature: Selected Essays*, trans. Jack Zipes and Frank Mecklenburg, Studies in Contemporary German Social Thought (Cambridge, MA: MIT Press, 1988).

53. Barbara Adam, "Memory of Futures," (2004), http://www.cardiff.ac.uk/socsi /futures/memoryofthefuture.pdf, accessed October 28, 2010.

54. Bloch, *The Principle of Hope*, Vol. 1. 7.

55. Daniel L. Schacter, Donna Rose Addis, and Randy L. Buckner, "Remembering the Past to Imagine the Future: The Prospective Brain," *Nature Reviews Neuroscience* 8 (2007): 657.

56. David H. Ingvar, "Memory of the Future: An Essay on the Temporal Organization of Conscious Awareness," *Human Neurobiology* 4, no. 3 (1985): 127–36; see also David H. Ingvar, "Motor Memory—A Memory of the Future," *Behavioral and Brain Sciences* 17 (1994): 210–11.

57. Barbara Adam, "Futurity from a Complexity Perspective," (2005), http://www .cardiff.ac.uk/socsi/futures/Web%20Complexity%20Futures.pdf, accessed October 28, 2010.

58. Katherine Marshall, "A Discussion with Reverend Canon Ted Karpf," Berkley Center for Religion, Peace and World Affairs, Georgetown University, Washington DC. Interview Conducted on November 13, 2010, http://berkleycenter.george-town.edu/interviews/a-discussion-with-reverend-canon-ted-karpf, accessed July 27, 2011.

59. David Harvey, *Spaces of Hope* (Berkeley, CA: University of California Press, 2000), 218.

60. See also chapter 8.

61. See, inter alia, Erik H. Erikson, *Childhood and Society*, 2nd ed. (New York: W. W. Norton & Company, 1963 [1950]); Jean Piaget, *Play, Dreams and Imitation in Childhood* (New York: Norton, 1962); Catherine Garvey, *Play* (Cambridge, MA: Harvard University Press, 1977); Lev Vygotsky, *Mind in Society*, trans. M. Cole (Cambridge, MA: Harvard University Press, 1978).

62. PN1 is a tool for researching psychoneuroimmunology, the interaction between nervous and immune system processes and how they are impacted by thoughts and emotions, a field that offers a potent body of research to be explored in terms of the effects of blessing or intergenerativity; see Michael Irwin and Kavita Vedhara, *Human Psychoneuroimmunology* (New York: Oxford University Press, 2005).

63. See, for example, Norman O. Brown, *Life against Death: The Psychoanalytical Meaning of History* (Middletown, CT: Wesleyan University Press, 1959); Robert Jay Lifton, *The Broken Connection: On Death and the Continuity of Life* (Washington: American Psychiatric Press, 1979). Also, A. R. Denham, "Rethinking Historical Trauma: Narratives of Resilience," *Transcultural Psychiatry* 45, no. 3 (2008): 391–414; M. S Micale and P. Lerner, *Traumatic Pasts: History, Psychiatry, and Trauma in the Modern Age, 1870–1930* (Cambridge, UK: Cambridge University Press, 2001); D. S. Schechter, "Intergenerational Communication of Violent Traumatic Experience within and by the Dyad: The Case of a Mother and Her Toddler," *Journal of Infant, Child, and Adolescent Psychotherapy* 3, no. 2 (2004): 203–32; Michelle Sotero, "A Conceptual Model of Historical Trauma: Implications for Public Health Practice

and Research," *Journal of Health Disparities Research and Practice*, 1, no. 1 (2006): 93–108; Cynthia C. Wesley-Esquimaux and Magdalena Smolewski, "Historic Trauma and Aboriginal Healing," (Ottawa, Ontario: Report for The Aboriginal Healing Foundation, 2004).

64. See ARHAP, "CHAMP/PC: Community Health Assets Mapping for Partnerships in Palliative Care—Facilitator's Guide," (Cape Town: ARHAP University of Cape Town, October 2009).

65. David Bohm, *Wholeness and the Implicate Order*, Routledge Classics (London ; New York: Routledge, 2002).

66. David Bohm, *On Dialogue* (London; New York: Routledge, 1996), 98–99.

67. Kenneth Wailoo, *Dying in the City of the Blues: Sickle Cell Anemia and the Politics of Race* (Chapel Hill, NC: University of North Carolina Press, 2001).

68. Bohm, *Wholeness and the Implicate Order*. 198.

69. Ibid., 194.

70. Ibid., 203.

5   Seeking Health: Persons, Bodies, and Choices

1. John L. McKnight, *The Careless Society: Community and Its Counterfeits* (New York: Basic Books, 1996), 10.

2. Not his real name.

3. James C. Scott, *Domination and the Arts of Resistance: Hidden Transcripts* (New Haven, CT: Yale University Press, 1991).

4. This true story comes from our close colleague in Memphis, Dr. Teresa Cutts. Names have been changed, but the story is not unusual.

5. Treating power/knowledge together, as designated by the copula, comes of course from Michel Foucault, *Power/Knowledge: Selected Writings and Other Interviews 1972–1977*, trans. Colin Gordon et al. (New York: Pantheon, 1980).

6. Institute of Medicine, *Crossing the Quality Chasm: A New Health System for the 21st Century*, Committee on Quality of Health Care in America (Washington, DC: National Academy Press, 2001).

7. Yvonne Denier, "Public Health, Well-Being and Reciprocity," *Ethical Perspectives: Journal of the European Ethics Network* 11, no. 1 (2005): 41–66.

8. Ted Karpf et al., eds., *Restoring Hope: Decent Care in the Midst of HIV/Aids* (London: Palgrave Macmillan, 2008).

9. World Health Organization, "A Cross-Cultural Study of Spirituality, Religion, and Personal Beliefs as Components of Quality of Life," *Social Science and Medicine* 62 (2006): 1486–97.

10. Institute of Medicine, *Crossing the Quality Chasm*. 4, 6.

11. It is not history in any deep sense of the term, and is more accurately seen only as an attempt to sketch an etiology, to try to discern a causal pattern, an instrumental and thus highly limited sense of "history."

12. The IOM proposes that health care should also be safe, effective, timely, efficient, and equitable; see Institute of Medicine, *Crossing the Quality Chasm*, Executive Summary. 5–6.

13. Denier, "Public Health, Well-Being and Reciprocity," 52.

14. H. Malm et al., "Ethics, Pandemics, and the Duty to Treat," *American Journal of Bioethics* 8, no. 8 (2008): 4–19.

15. See chapter 6.

16. Paul Ricoeur, *Oneself as Another* (Chicago: University of Chicago Press, 1992).

17. J. Todd Ferguson, "Introduction—Decent Care: A Proposal for the Future of HIV Care and Support," in Karpf et al., eds., *Restoring Hope*. xxv.
18. See Shoshanna Sofaer, "A Patient-centered Approach to Universal Decent Care," in ibid., 111–18.
19. Ibid., ix.
20. J. Todd Ferguson et al., "Decent Care: Living Values, Health Justice and Human Flourishing," WHO/Ford Foundation, http://www.wfmh.org/09DOCS /Decent%20Care%20Monograph%20for%20Ford%20Foundationr%20Final%20 24-8-09.pdf, accessed April 22, 2010.
21. George Lakoff and Mark Johnson, *Metaphors We Live By* (Chicago: University of Chicago Press, 2003).
22. Richard K. Thomas, *Society and Health: Sociology for Health Professionals* (New York: Kluwer Academic/Plenum Publishers, 2003), 213–45.
23. C. Leslie, "Medical Pluralism in World Perspective," *Social Science and Medicine* 14B, no. 4 (1980): 191–95.
24. Lucy Gilson, "Trust and the Development of Health Care as a Social Institution," *Social Science & Medicine* 56 (2003): 1453–68; Lucy Gilson, "Editorial: Building Trust and Value in Health Systems in Low- and Middle-Income Countries," *Social Science & Medicine* 61 (2005): 1381–84.
25. See Susanna Hausmann-Muela, Joan Muela Ribera, and Isaac Nyamongo, "Health-Seeking Behaviour and the Health System Response," *Disease Control Priorities Project* DCPP Working Paper No. 14 (Aug. 2003). The DCPP, "an ongoing effort to assess disease control priorities and produce evidence-based analysis and resource materials to inform health policymaking in developing countries," is a joint project of the Fogarty International Center of the National Institutes of Health, the World Health Organization, and The World Bank, funded by the Bill & Melinda Gates Foundation. (See http://www.dcp2.org/main/Home.html).
26. Ibid., 4.
27. Ibid., 5.
28. Citing A. Kleinman, "Concepts and a Model for the Comparison of Medical Systems as Cultural Systems," in *Concepts of Health, Illness and Disease*, ed. C. Currer and M. Stacey (New York: Berg Pub. Ltd, 1986), 27–50. See Hausmann-Muela, Ribera, and Nyamongo, "Health-Seeking Behaviour and the Health System Response," 6.
29. Hausmann-Muela, Ribera, and Nyamongo, "Health-Seeking Behaviour and the Health System Response," 9–18.
30. Ibid., 18.
31. Ibid., 30.
32. Jim Yong Kim, "Beyond Paradigm: Making Transcultural Connections in a Scientific Translation of Acupuncture," *Social Science & Medicine* 62 (2006): 2969–72. See also Joyce B. Flueckiger, *In Amma's Healing Room: Gender and Vernacular Islam in South India*. (Bloomington, IN: Indiana University Press, 2006).
33. A. Pickering, *The Mangle of Practice* (Chicago: University of Chicago Press, 1995).
34. Marie S. O'Neill et al., "Poverty, Environment, and Health the Role of Environmental Epidemiology and Environmental Epidemiologists," *Epidemiology* 18, no. 6 (2007): 664–68; CSDH, "Closing the Gap in a Generation: Health Equity through Action on the Social Determinants of Health," (Geneva: World Health Organization, Commission on Social Determinants of Health, 2008).
35. Paul Germond and James R. Cochrane, "Healthworlds: Conceptualizing Landscapes of Health and Healing," *Sociology* 44, no. 2 (2010): 307–24.
36. Ibid., 3.
37. See, for example, J. Csordas, "Ritual Healing and the Politics of Identity in Contemporary Navajo Society," *American Ethnologist* 26, no. 1 (1999): 3–23; John

M. Janzen, *Ngoma: Discourses of Healing in Central and Southern Africa* (Berkeley: University of California Press, 1992); T. Shoko, *Karanga Indigenous Religion in Zimbabwe: Health and Well-Being* (London: Ashgate, 2007); Paul U. Unschuld, "Traditional Chinese Medicine: Some Historical and Epistemological Reflections," *Social Science & Medicine* 24 (1987): 1023–29.

38. Jürgen Habermas, *Lifeworld and System: A Critique of Functionalist Reason*, trans. Thomas McCarthy, Vol. 2, The Theory of Communicative Action (Boston: Beacon Press, 1987).

39. See, for example, Christine A. Barry et al., "Giving Voice to the Lifeworld: More Humane, More Effective Medical Care? A Qualitative Study of Doctor-Patient Communication in General Practice," *Social Science & Medicine* 53 (2001): 487–505; Graham Scambler, ed. *Habermas, Critical Theory and Health* (London; New York: Routledge, 2001).

40. For a pertinent and profound articulation of these themes via psychoanalytic theory, see Ellie Ragland-Sullivan, *Jacques Lacan and the Philosophy of Psychoanalysis* (Urbana, IL; Chicago: University of Illinois Press, 1986).

41. Habermas, *Lifeworld and System: A Critique of Functionalist Reason*, 124.

42. Ibid., 140–48.

43. Ricoeur, *Oneself as Another*.

44. Ricoeur's philosophical ethics, built on his analysis of "oneself as another," is thus summarized by him as "living well together in just institutions"; cf. Ibid. The third, and last, irreducible realm to which Germond and Cochrane point, rooted in the tension between act and potentiality, is freedom, by which humans are capable of transcending their existing condition ("actuality") and creating another ("*homo faber*"—the creature that can make things), embodying through imagination and work a new possibility that did not exist before.

45. Candice Pert, *Molecules of Emotion* (New York: Touchstone, 1997), 141.

46. Michel Foucault, *Madness and Civilization: A History of Insanity in the Age of Reason*, trans. Richard Howard (New York: New York American Library (imprint: Mentor), 1967); Michel Foucault, *The Birth of the Clinic: An Archaeology of Medical Perception*, trans. A. M. Smith (New York: Random House (imprint: Vintage), 1975); Michel Foucault, *Discipline and Punishment: The Birth of the Prison*, trans. Alan Sheridan (New York: Random House (imprint: Vintage), 1979).

47. Foucault, *Power/Knowledge: Selected Writings*.

48. Graham Scambler, *Health and Social Change: A Critical Theory*, ed. Tim May, Issues in Society (Buckingham, UK; Philadelphia, PA: The Open University Press, 2002).

49. Paul Farmer, *Pathologies of Power: Health, Human Rights and the New War on the Poor* (Berkeley, CA: University of California Press, 2003); Jim Yong Kim et al., eds., *Dying for Growth: Global Inequality and the Health of the Poor* (Monroe, ME: Common Courage Press,2000).

50. As one example, see Kathryn M. Yount and Joel Gittelsohn, "Comparing Reports of Health-Seeking Behavior from the Integrated Illness History and a Standard Child Morbidity Survey," *Journal of Mixed Methods Research* 2, no. 1 (2008): 23–62.

6 PEOPLE WHO CONGREGATE: BUILDING ON STRENGTHS

1. Richard Dawkins, *The God Delusion* (Boston: Houghton Mifflin, 2006), 158ff; Christopher Hitchens, *God Is Not Great: How Religion Poisons Everything* (New York: Twelve/Warner Books, 2007).

2. William H. Foege, "Engaging Faith Communities as Partners in Improving Community Health," in *CDC/ATSDR Forum: Separation of Church and State, the Science Supporting Work with Faith Communities, and Exemplary Partnerships* (Atlanta, GA: US Department of Health & Human Services, Centers for Disease Control and Prevention, 1999), 4. See also William H. Foege, Robert W. Amler, and C. C. White, "Closing the Gap. Report of the Carter Center Health Policy Consultation," *Journal of the American Medical Association* 13, no. 254 (10) (1985): 1355–58.

3. James C. Scott, *Seeing Like a State: How Certain Schemes to Improve the Human Condition Have Failed* (New Haven, CT; London: Yale University Press, 1998).

4. H. Richard Niebuhr, *The Social Sources of Denominationalism* (Cleveland, OH: World Publishing, 1965).

5. James P. Wind and James W. Lewis, *American Congregations Volume 1: Portraits of Twelve Religious Communities* (Chicago: University of Chicago Press, 1998); James P. Wind and James W. Lewis, *American Congregations Volume 2: New Perspectives in the Study of Congregations* (Chicago: The University of Chicago Press, 1998).

6. Nancy Tatom Ammerman, *Pillars of Faith: American Congregations and Their Partners* (Berkeley, CA; Los Angeles: University of California Press, 2005); Nancy Tatom Ammerman et al., *Studying Congregations: A New Handbook* (Nashville, TN: Abingdon, 1998).

7. Scott Thumma and Warren Bird, "Not Who You Think They Are: The Real Story of People Who Attend America's Megachurches," (Hartford, CN: Hartford Institute for Religion Research & The Leadership Network, 2009).

8. Ram A. Cnaan and Stephanie C. Boddie, *The Invisible Caring Hand: American Congregations and the Provision of Welfare* (New York; London: New York University Press, 2002). See also Richard G. Bennett and W. Daniel Hale, *Building Healthy Communities through Medical-Religious Partnerships*, 2nd ed. (Baltimore, MD: Johns Hopkins University Press, 2009).

9. Gary R. Gunderson, *Deeply Woven Roots: Improving the Quality of Life in Your Community* (Minneapolis, MN: Fortress Press, 1997), 1.

10. Ibid., 15.

11. Zygmunt Bauman, *Liquid Modernity* (Cambridge, UK: Polity Press, 2000); Zygmunt Bauman, *Liquid Times: Living in an Age of Uncertainty* (Cambridge, UK: Polity Press, 2006).

12. Gunderson, *Deeply Woven Roots*. 24ff.

13. Nancy Tatom Ammerman, with et al., *Congregation and Community* (New Brunswick, NJ: Rutgers University Press, 1997), 354.

14. James R. Cochrane, "Sacred Crossings: Movement, Migration and the Fate of the Religious Body," in *Broken Bodies and Healing Communities: The Challenge of HIV and Aids in the South African Context*, ed. Neville Richardson (Pietermaritzburg: Cluster Publications, 2009), 72–85; Peggy Levitt, "Redefining the Boundaries of Belonging: The Institutional Character of Transnational Religious Life," *Sociology of Religion* 65, no. 1 (2004): 1–18.

15. Manuel A. Vásquez and Marie F. Marquardt, *Globalizing the Sacred: Religion across the Americas* (New Brunswick, NJ: Rutgers University Press, 2003), 149.

16. Ibid., 150.

17. John L. McKnight, *The Careless Society: Community and Its Counterfeits* (New York: Basic Books, 1996), 10ff.

18. Cnaan and Boddie, *The Invisible Caring Hand*. 80.

19. Christian Führer, *Und wir sind dabei gewesen: die Revolution, die aus der Kirche kam* (Berlin: Ullstein Buchverlage, 2009).

20. Cnaan and Boddie, *The Invisible Caring Hand*. 81.

21. Gunderson, *Deeply Woven Roots*. 39.

22. See Nan Lin, Karen Cook, and Ronald S. Burt, *Social Capital: Theory and Research* (New York: Aldine de Gruyter, 2001).
23. Gunderson, *Deeply Woven Roots*. 53.
24. Ammerman, *Pillars of Faith*. 158.
25. Ibid., 158ff.
26. Vásquez and Marquardt, *Globalizing the Sacred*. 63.
27. Ammerman, *Pillars of Faith*. 158.
28. Ibid., 160.
29. Ibid., 172.
30. Ibid., 176.
31. Community mosque.
32. Cnaan and Boddie, *The Invisible Caring Hand*. 166ff.
33. Ibid., 177.
34. Gunderson, *Deeply Woven Roots*. 68.
35. Paul Ricoeur, *Time and Narrative, Volume 1*, trans. Kathleen McLaughlin and David Pellauer (Chicago: University of Chicago Press, 1984). See especially chapters 4 ("Eclipse of the Narrative"), 5 ("Defenses of Narrative"), and 6 ("Historical Intentionality").
36. Ammerman, *Pillars of Faith*. 268–69 passim.
37. Ted Karpf, "The Vital Lie," in *The Gospel Imperative in the Midst of Aids*, ed. Robert H. Iles (Wilton, CT: Morehouse Publications, 1989).
38. Ibid., 186–87.
39. Rosalyn Carter, "Reweaving the Fabric of Care: Mind, Body, Spirit and Community," in *Faith & Health* (Atlanta, GA: Interfaith Health Program, 1999), 2.
40. Wendell Berry, *What Are People For?* (New York: North Point Press, 1990), 78.
41. Ammerman et al., *Congregation and Community*. 145ff.
42. Gunderson, *Deeply Woven Roots*. 86.
43. James R. Cochrane, *Circles of Dignity: Community Wisdom and Theological Reflection* (Minneapolis, MN: Fortress Press, 1999).
44. Ben Sherwood, *The Survivors Club: The Secrets and Science That Could Save Your Life* (New York: Grand Central Publishing, 2009), 144ff.
45. Gunderson, *Deeply Woven Roots*. 95.
46. See chapter 5 on "Seeking Health."
47. Story by Dr. Teresa Cutts.
48. Liz Thomas et al., "'Let Us Embrace': Role and Significance of an Integrated Faith-Based Initiative for HIV and Aids: Masangane Case Study," (Cape Town: African Religious Health Assets Programme, University of Cape Town, 2006).
49. Sherwood, *The Survivors Club*. 140.
50. Gunderson, *Deeply Woven Roots*. 95.
51. Ammerman, *Pillars of Faith*. 23.
52. Ibid., 25.
53. Vásquez and Marquardt, *Globalizing the Sacred*. 1.
54. Ibid.
55. Amy Greene, "The Spiritual Dimension," in *Faith and Health* (Atlanta, GA: Interfaith Health Program, The Carter Center, 1994), 6.
56. Manuel Castells, *The Rise of the Network Society* (Oxford, UK: Blackwell Publishers, 1996); David Harvey, "Time-Space Compression and the Rise of Modernism as a Cultural Force," in *The Globalization Reader*, ed. Frank Lechner and John Boli (Oxford, UK: Blackwell Publishers, 2000), 134–40.
57. Vásquez and Marquardt, *Globalizing the Sacred*. 225.
58. See, for example, Peggy Levitt, "'You Know, Abraham Was Really the First Immigrant': Religion and Transnational Migration," *International Migration Review* 37, no. 3 (2003): 847–73; Levitt, "Redefining the Boundaries of Belonging," 1–18.

59. Ammerman et al., *Congregation and Community*. 346ff.
60. Stephen F. Jencks, Mark V. Williams, and Eric Coleman, "Rehospitalizations among Patients in the Medicare Fee-for-Service Program," *New England Journal of Medicine* 360 (2009): 1418–28.
61. Dave Hilton, "Calling for the Church to Bring Whole Person Health to All" (presentation, "Faith and Health: Making the Connection," Annual Spring Conference, Church Health Center and Methodist Le Bonheur Healthcare, Memphis, TN, 2006).
62. Teresa Cutts and Gary Gunderson, "The Memphis Model: Finding Life in a Tough Town," Conference Paper at the Grand Rounds (Memphis, TN: University of Memphis School of Public Health, 2009).

7   Boundary Leadership: Embodying Complexity in Turbulence

1. For a more detailed picture, see James R. Cochrane, "Agapé: The Cape Office of the Christian Institute," *Journal of Theology for Southern Africa* 118 (2004): 53–68. See also Peter Walshe, *Church Versus State in South Africa: The Case of the Christian Institute* (London; Maryknoll, NY: C. Hurst; Orbis, 1983).
2. See chapter 3.
3. James C. Scott, *Seeing Like a State: How Certain Schemes to Improve the Human Condition Have Failed* (New Haven, CT; London: Yale University Press, 1998).
4. Discussed in chapter one, ibid.
5. Wendell Berry, *Sex, Economy, Freedom & Community* (New York; San Francisco: Pantheon, 1992), 4ff.
6. Wendell Berry, *Home Economics: Fourteen Essays* (San Francisco: North Point Press, 1987), 79. See also Wendell Berry, *Life Is a Miracle* (Washington, DC: Counterpoint, 2000), 48–50.
7. David Bohm and Lee Nichol, *On Dialogue* (London; New York: Routledge, 2004), 95.
8. Ibid., 96–97.
9. No one has made this clearer than Immanuel Kant has, through his various critiques of pure and practical reason, judgment, and religion.
10. Site visit, research conducted as part of the World Council of Churches International Consultation on Mental Health and Faith Communities, Tirupattur, India, Helping Hearts ministry, December 2, 2007. See also http://udavumullangal.org/.
11. See Hattie Elie Jackson, *65 Dark Days in '68: Reflections: Memphis Sanitation Strike* (Southaven, MS: The King's Press, 2004).
12. Tracy E. K'Meyer, *Interracialism and Christian Community in the Postwar South: The Story of Koinonia Farm* (Charlottesville, VA: University Press of Virginia, 1997); Dallas Lee, *The Cotton Patch Evidence: The Story of Clarence Jordan and the Koinonia Farm Experiment* (New York: Harper and Row, 1971).
13. IHP, "The Case for Health and Faith: An Open Letter," in *Faith & Health* (Atlanta, GA: Interfaith Health Program, Rollins School of Public Health, Emory University, 2001).
14. Ibid.
15. Gary R. Gunderson, *Boundary Leaders: Leadership Skills for People of Faith* (Minneapolis, MN: Fortress, 2004).
16. Miriam Kiser, Deborah L. Jones, and Gary R. Gunderson, "Faith and Health: Leadership Aligning Assets to Transform Communities," *International Review of Mission* 95 no. 376/377 (2006): 50–58.

17. See for example, The Church of Scotland, "Church Without Walls," http://www
.churchofscotland.org.uk/connect/church_without_walls, accessed October 23,
2011; and Jim Petersen, *Church without Walls: Moving Beyond Traditional Boundaries*
(Colorado Springs, CO: Nav Press, 1992).
18. Personal history, James R Cochrane.
19. See Kate Wright et al., "Competency Development in Public Health Leadership,"
American Journal of Public Health 90, no. 8 (2000): 1202–07.
20. Ibid.
21. Notes from Gunderson, meeting at CTS, January 14, 2002.
22. Bohm and Nichol, *On Dialogue*, 2–3.
23. For a fuller discussion, see Gunderson, *Boundary Leaders*. 83–104.
24. Albert Camus, *The Rebel: An Essay on Man in Revolt* (New York: Vintage, 1992).
25. James R. Cochrane, "Religion as Social Capital in the Context of Health: Mapping
the Field," in *Assets and Agency: Papers and Proceedings of the ARHAP International
Colloquium*, ed. James R Cochrane and Barbara Schmid (Cape Town: African
Religious Health Assets Programme, 2003).
26. Phone Survey of Indigent Patients at Methodist Le Bonheur Healthcare, conducted
by Marketing Research Department, unpublished, 2006.
27. See Teresa Cutts, "The Memphis Congregational Health Network Model:
Grounding ARHAP Theory " in *When Religion and Health Align: Mobilizing
Religious Health Assets for Transformation*, ed. James R. Cochrane, Barbara Schmid,
and Teresa Cutts (Pietermaritzburg: Cluster Publications, 2010), 193–209.
28. R. B. Aviram, B. S. Brodsky, and B. Stanley, "Borderline Personality Disorder,
Stigma, and Treatment Implications," *Harvard Review of Psychiatry* 14, no. 5
(2006): 249–56; on valence theory, see L. K. Guerrero and M. L. Hecht, eds., *The
Nonverbal Communication Reader: Classic and Contemporary Readings*, 3rd ed.
(Long Grove, IL: Waveland Press,2008), especially 511–20.
29. Personal communication, Dr. Teresa Cutts. See also M. M. Linehan and L. Dimeff,
" Dialectical Behavior Therapy in a Nutshell," *The California Psychologist* 34
(2001): 10–13.
30. See James R. Cochrane, "'Damned If You Do, Damned If You Don't': Rereading
the Public Theology of the Christian Institute for the Contemporary Practitioner,"
in *Christian in Public: Aims, Methodologies and Issues in Public Theology*, ed. Len
Hansen, Beyers Naudé Centre Series on Public Theology (Stellenbosch: Stellenbosch
University, SUN Press, 2007), 165–76.
31. Referring to Habermas's understanding of our contemporary condition, as discussed
in Jürgen Habermas, *The Postnational Constellation: Political Essays* (Cambridge,
UK: Polity Press, 2001).
32. See Jackson, *65 Dark Days in '68*.
33. Cochrane, "Agapé: The Cape Office of the Christian Institute."
34. See the chapter, "The Face that Speaks," in Emmanuel Lévinas, *Totality and
Infinity: An Essay on Exteriority*, trans. Alphonso Lingis (Pittsburgh, PA: Duquesne
University Press, 1969).
35. We discuss the CHN further in the concluding chapter.
36. On organizational dynamics, see Marco Iansiti and Roy Levien, *The Keystone
Advantage: What the New Dynamics of Business Ecosystems Mean for Strategy,
Innovation and Sustainability* (Boston: Harvard Business School Press, 2004).
More generally, see also Manuel Castells, *The Rise of the Network Society* (Oxford,
UK: Blackwell Publishers, 1996).
37. Here and in what follows, we depend upon work done at the Center for Turbulence
Studies, Stanford University, http://www.stanford.edu/group/ctr/gallery.html,
accessed November 15, 2009.
38. Beverly J. McKeon, "Controlling Turbulence," *Science* 327 (2010): 1462–63.

39. John M. Barry, *Rising Tide: The Great Mississippi Flood of 1927 and How It Changed America* (New York: Simon & Schuster, 1998), 38.

8 THE CHALLENGE OF SYSTEMS

1. Richard Wilkinson and Kate Pickett, *The Spirit Level: Why Greater Equality Makes Societies Stronger* (London; New York: Penguin & Bloomsbury Press, 2009), 8.
2. Ibid., 12.
3. Ibid., 263.
4. Ibid., 39.
5. See chapter 2, on Religious Health Assets.
6. Recognizing Foucault's work on these themes, including health, we nevertheless frame them somewhat differently; see Michel Foucault, *The Birth of the Clinic: An Archaeology of Medical Perception*, trans. A. M. Smith (New York: Random House (imprint: Vintage), 1975); Michel Foucault, *Power/knowledge: selected writings and other interviews 1972–1977*, trans. Colin Gordon, et al. (New York: Pantheon, 1980).
7. United Nations Development Programme, "Human Development Report: International Cooperation at a Crossroads—Aid, Trade and Security in an Unequal World," (New York: United Nations, 2005), 55.
8. B. P. Mpepo, "The Path Away from Poverty: An Easy Look at Zambia's Poverty Reduction Strategy Paper, 2002–2004," (Lusaka: Civil Society for Poverty Reduction, 2004), 9.
9. African Religious Health Assets Programme, "Appreciating Assets: The Contribution of Religion to Universal Access in Africa," (Cape Town: ARHAP, Report for the World Health Organization, 2006), Appendix D.
10. For details and resources, see the World Bank's website, http://www.povertynet.org/.
11. The PRSPs include a requirement that all stakeholders should be consulted in the process of defining and developing policy, for example.
12. See the section on "Assets and Capabilities" in chapter 3.
13. Mahmood Mamdani, *Citizen and Subject: Contemporary Africa and the Legacy of Late Colonialism* (Cape Town; Kampala: David Philip; Fountain Publishers, 1996).
14. See Martha C. Nussbaum and Jonathan Glover, eds., *Women, Culture, and Development: A Study of Human Capabilities* (Oxford, UK: Oxford University Press, 1995).
15. Paul Farmer, *Pathologies of Power: Health, Human Rights and the New War on the Poor* (Berkeley, CA: University of California Press, 2003).
16. Suki Ali, Kelly Coate, and Wangui wa Goro, eds., *Global Feminist Politics: Identities in a Changing World* (London: Routledge, 2000), 13–14.
17. Farmer, *Pathologies of Power*. Foreword, xvi.
18. See, inter alia, Robert H. Bates, *When Things Fell Apart: State Failure in Late-Century Africa*, Cambridge Studies in Comparative Politics (New York: Cambridge University Press, 2008); Mark Findlay, *The Globalisation of Crime: Understanding Transitional Relationships in Context* (Cambridge, UK: Cambridge University Press, 1999); Jonathan Glennie, *The Trouble with Aid: Why Less Could Mean More for Africa* (London: Zed Books, in association with International African Institute, Royal African Society, and the Social Science Research Council, 2008); Misha Glenny, *McMafia: Seriously Organized Crime* (London: Vintage Books, 2009); Caroline Thomas and Peter Wilkin, *Globalization, Human Security, and the African Experience*, Critical Security Studies (Boulder, CO: Lynne Rienner Publishers, 1998).

19. Jean Grugel and Hout Wil, *Regionalism across the North-South Divide: State Strategies and Globalization*, European Political Science Series (New York: Routledge, 1999); Jürgen Habermas, *The Postnational Constellation: Political Essays* (Cambridge, UK: Polity Press, 2001); R. J. Holton, *Globalization and the Nation-State*, 2nd edition (New York: Palgrave Macmillan, 2011).

20. Geoffrey Garrett, "The Causes of Globalization," *Comparative Political Studies* 33, no. 6–7 (2000): 941–91.

21. Chris Simms, Mike Rowson, and Siobhan Peattie, "The Bitterest Pill of All: The Collapse of Africa's Health Systems," (London: Save the Children Fund (UK), 2001; An Eldis Document, http://www.eldis.org/assets/Docs/29246.html, accessed July 31, 2011).

22. See, for example, the recent WHO-backed First Global Symposium on Health Systems Research held in Montreux, Switzerland, in 2010: http://www.hsr-symposium.org/, accessed June 21, 2011.

23. Habermas, *Postnational Constellation*. 95.

24. Ibid.

25. Paul Farmer, *Infections and Inequalities: The Modern Plagues* (Berkeley, CA; Los Angeles: University of California, 1999). See also Graham Scambler, *Health and Social Change: A Critical Theory*, ed. Tim May (Buckingham and Philadelphia: The Open University Press, 2002). 86ff.

26. Laurie Garrett, *Betrayal of Trust: The Collapse of Global Public Health* (New York: Hyperion, 2000).

27. Lucy Gilson, "Trust and the Development of Health Care as a Social Institution," *Social Science & Medicine* 56 (2003): 1464.

28. John J. Hall and Richard Taylor, "Health for All Beyond 2000: The Demise of the Alma-Ata Declaration and Primary Health Care in Developing Countries," *Medical Journal of Australia* 178 (2003): 17–20.

29. Marcos Cueto, "The Origins of Primary Health Care and Selective Primary Health Care," *American Journal of Public Health* 94, no. 11 (2004): 1864–74; S. Macfarlane, M. Racelis, and F. Muli-Musiime, "Public Health in Developing Countries," *Lancet* 356, no. 9232 (2000): 843.

30. Hall and Taylor, "Health for all," 18–19.

31. World Bank, *World Development Report 1993: Investing in Health* (New York: Oxford University Press, 1993).

32. Hall and Taylor, "Health for all," 18.

33. Michael E. Porter and Elizabeth Olmsted Teisberg, *Redefining Health Care: Creating Value-Based Competition on Results* (Boston: Harvard Business School Press, 2006).

34. Ibid., 381–86.

35. Ibid., 379.

36. See www.IHI.org.

37. C. Craig, D. Eby, and J. Whittington, "Care Coordination Model: Better Care at Lower Cost for People with Multiple Health and Social Needs," (Cambridge, MA: Institute for Healthcare Improvement, 2011).

38. Ibid., 3.

39. James C. Scott, *Seeing Like a State: How Certain Schemes to Improve the Human Condition Have Failed* (New Haven, CT; London: Yale University Press, 1998), 80.

40. Ibid., 340–44f passim.

41. Ibid., 6.

42. Ibid., 11.

43. Mark A. Smith, "Sap Opens Road for Hana and Big Data at Sapphire Now," in *Information Management Blogs*, May 27, 2011, http://www.information-management

.com/blogs/big_data_analytics_business_intelligence_SAP-10020453-1.html, accessed July 12, 2011.

44. James C. Scott, *Domination and the Arts of Resistance: Hidden Transcripts* (New Haven, CT: Yale University Press, 1991).

45. Robert Chambers and G. R. Conway, *Sustainable Rural Livelihoods: Practical Concepts for the 21st Century*, DP 296 (Brighton, UK: Institute of Development Studies, University of Sussex, 1991); I. Scoones, *Sustainable Rural Livelihoods: A framework for Analysis*, WP 72 (Brighton, UK: Institute of Development Studies, University of Sussex, 1998).

46. Charles Elliot, *Locating the Energy for Change: An Introduction to Appreciative Inquiry* (Winnipeg: International Institute for Sustainable Development, 1999).

47. Nan Lin, Karen Cook, and Ronald S. Burt, *Social Capital: Theory and Research* (New York: Aldine de Gruyter, 2001); Corwin Smidt, ed., *Religion as Social Capital: Producing the Common Good* (Waco, TX: Baylor University Press, 2003).

48. Harro Albrecht, "Rudolf Virchow," *Die Zeit*, November 12, 2009. Available at http://www.zeit.de/2009/47/Vorbilder-Virchow, accessed June 29, 2011; our translations, original citations in German are: "Die medizinische Wissenschaft is in ihrem innersten Kern und Wesen eine social Wissenschaft" and "Die Politik sei weiter nichts 'als Medicin im Grossen."

49. Scambler, *Health and Social Change*.

50. Cited in Richard Hofrichter, ed. *Health and Social Justice: Politics, Ideology, and Inequity in the Distribution of Disease* (San Francisco: Jossey-Bass [John Wiley & Sons], 2003), 6.

51. Farmer, *Infections and Inequalities*.

52. See EQUINET, <<http://www.equinetafrica.org/workequity.php>>, and also the discussion on these principles in EQUINET Steering Committee, "Equity in Health in Southern Africa: Overview and Issues from an Annotated Bibliography," (Harare, Zimbabwe: Regional Network for Equity in Health in Southern Africa, 1998).

53. World Bank, *Investing in health*.

54. Fabienne Peter, "Health Equity and Social Justice," *Journal of Applied Philosophy* 18, no. 2 (2001): 159–70.

55. EQUINET Steering Committee, "Equity in Health in Southern Africa: Turning Values into Practice" (Harare, Zimbabwe: Regional Network for Equity in Health in Southern Africa, 2000), 2.

56. Ibid., 3.

57. Macfarlane, Racelis, and Muli-Musiime, "Public Health in Developing Countries."

58. Ibid., 842.

59. See James R. Cochrane, "'Fire from Above, Fire from Below': Health, Justice and the Persistence of the Sacred," *Theoria* 116 (2008): 67; also James R. Cochrane, "Health and the Uses of Religion: Recovering the Political Proper?" in *Development and Politics from Below: Exploring Religious Spaces in the African State*, ed. Barbara Bompani and Maria Frahm-Aarp (London: Palgrave-MacMillan, 2010).

60. One thing most religious leaders from various traditions around the world agree on is this maxim; see Nancy Hodes and Michael Hays, eds., *The United Nations and the World's Religions: Prospects for a Global Ethic* (Cambridge, MA: Boston Research Center for the 21st Century, 1995); Patricia M. Mische and Melissa Merkling, eds., *Toward a Global Civilization? The Contribution of Religions* (New York: Peter Lang, 2001).

61. Paul Ricoeur, *Oneself as Another* (Chicago: University of Chicago Press, 1992), 330.

62. See chapter 5.

63. Ricoeur, *Oneself as Another*, 320.

64. Alice O'Connor, *Poverty Knowledge: Social Science, Social Policy and the Poor in Twentieth-Century U.S. History* (Princeton, NJ; Oxford, UK: Princeton University Press, 2001).
65. Ibid., 4.
66. Ibid., 6–7.
67. Alexander Bird, *Thomas Kuhn* (Princeton, NJ: Princeton University Press, 2000); Thomas S. Kuhn, *The Structure of Scientific Revolutions*, 3rd ed., Foundations of the Unity of Science (Chicago: University of Chicago Press, 1996).
68. John Berger, *Ways of Seeing* (Harmondsworth, Middlesex, UK: Penguin, 1972).
69. Raj Bophal, "Paradigms in Epidemiology Textbooks: In the Footsteps of Thomas Kuhn," *American Journal of Public Health* 89, no. 8 (1999): 1162.
70. O'Connor, *Poverty knowledge*. 292.
71. Jürgen Habermas, *Between Facts and Norms: Contributions to a Discourse Theory of Law and Democracy*, trans. William Rehg (Cambridge, MA: MIT Press, 1998), 365. Emphasis in the original.
72. See chapter 5 for a discussion on this concept.

9 Religion and the Health of the Public: Deep Accountability

1. James Gleick, *Chaos: Making a New Science* (New York: Penguin Books, 1988), 3.
2. Ibid.
3. Ibid., 298.
4. Ibid., 44.
5. Ibid., 299.
6. Linda M. Chatters, "Religion and Health: Public Health Research and Practice," *Annual Review of Public Health* 21 (2000): 336.
7. Mark L. Rosenberg, *Real Collaboration: What It Takes for Global Health to Succeed*, California/Milbank Books on Health and the Public (Berkeley, CA: University of California Press, 2010), 29.
8. Ibid., 211–21.
9. CoE, "The Memphis Model: Mapping Research Opportunities at the Intersection of Faith and Health in Memphis," (Memphis, TN: Center of Excellence in Faith and Health, Methodist Le Bonheur Healthcare, 2010), 1.
10. Institute of Medicine, *Crossing the Quality Chasm: A New Health System for the 21st Century*, Committee on Quality of Health Care in America (Washington, DC: National Academy Press, 2001).
11. Teresa Cutts, "The Memphis Congregational Health Network Model: Grounding ARHAP Theory " in *When Religion and Health Align: Mobilizing Religious Health Assets for Transformation*, ed. James R. Cochrane, Barbara Schmid, and Teresa Cutts (Pietermaritzburg: Cluster Publications, 2010), 193–209.
12. For a description and analysis of the Masangane programme, see Liz Thomas et al., "'Let Us Embrace': Role and Significance of an Integrated Faith-Based Initiative for HIV and Aids: Masangane Case Study," (Cape Town: African Religious Health Assets Programme, University of Cape Town, 2006).
13. Margaret Thatcher, "Interview (Douglas Keay)," *Women's Own*, October 31, 1987.
14. See, for example, Gary S. Becker, *The Economic Approach to Human Behavior* (Chicago: University of Chicago Press, 1978); Jon Elster, *Nuts and Bolts for the Social Sciences* (Cambridge, UK: Cambridge University Press, 1989).
15. Margaret Jane Radin, "Response: Persistent Perplexities," *Kennedy Institute of Ethics Journal* 11, no. 3 (2001): 308; see also Margaret Jane Radin, *Contested Commodities* (Cambridge, MA: Harvard University Press, 1996).

BIBLIOGRAPHY

Adam, Barbara. "Futurity from a Complexity Perspective." (2005). Accessed October 28, 2010. http://www.cardiff.ac.uk/socsi/futures/Web%20Complexity%20Futures.pdf.
———. "Memory of Futures." (2004). Accessed October 28, 2010. http://www.cardiff.ac.uk/socsi/futures/memoryofthefuture.pdf.
African Religious Health Assets Programme. "Appreciating Assets: The Contribution of Religion to Universal Access in Africa." Cape Town: ARHAP, Report for the World Health Organization, 2006.
———. "CHAMP/PC: Community Health Assets Mapping for Partnerships in Palliative Care—Facilitator's Guide." Cape Town: ARHAP University of Cape Town, October 2009.
Agamben, Giorgio. *Homo Sacer: Sovereign Power and Bare Life.* Stanford, CA: Stanford University Press, 1998.
Agrimi, Jole, and Chiara Crisciani. "Charity and Aid in Medieval Christian Civilization." In *Western Medical Thought from Antiquity to the Middle Ages,* edited by Mirko D. Grmek. 170–96. Cambridge, MA; London: Harvard University Press, 1998.
Albrecht, Harro. "Rudolf Virchow." *Die Zeit* (Nov. 12, 2009).
Ali, Suki, Kelly Coate, and Wangui wa Goro, eds. *Global Feminist Politics: Identities in a Changing World.* London: Routledge, 2000.
Almond, Gabriel A., R. Scott Appleby, and Emmanuel Sivan. *Strong Religion: The Rise of Fundamentalism around the World.* Chicago: University of Chicago Press, 2003.
Amler, Robert W., and H. Bruce Dull, eds. *Closing the Gap: The Burden of Unnecessary Illness.* New York: Oxford University Press, 1987.
Ammerman, Nancy Tatom. *Pillars of Faith: American Congregations and Their Partners.* Berkeley, CA; Los Angeles: University of California Press, 2005.
Ammerman, Nancy Tatom, Jackson W. Carroll, Carl S. Dudley, and William McKinney. *Studying Congregations: A New Handbook.* Nashville, TN: Abingdon, 1998.
Ammerman, Nancy Tatom, with, Arthur E. Farnsley, Tammy Adams, and et. al. *Congregation and Community.* New Brunswick, NJ: Rutgers University Press, 1997.
Antonovsky, Aaron. *Health, Stress and Coping.* San Francisco: Jossey-Bass Publishers, 1979.
———. *Unraveling the Mystery of Health: How People Manage Stress and Stay Well.* San Francisco: Jossey-Bass Publishers, 1987.
Arjomand, Said Amir. "Religion and the Diversity of Normative Orders." In *The Political Dimensions of Religion,* edited by Said Amir Arjomand. 45–68. New York: State University of New York Press, 1993.
Aron, Raymond. *Progress and Disillusion: The Dialectics of Modern Society.* The Britannica Perspectives. New York: New American Library, 1968.
Aviram, R. B., B. S. Brodsky, and B. Stanley. "Borderline Personality Disorder, Stigma, and Treatment Implications." *Harvard Review of Psychiatry* 14, no. 5 (Sept.-Oct. 2006): 249–56.

Bandura, Albert. "Self Efficacy Mechanism in Human Agency."*American Psychologist* 37, no. 2 (Feb. 1982): 122–47.

Barry, Christine A., Fiona A. Stevenson, Nicky Britten, Nick Barber, and Colin P. Bradley. "Giving Voice to the Lifeworld: More Humane, More Effective Medical Care? A Qualitative Study of Doctor-Patient Communication in General Practice." *Social Science & Medicine* 53 (2001): 487–505.

Barry, John M. *Rising Tide: The Great Mississippi Flood of 1927 and How It Changed America.* New York: Simon & Schuster, 1998.

Bates, Robert H. *When Things Fell Apart: State Failure in Late-Century Africa.* Cambridge Studies in Comparative Politics. New York: Cambridge University Press, 2008.

Bauman, Zygmunt. *Globalization: The Human Consequences.* Cambridge, UK: Polity Press, 1998.

———. *Liquid Modernity.* Cambridge, UK: Polity Press, 2000.

———. *Liquid Times: Living in an Age of Uncertainty.* Cambridge, UK: Polity Press, 2006.

Becker, Gary S. *The Economic Approach to Human Behavior.* Chicago: University of Chicago Press, 1978.

Bellamy, Peter. "The Significance of Bob Lambourne's Writing Today." *Contact* 81 (1984): 12–15.

Benn, Christoph. "The Influence of Cultural and Religious Frameworks on the Future Course of the HIV/Aids Pandemic." *Journal of Theology for Southern Africa* 113 (July 2002): 3–18.

Bennett, Richard G., and W. Daniel Hale. *Building Healthy Communities through Medical-Religious Partnerships.* 2nd ed. Baltimore, MD: Johns Hopkins University Press, 2009.

Berger, John. *Ways of Seeing.* Harmondsworth, Middlesex, UK: Penguin, 1972.

Berger, Peter L. "Reflections on the Sociology of Religion Today: The 2000 Paul Hanly Furfey Lecture." *Sociology of Religion* 62, no. 4 (2001): 443–54.

Berger, Peter L., and Robert W. Hefner. "Spiritual Capital in Comparative Perspective." Institute for the Study of Economic Culture. Accessed June 6, 2011. http://www.spiritualcapitalresearchprogram.com/pdf/Berger.pdf.

Berry, Wendell. *Home Economics: Fourteen Essays.* San Francisco: North Point Press, 1987.

———. *Life Is a Miracle.* Washington, DC: Counterpoint, 2000.

———. *Sex, Economy, Freedom & Community.* New York; San Francisco: Pantheon, 1992.

———. *What Are People For?* New York: North Point Press, 1990.

Bhattacharya, S., and R. Dasgupta. "A Tale of Two Global Health Programs: Smallpox Eradication's Lessons for the Antipolio Campaign in India." *American Journal of Public Health* 99, no. 7 (July 2009): 1176–84.

Bird, Alexander. *Thomas Kuhn.* Princeton, NJ: Princeton University Press, 2000.

Bloch, Ernst. *The Principle of Hope.* Translated by Neville Plaice, Stephen Plaice, and Paul Knight. Vol. 1, Cambridge, MA: MIT Press, 1986.

Bloch, Ernst. *The Principle of Hope.* Translated by Neville Plaice, Stephen Plaice, and Paul Knight. Vol. 2, Cambridge, MA: MIT Press, 1986.

———. *The Utopian Function of Art and Literature: Selected Essays.* Translated by Jack Zipes and Frank Mecklenburg. Studies in Contemporary German Social Thought. Cambridge, MA: MIT Press, 1988.

Bohm, David. *On Dialogue.* London; New York: Routledge, 1996.

———. *Wholeness and the Implicate Order.* Routledge Classics. London; New York: Routledge, 2002.

Bohm, David, and Lee Nichol. *On Dialogue.* London; New York: Routledge, 2004.

Bophal, Raj. "Paradigms in Epidemiology Textbooks: In the Footsteps of Thomas Kuhn." *American Journal of Public Health* 89, no. 8 (Aug. 1999): 1162–65.

Bordo, Michael D., Alan M. Taylor, and Jeffrey G. Williamson, eds. *Globalization in Historical Perspective*. Chicago: University of Chicago Press, 2003.

Bourdieu, Pierre. *The Logic of Practice*. Cambridge, UK: Polity Press, 1990.

Braudel, Fernand. *On History*. Translated by Sarah Matthews. Chicago: University of Chicago Press, 1980.

Brown, Norman O. *Life against Death: The Psychoanalytical Meaning of History*. Middletown, CT: Wesleyan University Press, 1959.

Bryant, John H. "Five Challenges to the Churches in Health Work." *Contact* 42 (1977): 1–4.

———. *Health and the Developing World*. Ithaca, NY: Cornell University Press, 1970.

Bryant, J. H., and David Jenkins. "Moral Issues and Health Care." *Contact* 4 (July 1971): 1–35.

Burt, Ronald S. "Social Holes Versus Network Closure as Social Capital." In *Social Capital: Theory and Research*, edited by Nan Lin, Karen Cook, and Ronald S. Burt. Sociology and Economics: Controversy and Integration, 31–56. New York: Aldine de Gruyter, 2001.

Cameron, Elaine, Jonathan Mathers, and Jayne Parry. "'Health and Well-Being': Questioning the Use of Health Concepts in Public Health Policy and Practice." *Critical Public Health* 18, no. 2 (2008): 225–32.

Camus, Albert. *The Rebel: An Essay on Man in Revolt*. New York: Vintage, 1992.

Carlisle, Sandra, and Phil Hanlon. "'Well-Being' as a Focus for Public Health? A Critique and Defence." *Critical Public Health* 18, no. 3 (2008): 263–70.

Carrin, Guy, Aviva Ron, Yang Huib, Wang Hongb, Zhang Tuohongb, Zhang Lichengb, Zhang Shuob, *et al.* "The Reform of the Rural Cooperative Medical System in the People's Republic of China: Interim Experience in 14 Pilot Counties." *Social Science & Medicine* 48, no. 7 (1999): 961–67.

Carroll, Lewis. *Through the Looking Glass and What Alice Found There*. New York: Random House, 1946.

Carroll, Thomas F. *Intermediary NGOs: The Supporting Link in Grassroots Development*. Library of Management for Development. West Hartford, CT: Kumarian Press, 1992.

Carter, Rosalyn. "Reweaving the Fabric of Care: Mind, Body, Spirit and Community." *Faith & Health*. Atlanta, GA: Interfaith Health Program, 1999.

Casanova, José. *Public Religions in the Modern World*. Chicago: University of Chicago Press, 1994.

Castells, Manuel. *The Rise of the Network Society*. Oxford, UK: Blackwell Publishers, 1996.

Center for Turbulence Studies. Stanford University. Accessed November 15, 2009. http://www.stanford.edu/group/ctr/gallery.html.

Chambers, Robert, and G. R. Conway. *Sustainable Rural Livelihoods: Practical Concepts for the 21st Century*. Dp 296. Brighton, UK: Institute of Development Studies, University of Sussex, 1991.

Chaskin, R. J., P. Brown, S. Venkatesh, and A. Vidal. *Building Community Capacity*. New York: Aldine de Gruyter, 2001.

Chatters, Linda M. "Religion and Health: Public Health Research and Practice." *Annual Review of Public Health* 21 (2000): 335–67.

Chave, S. P. W. "Henry Whitehead and Cholera in Broad Street." *Medical History* 2, no. 2 (1958): 92–109.

Church of Scotland, The. "Church Without Walls." Accessed October 23, 2011. http://www.churchofscotland.org.uk/connect/church_without_walls.

Cnaan, Ram A., and Stephanie C. Boddie. *The Invisible Caring Hand: American Congregations and the Provision of Welfare*. New York; London: New York University Press, 2002.

Cochrane, James R. "Agapé: The Cape Office of the Christian Institute." *Journal of Theology for Southern Africa* 118 (2004): 53–68.

Cochrane, James R. *Circles of Dignity: Community Wisdom and Theological Reflection*. Minneapolis, MN: Fortress Press, 1999.

———. "'Damned If You Do, Damned If You Don't': Rereading the Public Theology of the Christian Institute for the Contemporary Practitioner." In *Christian in Public: Aims, Methodologies and Issues in Public Theology*, edited by Len Hansen. Beyers Naudé Centre Series on Public Theology, 165–76. Stellenbosch: Stellenbosch University, SUN Press, 2007.

———. "'Fire from Above, Fire from Below': Health, Justice and the Persistence of the Sacred." *Theoria* 116 (Aug. 2008): 67–96.

———. "Health and the Uses of Religion: Recovering the Political Proper?" In *Development and Politics from Below: Exploring Religious Spaces in the African State*, edited by Barbara Bompani and Maria Frahm-Aarp.175–96. London: Palgrave-MacMillan, 2010.

———. "A Model of Integral Development: Assessing and Working with Religious Health Assets." In *Religion and Development: Ways of Transforming the World*, edited by Gerrie ter Haar. 231–52. London; New York: Hurst & Co; Columbia University Press, 2011.

———. "Religion as Social Capital in the Context of Health: Mapping the Field." In *Assets and Agency: Papers and Proceedings of the ARHAP International Colloquium*, edited by James R. Cochrane and Barbara Schmid. 42–48. Cape Town: African Religious Health Assets Programme, 2003.

———. "Religion in the Health of Migrant Communities: Cultural Assets or Medical Deficits?" *Journal of Ethnic and Migration Studies* 32, no. 4 (May 2006): 715–36.

———. "Sacred Crossings: Movement, Migration and the Fate of the Religious Body." In *Broken Bodies and Healing Communities: The Challenge of HIV and Aids in the South African Context*, edited by Neville Richardson. 72–85. Pietermaritzburg: Cluster Publications, 2009.

———. *Servants of Power: The Role of English-Speaking Churches, 1903–1930*. Johannesburg: Ravan Press, 1987.

———. "Trustworthy Intermediaries: Role of Religious Agents on the Boundaries of Public Health." In *When Religion and Health Align: Mobilising Religious Health Assets for Transformation*, edited by James R. Cochrane, Barbara Schmid, and Teresa Cutts. 150–63. Pietermaritzburg: Cluster Publications, 2011.

CoE. "The Memphis Model: Mapping Research Opportunities at the Intersection of Faith and Health in Memphis." Memphis, TN: Center of Excellence in Faith and Health, Methodist Le Bonheur Healthcare, 2010.

Coleman, James S. *Foundations of Social Theory*. Cambridge, MA: Harvard University Press, 1990.

Craig, C., D. Eby, and J. Whittington. "Care Coordination Model: Better Care at Lower Cost for People with Multiple Health and Social Needs." Cambridge, MA: Institute for Healthcare Improvement, 2011.

Crosby, Molly Caldwe. *The American Plague: The Untold Story of Yellow Fever, the Epidemic That Shaped Our History*. New York: Berkley Books, 2007.

CSDH. "Closing the Gap in a Generation: Health Equity through Action on the Social Determinants of Health." Geneva: World Health Organization, Commission on Social Determinants of Health, 2008.

Csordas, J. "Ritual Healing and the Politics of Identity in Contemporary Navajo Society." *American Ethnologist* 26, no. 1 (1999): 3–23.

Cueto, Marcos. "The Origins of Primary Health Care and Selective Primary Health Care." *American Journal of Public Health* 94, no. 11 (Nov. 2004): 1864–74.

Cutts, Teresa. "The Memphis Congregational Health Network Model: Grounding ARHAP Theory ". In *When Religion and Health Align: Mobilizing Religious Health*

Assets for Transformation, edited by James R. Cochrane, Barbara Schmid, and Teresa Cutts. 193–209. Pietermaritzburg: Cluster Publications, 2010.

Cutts, Teresa, and Gary Gunderson. "The Memphis Model: Finding Life in a Tough Town." Conference Paper at the Grand Rounds. Memphis, TN: University of Memphis School of Public Health, 2009.

Dawkins, Richard. *The God Delusion*. Boston: Houghton Mifflin, 2006.

de Gruchy, Steve. "Of Agency, Assets and Appreciation: Seeking Some Commonalities between Theology and Development." *Journal of Theology for Southern Africa* 117 (Nov. 2003): 20–39.

de Gruchy, Steve, James R. Cochrane, Jill Olivier, and Sinatra Matimelo. "Participatory Inquiry on the Interface between Religion and Health: What Does It Achieve, and What Not?" In *When Religion and Health Align: Mobilizing Religious Health Assets for Transformation*, edited by James R. Cochrane, Barbara Schmid, and Teresa Cutts. 43–61. Pietermaritzburg: Cluster Publications, 2011.

de Waal, Frans. *The Age of Empathy: Nature's Lessons for a Kinder Society*. New York: Harmony Books, 2009.

Denham, A. R. "Rethinking Historical Trauma: Narratives of Resilience." *Transcultural Psychiatry* 45, no. 3 (Sep. 2008): 391–414.

Denier, Yvonne. "Public Health, Well-Being and Reciprocity." *Ethical Perspectives: Journal of the European Ethics Network* 11, no. 1 (2005): 41–66.

Department of Health. "A Policy for the Development of a District Health System for South Africa." Pretoria: Government of South Africa, 1996.

———. "Restructuring the National Health System for Universal Primary Health Care." Pretoria: Government of South Africa, 1996.

Derrida, Jacques. "Faith and Knowledge: The Two Sources of 'Religion' at the Limits of Reason Alone." In *Religion*, edited by Jacques Derrida and Gianni Vattimo. Cultural Memory in the Present, 1–78. Cambridge, UK: Polity Press, 1998.

Droege, Thomas A. "Congregations as Communities of Health and Healing." *Interpretation* 69, no. 2 (1995): 117–29.

Duffy, John. *The Sanitarians: A History of American Public Health*. Urbana, IL; Chicago: University of Illinois Press, 1992.

Eason, Andrew M. "'All Things to All People to Save Some': Salvation Army Missionary Work among the Zulus of Victorian Natal." *Journal of Southern African Studies* 35, no. 1 (2009): 7–27.

Eger, E., S. R. Schweinberger, R. J. Dolan, and R. N. Henson. "Familiarity Enhances Invariance of Face Representations in Human Ventral Visual Cortex: Fmri Evidence." *Neuroimage* 26, no. 4 (July 15, 2005): 1128–39.

Elliot, Charles. *Locating the Energy for Change: An Introduction to Appreciative Inquiry*. Winnipeg: International Institute for Sustainable Development, 1999.

Elster, Jon. *Nuts and Bolts for the Social Sciences*. Cambridge, UK: Cambridge University Press, 1989.

EQUINET Steering Committee. "Equity in Health in Southern Africa: Overview and Issues from an Annotated Bibliography." Harare, Zimbabwe: Regional Network for Equity in Health in Southern Africa, 1998.

———. "Equity in Health in Southern Africa: Turning Values into Practice." Harare, Zimbabwe: Regional Network for Equity in Health in Southern Africa, 2000.

Erikson, Erik H. *Childhood and Society*. 2nd ed. New York: W. W. Norton & Company, 1963 [1950].

Eriksson, Monica, and Bengt Lindström. "A Salutogenic Interpretation of the Ottawa Charter." *Health Promotion International* 23, no. 2 (2008): 190–99.

———. "Validity of Antonovsky's Sense of Coherence Scale: A Systematic Review." *Journal of Epidemiology and Community Health* 59 (2005): 460–66.

Farmer, Paul. *Infections and Inequalities: The Modern Plagues*. Berkeley, CA; Los Angeles: University of California, 1999.

———. *Pathologies of Power: Health, Human Rights and the New War on the Poor*. Berkeley, CA: University of California Press, 2003.

Farquhar, Judith, and Zhang Qicheng. "Biopolitical Beijing: Pleasure, Sovereignty, and Self-Cultivation in China's Capital." *Cultural Anthropology* 20, no. 3 (2005): 303–27.

———. *Ten Thousand Things: Nurturing Life in Contemporary Beijing*. New York: Zone Books, 2012.

Febvre, Lucien. *A New Kind of History and Other Essays*. Translated by Peter Burke and K. Folca. New York: Harper & Row (Harper Torchbooks), 1973.

Felix-Burdine & Associates. "Model of Community Capacity for Health Improvement." Allentown, PA: Report for the Robert Wood Johnson Foundation, 2000.

Ferguson, J. Todd, Ted Karpf, Matthew Weait, and Robin Y. Swift. "Decent Care: Living Values, Health Justice and Human Flourishing." WHO/Ford Foundation. Accessed April 22, 2010. http://www.wfmh.org/09DOCS/Decent%20Care%20Monograph%20for%20Ford%20Foundationr%20Final%2024-8-09.pdf.

Ferlander, Sarah. "The Importance of Different Forms of Social Capital for Health." *Acta Sociologica* 50, no. 2 (2007): 115–28.

Findlay, Mark. *The Globalisation of Crime: Understanding Transitional Relationships in Context*. Cambridge, UK: Cambridge University Press, 1999.

Fleßa, Steffen. *Gesundheitsreformen in Entwicklungsländern: Eine kritische Analyse aus Sicht der kirchlichen Entwicklungshilfe*. Frankfurt am Main: Verlag Otto Lembeck, 2002.

Flueckiger, Joyce B. *In Amma's Healing Room: Gender and Vernacular Islam in South India*. Bloomington, IN: Indiana University Press, 2006.

Foege, William H. "Engaging Faith Communities as Partners in Improving Community Health." In *CDC/ATSDR Forum: Separation of Church and State, the Science Supporting Work with Faith Communities, and Exemplary Partnerships*. Atlanta, GA: US Department of Health & Human Services, Centers for Disease Control and Prevention, 1999.

———. "Keynote Speech, the Thomas Francis Jr. Medal in Global Public Health." University of Michigan. Accessed October 26, 2010. www.polio.umich.edu/program/foege.html.

———. "Smallpox Eradication: William Foege Oral History—Interviewed by Victoria Harden." Centers for Disease Control and Prevention. Accessed October 26, 2010. http://www.globalhealthchronicles.org/smallpox/record/view/pid/emory:15jvg.

Foege, William H., Donald Millar, and J. Michael Lane. "Selective Epidemiologic Control in Smallpox Eradication." *American Journal of Epidemiology* 94, no. 4 (1971): 311–15.

Foege, William H., J. D. Millar, and D. A. Henderson. "Smallpox Eradication in West and Central Africa." *Bulletin of the World Health Organization* 52, no. 2 (1975): 209–22.

Foege, William H., Robert W. Amler, and C. C. White. "Closing the Gap. Report of the Carter Center Health Policy Consultation." *Journal of the American Medical Association* 13, no. 254 (10) (1985): 1355–58.

Foster, Geoff. "Study of the Response by Faith-Based Organizations to Orphans and Vulnerable Children: Preliminary Summary Report." 36. Nairobi: World Conference of Religions for Peace; United Nations Children Fund—UNICEF, 2003.

Foucault, Michel. *The Birth of the Clinic: An Archaeology of Medical Perception*. Translated by A. M. Smith. New York: Random House (imprint: Vintage), 1975.

———. *Discipline and Punishment: The Birth of the Prison*. Translated by Alan Sheridan. New York: Random House (imprint: Vintage), 1979.

————. *Madness and Civilization: A History of Insanity in the Age of Reason*. Translated by Richard Howard. New York: New York American Library (imprint: Mentor), 1967.

————. *Power/Knowledge: Selected Writings and Other Interviews 1972–1977*. Translated by Colin Gordon, Leo Marshal, John Mepham, and Kate Soper. New York: Pantheon, 1980.

Frankl, Viktor E. *The Doctor and the Soul, from Psychotherapy to Logotherapy*. Translated by Richard Winston and Clara Winston. New York: Bantam, 1971.

————. *Man's Search for Meaning*. Revised & updated ed. New York: Washington Square Press, 1997 [1946]. Ein Psycholog erlebt das Konzentrationslager [1946].

Fricchionne, Gregory L. "Separation, Attachment and Altruistic Love: The Evolutionary Basis for Medical Caring." In *Altruism and Altruistic Love*, edited by Stephen G. Post and Lynn G. Underwood. 346–61. Oxford, UK: Oxford University Press, 2002.

Friedman, Thomas L. "Global Weirding Is Here." *New York Times*, February 17, 2010.

Froestad, Jan. "Environmental Health Problems in Hout Bay: The Challenge of Generalising Trust in South Africa." *Journal of Southern African Studies* 31, no. 2 (June 2005): 333–56.

————. "Health, Democracy and Governance in South Africa: Two Case Studies." Unpublished paper, Bergen, Norway: University of Bergen, 2002.

————. "The Incapacitating Impact of Distrust: Observations from the Health Sector." In *Trust in Public Institutions in South Africa*, edited by Steinar Askvik and Nelleke Baak. 167–80. Aldershot, UK: Ashgate Publishing, 2005.

Führer, Christian. *Und wir sind dabei gewesen: die Revolution, die aus der Kirche kam*. Berlin: Ullstein Buchverlage, 2009.

Garrett, Geoffrey. "The Causes of Globalization." *Comparative Political Studies* 33, no. 6–7 (2000): 941–91.

Garrett, Laurie. *Betrayal of Trust: The Collapse of Global Public Health*. New York: Hyperion, 2000.

Garvey, Catherine. *Play*. Cambridge, MA: Harvard University Press, 1977.

Germond, Paul, and James R. Cochrane. "Healthworlds: Conceptualizing Landscapes of Health and Healing." *Sociology* 44, no. 2 (Apr. 2010): 307–24.

Germond, Paul, and Sepetla Molapo. "In Search of *Bophelo* in a Time of AIDS: Seeking a Coherence of Economies of Health and Economies of Salvation." *Journal of Theology for Southern Africa* 126 (2006): 27–47.

Gilson, Lucy. "Editorial: Building Trust and Value in Health Systems in Low- and Middle-Income Countries." *Social Science & Medicine* 61 (2005): 1381–84.

————. "In Defence and Pursuit of Equity," *Social Science and Medicine* 47, no. 12 (1998): 1891–96.

————. "Trust and the Development of Health Care as a Social Institution." *Social Science & Medicine* 56 (2003): 1453–68.

Gilson, Lucy, Jane Doherty, Rene Loewenson, Victoria Francis, and Members of the Knowledge Network. "Challenging Inequity through Health Systems." Geneva: WHO Commission on the Social Determinants of Health, 2007.

Gleick, James. *Chaos: Making a New Science*. New York: Penguin Books, 1988.

Glennie, Jonathan. *The Trouble with Aid: Why Less Could Mean More for Africa*. London: Zed Books, in association with International African Institute, Royal African Society, and the Social Science Research Council, 2008.

Glenny, Misha. *McMafia: Seriously Organized Crime*. London: Vintage Books, 2009.

Greene, Amy. "The Spiritual Dimension." In *Faith and Health*. 1–6. Atlanta, GA: Interfaith Health Program, The Carter Center, 1994.

Grugel, Jean, and Hout Wil. *Regionalism across the North-South Divide: State Strategies and Globalization*. European Political Science Series. New York: Routledge, 1999.

Grundmann, Christoffer H. "Mission and Healing in Historical Perspective." *International Bulletin of Missionary Research* 32, no. 4 (2008): 185–88.

———. *Sent to Heal!: Emergence and Development of Medical Missions.* Lanham, MD: University Press of America, 2005.

Guerrero, L. K., and M. L. Hecht, eds. *The Nonverbal Communication Reader: Classic and Contemporary Readings.* 3rd ed. Long Grove, IL: Waveland Press, 2008.

Gunderson, Gary R. *Boundary Leaders: Leadership Skills for People of Faith.* Minneapolis, MN: Fortress, 2004.

———. *Deeply Woven Roots: Improving the Quality of Life in Your Community.* Minneapolis, MN: Fortress Press, 1997.

———. "The Task Ahead." In *Faith and Health.* Atlanta, GA: Interfaith Health Program, Carter Center, 1994.

Gunderson, Gary R., and Larry Pray. *Leading Causes of Life.* Memphis, TN: The Center of Excellence in Faith and Health, Methodist Le Bonheur Healthcare, 2006.

Habermas, Jürgen. *Between Facts and Norms: Contributions to a Discourse Theory of Law and Democracy.* Translated by William Rehg. Cambridge, MA: MIT Press, 1998.

———. *Lifeworld and System: A Critique of Functionalist Reason.* Translated by Thomas McCarthy. The Theory of Communicative Action. Vol. 2, Boston: Beacon Press, 1987.

———. *The Postnational Constellation: Political Essays.* Cambridge, UK: Polity Press, 2001.

Hall, John J., and Richard Taylor. "Health for All Beyond 2000: The Demise of the Alma-Ata Declaration and Primary Health Care in Developing Countries." *Medical Journal of Australia* 178, (Jan. 6, 2003): 17–20.

Harvey, David. *Spaces of Hope.* Berkeley, CA: University of California Press, 2000.

———. "Time-Space Compression and the Rise of Modernism as a Cultural Force." In *The Globalization Reader,* edited by Frank Lechner and John Boli. 134–40. Oxford, UK: Blackwell Publishers, 2000.

Hausmann-Muela, Susanna, Joan Muela Ribera, and Isaac Nyamongo. "Health-Seeking Behaviour and the Health System Response." *Disease Control Priorities Project* DCPP Working Paper No. 14 (Aug. 2003).

Hilton, Dave. "Calling for the Church to Bring Whole Person Health to All." Presentation at "Faith and Health: Making the Connection," Annual Spring Conference, Church Health Center and Methodist Le Bonheur Healthcare, Memphis, TN, 2006.

Hitchens, Christopher. *God Is Not Great: How Religion Poisons Everything.* New York: Twelve/Warner Books, 2007.

Hodes, Nancy, and Michael Hays, eds. *The United Nations and the World's Religions: Prospects for a Global Ethic.* Cambridge, MA: Boston Research Center for the 21st Century, 1995.

Hofrichter, Richard, ed. *Health and Social Justice: Politics, Ideology, and Inequity in the Distribution of Disease.* San Francisco: Jossey-Bass [John Wiley & Sons], 2003.

Holton, R. J. *Globalization and the Nation-State.* 2nd ed. New York: Palgrave Macmillan, 2011.

Horden, Peregrine. "The Earliest Hospitals in Byzantium, Western Europe, and Islam." *Journal of Interdisciplinary History* xxxv, no. 3 (Winter 2005): 361–89.

Hout Bay Resident's Association. "Poisoned Earth." *Hout and About.* Accessed October 22, 2011. http://www.houtbay.org.za/Newsletters/200809_HoutAbout.htm.

Iannaccone, Laurence R. "Religious Practice: A Human Capital Approach." *Journal for the Scientific Study of Religion* 29, no. 3 (Sep. 1990): 297–314.

Iannaccone, Laurence R., and Jonathan Klick. "Spiritual Capital: An Introduction and Literature Review." Cambridge, MA: Paper Presented in the Spiritual Capital Planning Meeting, 2003.

Iansiti, Marco, and Roy Levien. *The Keystone Advantage: What the New Dynamics of Business Ecosystems Mean for Strategy, Innovation and Sustainability.* Boston: Harvard Business School Press, 2004.

Idler, Ellen L. "Religion and Aging." In *Handbook of Aging and the Social Sciences,* edited by Robert H. Binstock and Linda K. George. 277–300. San Diego: Elsevier, 2006.

———. "Religious Involvement and the Health of the Elderly: Some Hypotheses and an Initial Test." *Social Forces* 66, no. 1 (1987): 226–38.

IHP. "The Case for Health and Faith: An Open Letter." In *Faith & Health.* Atlanta, GA: Interfaith Health Program, Rollins School of Public Health, Emory University, 2001.

Illich, Ivan. *Medical Nemesis: The Expropriation of Health.* Toronto: Bantam, 1979.

Ingvar, David H. "Memory of the Future: An Essay on the Temporal Organization of Conscious Awareness." *Human Neurobiology* 4, no. 3 (1985): 127–36.

———. "Motor Memory—A Memory of the Future." *Behavioral and Brain Sciences* 17 (1994): 210–11.

Institute of Medicine. *Crossing the Quality Chasm: A New Health System for the 21st Century.* Committee on Quality of Health Care in America.Washington, DC: National Academy Press, 2001.

———. "The Future of Public Health." Washington, DC: National Academy Press, 1988.

Ion, Heather Wood. "Creating an Epidemic of Health." Presentation at the Epidemic of Health Meeting, Center of Excellence in Faith and Health, Methodist Le Bonheur Healthcare, Memphis, TN, 2011.

Irwin, Michael, and Kavita Vedhara. *Human Psychoneuroimmunology.* New York: Oxford University Press, 2005.

Jackson, Hattie Elie. *65 Dark Days in '68: Reflections: Memphis Sanitation Strike.* Southaven, MS: The King's Press, 2004.

Janzen, John M. *Ngoma: Discourses of Healing in Central and Southern Africa.* Berkeley, CA: University of California Press, 1992.

Jasek-Rysdahl, Kelvin. "Applying Sen's Capabilities Framework to Neighborhoods: Using Local Asset Maps to Deepen Our Understanding of Well-Being." *Review of Social Economy* LIX, no. 3 (2001): 313–29.

Jencks, Stephen F., Mark V. Williams, and Eric Coleman. "Rehospitalizations among Patients in the Medicare Fee-for-Service Program." *New England Journal of Medicine* 360 (2009): 1418–28.

Johnson, Steven. *The Ghost Map: The Story of London's Most Terrifying Epidemic—And How It Changed Science, Cities, and the Modern World.* New York: Riverhead Books (Penguin), 2006.

Jones, R. "Cognitive Frames and Cultural Responses to Aids Education." Paper presented at the 12th International Conference on AIDS, Geneva, 1998.

K'Meyer, Tracy E. *Interracialism and Christian Community in the Postwar South: The Story of Koinonia Farm.* Charlottesville, VA: University Press of Virginia, 1997.

Kaplan, Edward H., and Lawrence M. Wein. "Smallpox Eradication in West and Central Africa: Surveillance-Containment or Herd Immunity?" *Epidemiology* 14, no. 1 (Jan. 2003): 90–92.

Karpf, Ted. "The Vital Lie." In *The Gospel Imperative in the Midst of Aids,* edited by Robert H. Iles. 185–92. Wilton, CT: Morehouse Publications, 1989.

Karpf, Ted, J. Todd Ferguson, Robin Swift, and Jeffrey V. Lazarus, eds. *Restoring Hope: Decent Care in the Midst of HIV/Aids.* London: Palgrave Macmillan, 2008.

Keyes, Corey L. M. "Complete Mental Health: An Agenda for the 21st Century." In *Flourishing: Positive Psychology and the Life Well-Lived,* edited by Corey L. M. Keyes and Jonathan Haidt. 293–312. Washington DC: American Psychological Association, 2003.

Keyes, Corey L. M. "The Mental Health Continuum: From Languishing to Flourishing in Life." *Journal of Health and Social Behavior* 43 (2002): 207–22.

Kim, Jim Yong. "Beyond Paradigm: Making Transcultural Connections in a Scientific Translation of Acupuncture." *Social Science & Medicine* 62 (2006): 2960–72.

Kim, Jim Yong, Joyce V. Millen, Alec Irwin, and John Gershman, eds. *Dying for Growth: Global Inequality and the Health of the Poor*. Monroe, ME: Common Courage Press, 2000.

Kinsley, David R. *Health, Healing and Religion: A Cross Cultural Perspective*. Upper Saddle River, NJ: Prentice Hall, 1995.

Kiser, Miriam, Deborah L. Jones, and Gary R. Gunderson. "Faith and Health: Leadership Aligning Assets to Transform Communities." *International Review of Mission* 95 no. 376/377 (Jan./Apr. 2006): 50–58.

Kleinman, A. "Concepts and a Model for the Comparison of Medical Systems as Cultural Systems." In *Concepts of Health, Illness and Disease*, edited by C. Currer and M. Stacey. 27–50. New York: Berg Pub. Ltd., 1986.

Koenig, Harold G., Michael E. McCullough, and David B. Larson. *Handbook of Religion and Health*. Oxford: Oxford University Press, 2001.

Korten, David. *Getting to the 21st Century: Voluntary Action and the Global Agenda*. West Hartford, CT: Kumarian Press, 1990.

Kretzmann, John P., and John L. McKnight. *Building Communities from the Inside Out: A Path toward Finding and Mobilizing a Community's Assets*. Chicago: ACTA Publications, 1993.

Kreuter, Marshall, Christopher DeRosa, Elizabeth Howze, and Grant Baldwin. "Understanding Wicked Problems: A Key to Advancing Environmental Health Promotion." *Health Education & Behavior* 31, no. 4 (2004): 441–54.

Kreuter, Marshall W., Nicole A. Lezin, Laura Young, and Adam N. Koplan. "Social Capital: Evaluation Implications for Community Health Promotion." In *Evaluation in Health Promotion: Principles and Perspectives*, edited by Irving Rootman, Michael Goodstadt, Brian Hyndman, David V. McQueen, Louise Potvin, Jane Springett and Ziglio Erio. 439–62. Copenhagen: World Health Organization Regional Publications, European Series, No. 92, 2001.

Krieger, Nancy. "Proximal, Distal, and the Politics of Causation: What's Level Got to Do with It?" *American Journal of Public Health* 98 (2008): 221–30.

———. "Why Epidemiologists Cannot Afford to Ignore Poverty." *Epidemiology* 18 (2007): 658–63.

Kuhn, Thomas S. *The Structure of Scientific Revolutions*. Foundations of the Unity of Science. 3rd ed. Chicago: University of Chicago Press, 1996.

Lakoff, George, and Mark Johnson. *Metaphors We Live By*. 2nd ed. Chicago: University of Chicago Press, 2003 (1980).

Lakoff, George, and with Mark Johnson. *Philosophy in the Flesh: The Embodied Mind and Its Challenge to Western Thought*. New York: Basic Books, 1999.

Lambourne, Robert A. "Secular and Christian Models of Health and Salvation." *Contact* 1 (1970): 1–11.

Lee, Dallas. *The Cotton Patch Evidence: The Story of Clarence Jordan and the Koinonia Farm Experiment*. New York: Harper and Row, 1971.

Leslie, C. "Medical Pluralism in World Perspective." *Social Science and Medicine* 14B, no. 4 (1980): 191–95.

Lévinas, Emmanuel. *Totality and Infinity: An Essay on Exteriority*. Translated by Alphonso Lingis. Pittsburgh, PA: Duquesne University Press, 1969.

Levitt, Peggy. "Redefining the Boundaries of Belonging: The Institutional Character of Transnational Religious Life." *Sociology of Religion* 65, no. 1 (2004): 1–18.

———. "'You Know, Abraham Was Really the First Immigrant': Religion and Transnational Migration." *International Migration Review* 37, no. 3 (Fall 2003): 847–73.

Lifton, Robert Jay. *The Broken Connection: On Death and the Continuity of Life.* Washington: American Psychiatric Press, 1979.

Lin, Nan, Karen Cook, and Ronald S. Burt. *Social Capital: Theory and Research.* New York: Aldine de Gruyter, 2001.

Lindström, Bengt , and Monica Eriksson. "Contextualizing Salutogenesis and Antonovsky in Public Health Development." *Health Promotion International* 21, no. 3 (2006): 238–44.

Linehan, M. M., and L. Dimeff. "Dialectical Behavior Therapy in a Nutshell." *The California Psychologist* 34 (2001): 10–13.

Lomas, Jonathan. "Social Capital and Health: Implications for Public Health and Epidemiology." *Social Science and Medicine* 47, no. 9 (1998): 1181–88.

Macfarlane, S., M. Racelis, and F. Muli-Musiime. "Public Health in Developing Countries." *Lancet* 356, no. 9232 (2000): 841–46.

Malm, H., T. May, L. P. Francis, S. B. Omer, D. A. Salmon, and R. Hood. "Ethics, Pandemics, and the Duty to Treat." *American Journal of Bioethics* 8, no. 8 (Aug. 2008): 4–19.

Mamdani, Mahmood. *Citizen and Subject: Contemporary Africa and the Legacy of Late Colonialism.* Cape Town; Kampala: David Philip; Fountain Publishers, 1996.

Marcel, Gabriel. *Homo Viator: Introduction to a Metaphysics of Hope.* Translated by Martha Crauford. New York: Harper and Row (imprint: Harper Torchbooks /Cathedral Library), 1962.

Marennikova, Svetlana S. "Commentary: Perspectives on Smallpox Eradication." *Epidemiology* 14, no. 1 (2003): 93.

Marshall, Katherine. "A Discussion with Reverend Canon Ted Karpf," Berkley Center for Religion, Peace and World Affairs, Georgetown University, Washington DC. Interview conducted on November 13, 2010. Accessed July 27, 2011. http://berkleycenter.georgetown.edu/interviews/a-discussion-with-reverend-canon-ted-karpf.

McGilvray, James C. "The Church and Health: Reflections and Possibilities." *Contact* 81 (Oct. 1984): 2–11.

———. *The Quest for Health and Wholeness.* Tübingen: German Institute for Medical Mission, 1981.

McKeon, Beverly J. "Controlling Turbulence." *Science* 327 (Mar. 19, 2010): 1462–63.

McKnight, John L. *The Careless Society: Community and Its Counterfeits.* New York: Basic Books, 1996.

Micale, M. S, and P. Lerner. *Traumatic Pasts: History, Psychiatry, and Trauma in the Modern Age, 1870–1930.* Cambridge, UK: Cambridge University Press, 2001.

Miller, S. M. "Thinking Strategically About Society and Health." In *Society and Health*, edited by Benjamin C. Amick III, Sol Levine, Alvin R. Tarlov, and Diana Chapman Walsh. 342–58. New York; Oxford, UK: Oxford University Press, 1995.

Mische , Patricia M., and Melissa Merkling, eds. *Toward a Global Civilization? The Contribution of Religions.* New York: Peter Lang, 2001.

Moltmann, Jürgen. *Theology of Hope: On the Ground and the Implications of a Christian Eschatology.* New York: Harper and Row, 1967.

Morris, Robert D. *The Blue Death: Disease, Disaster, and the Water We Drink.* New York: Harper Collins, 2007.

Moyers, Bill. *A World of Ideas II.* New York: Doubleday, 1990.

Mpepo, B. P. "The Path Away from Poverty: An Easy Look at Zambia's Poverty Reduction Strategy Paper, 2002–2004." Lusaka: Civil Society for Poverty Reduction, 2004.

Munnecke, Tom. "Ensembles and Transformations." San Diego, CA: Report for the Science Applications International Corporation, 2000.

Murphy, E., and R. Dingwall. *Qualitative Methods and Health Policy Research.* New York: Aldine de Gruyter, 2003.

Newsom, S. W. B. "Pioneers in Infection Control: John Snow, Henry Whitehead, the Broad Street Pump, and the Beginnings of Geographical Epidemiology." *Journal of Hospital Infection* 64, no. 6 (2006): 210–21.

Niebuhr, H. Richard. *The Social Sources of Denominationalism.* Cleveland, OH: World Publishing, 1965.

Nisbet, Robert. *History of the Idea of Progress.* New York: Basic, 1980.

Norton, Barbara L., Kenneth R. McLeroy, James N. Burdine, Michael R. J. Felix, and Alicia M. Dorsey. "Community Capacity: Concept, Theories, and Methods." In *Emerging Theories in Health Promotion Practice and Research: Strategies for Improving Public Health,* edited by Ralph J. DiClemente, Richard A. Crosby, and Michelle C. Kegler. 194–227. San Francisco: Jossey-Bass [John Wiley & Sons], 2002.

Nürnberger, Klaus. *Prosperity, Poverty and Pollution: Managing the Approaching Crisis.* London: Zed Books, 1999.

Nussbaum, Martha C. "Adaptive Preferences and Women's Options." *Economics and Philosophy* 17, no. 5 (2001): 67–88.

———. "Human Capabilities, Female Human Beings." In *Women, Culture and Development: A Study of Human Capabilities,* edited by Martha C. Nussbaum and Jonathan Glover. 61–104. Oxford, UK: Clarendon Press, 1995.

———. *Women and Human Development: The Capabilities Approach.* Cambridge, UK: Cambridge University Press, 2000.

Nussbaum, Martha C., and Jonathan Glover, eds. *Women, Culture, and Development: A Study of Human Capabilities.* Oxford, UK:Oxford University Press, 1995.

Nutton, Vivian. "The Medical Meeting Place." In *Ancient Medicine in Its Socio-Cultural Context, Volume 1,* edited by Ph. J. van der Eijk, H. F. J. Horstmanshoff, and P. H. Schrijvers. The Wellcome Institute Series in the History of Medicine, 3–25. Amsterdam; Atlanta, GA: Rodopi, 1995.

O'Connor, Alice. *Poverty Knowledge: Social Science, Social Policy and the Poor in Twentieth-Century U.S. History.* Princeton, NJ; Oxford, UK: Princeton University Press, 2001.

O'Neill, Marie S., Anthony J. McMichael, Joel Schwartz, and Wartenberg. Daniel. "Poverty, Environment, and Health: The Role of Environmental Epidemiology and Environmental Epidemiologists." *Epidemiology* 18, no. 6 (Nov. 2007): 664–68.

Offe, Claus. "How Can We Trust Our Fellow Citizens?" In *Democracy and Trust,* edited by Mark E. Warren. 42–87. Cambridge, UK: Cambridge University Press, 1999.

Pargament, Kenneth I. *The Psychology of Religion and Coping: Theory, Research, Practice.* New York: The Guilford Press, 2001.

Paterson, Gillian. "The CMC Story, 1968–1998." *Contact* 161/162 (1998): 3–52.

Pennebaker, James. *Opening Up: The Healing Power of Expressing Emotions.* New York: Guilford Press, 1997.

Pert, Candice. *Molecules of Emotion.* New York: Touchstone, 1997.

Peter, Fabienne. "Health Equity and Social Justice." *Journal of Applied Philosophy* 18, no. 2 (2001): 159–70.

Petersen, Jim. *Church without Walls: Moving Beyond Traditional Boundaries.* Colorado Springs, CO: Nav Press, 1992.

Piaget, Jean. *Play, Dreams and Imitation in Childhood.* New York: Norton, 1962.

Pickering, A. *The Mangle of Practice.* Chicago: University of Chicago Press, 1995.

Porter, Dorothy. *Health, Civilization and the State: A History of Public Health from Ancient to Modern Times.* New York: Routledge, 1994.

Porter, Michael E., and Elizabeth Olmsted Teisberg. *Redefining Health Care: Creating Value-Based Competition on Results.* Boston: Harvard Business School Press, 2006.

Radin, Margaret Jane. *Contested Commodities.* Cambridge, MA: Harvard University Press, 1996.

———. "Response: Persistent Perplexities." *Kennedy Institute of Ethics Journal* 11, no. 3 (2001): 305–15.

Ragland-Sullivan, Ellie. *Jacques Lacan and the Philosophy of Psychoanalysis*. Urbana, IL; Chicago: University of Illinois Press, 1986.

Ramo, Joshua Cooper. *The Age of the Unthinkable: Why the New World Disorder Constantly Surprises Us and What We Can Do About It*. New York: Little, Brown and Company, 2009.

Rannan-Eliya, Ravi P., and Nishan De Mel. "Resource Mobilization in Sri Lanka's Health Sector." Institute of Policy Studies, Harvard School of Public Health & Health Policy Programme. Accessed April 21, 2010. http://www.hsph.harvard.edu/ihsg/publications/pdf/No-42.pdf.

Ricoeur, Paul. *Oneself as Another*. Chicago: University of Chicago Press, 1992.

———. *The Rule of Metaphor: Multi-Disciplinary Studies of the Creation of Meaning in Language*. Translated by Robert Czerny, Kathleen McLaughlin, and John Costello. Toronto: University of Toronto Press, 1977.

———. *Time and Narrative, Volume 1*. Translated by Kathleen McLaughlin and David Pellauer. Chicago: University of Chicago Press, 1984.

———. *Time and Narrative, Volume 3*. Translated by Kathleen McLaughlin and David Pellauer. Chicago: University of Chicago Press, 1988.

Robertson, Roland, and JoAnn Chirico. "Humanity, Globalization and Worldwide Religious Resurgence." In *The Globalization Reader*, edited by Frank Lechner and John Boli. 93–98. Oxford, UK: Blackwell Publishers, 2000.

Rosen, George. *A History of Public Health*. Baltimore, MD: Johns Hopkins University Press, 1999.

Rosenberg, Mark L. *Real Collaboration: What It Takes for Global Health to Succeed*. California/Milbank Books on Health and the Public. Berkeley, CA: University of California Press, 2010.

Roy, Jean. "Smallpox Eradication: Jean Roy Oral History—Interviewed by Victoria Harden." Centers for Disease Control and Prevention. Accessed January 24, 2010. http://www.globalhealthchronicles.org/smallpox/record/view/pid/emory:15n9k.

Salk, Jonas. *The Survival of the Wisest*. New York: Harper & Row, 1973.

Scambler, Graham, ed. *Habermas, Critical Theory and Health*. London; New York: Routledge, 2001.

———. *Health and Social Change: A Critical Theory*. Issues in Society, edited by Tim May. Buckingham, UK; Philadelphia, PA: The Open University Press, 2002.

Scanlon, T. M. "Value, Desire and Quality of Life." In *The Quality of Life*, edited by Martha C. Nussbaum and Amartya Sen. 201–07 New York: Clarendon Press, 1993.

Schacter, Daniel L., Donna Rose Addis, and Randy L. Buckner. "Remembering the Past to Imagine the Future: The Prospective Brain." *Nature Reviews Neuroscience* 8 (Sep. 2007): 657–61.

Schechter, D. S. "Intergenerational Communication of Violent Traumatic Experience within and by the Dyad: The Case of a Mother and Her Toddler." *Journal of Infant, Child, and Adolescent Psychotherapy* 3, no. 2 (2004): 203–32.

Schweitzer, Albert. *Zwischen Wasser und Urwald: Erlebnisse und Beobachtungen eines Arztes in Urwalde Äquatorialafrikas*. München: Verlag C. H. Beck, 1963.

Scoones, I. *Sustainable Rural Livelihoods: A Framework for Analysis*. Wp 72. Brighton, UK: Institute of Development Studies, University of Sussex, 1998.

Scott, Catherine, and Anne Hofmeyer. "Networks and Social Capital: A Relational Approach to Primary Healthcare Reform." *Health Research Policy and Systems* 5, no. 9 (2007): 1–27.

Scott, James C. *Domination and the Arts of Resistance: Hidden Transcripts*. New Haven, CT: Yale University Press, 1991.

———. *Seeing Like a State: How Certain Schemes to Improve the Human Condition Have Failed*. New Haven, CT; London: Yale University Press, 1998.

Seligman, Martin E. P. *Learned Optimism: How to Change Your Mind and Your Life.* New York: Knopf; Penguin Books, 1991, 1998.
Seligman, Martin E. P. *Flourish: A Visionary New Understanding of Happiness and Well-Being.* New York: Free Press, 2011.
Shapiro, Susan P. "Agency Theory." *Annual Review of Sociology* 31 (2005): 263–84.
Sherwood, Ben. *The Survivors Club: The Secrets and Science That Could Save Your Life.* New York: Grand Central Publishing, 2009.
Shoko, T. *Karanga Indigenous Religion in Zimbabwe: Health and Well-Being.* London: Ashgate, 2007.
Simms, Chris, Mike Rowson, and Siobhan Peattie. "The Bitterest Pill of All: The Collapse of Africa's Health Systems." London: Save the Children Fund (UK), 2001. An Eldis Document. Accessed July 31, 2011. http://www.eldis.org/assets/Docs/29246.html.
Skidelsky, Robert. "The Remedist: Why John Maynard Keynes Is the Man of the Year." *The New York Times Magazine,* December 14, 2008, 21–22.
Smidt, Corwin, ed. *Religion as Social Capital: Producing the Common Good.* Waco, TX: Baylor University Press, 2003.
Smith, George Davey, and John Lynch. "Commentary: Social Capital, Social Epidemiology and Disease Aetiology." *International Journal of Epidemiology* 33 (2004): 691–700.
Smith, Mark A. "Sap Opens Road for Hana and Big Data at Sapphire Now." In *Information Management Blogs.* May 27, 2011. Accessed July 12, 2011. http://www.information-management.com/blogs/big_data_analytics_business_intelligence_SAP-10020453-1.html.
Sotero, Michelle. "A Conceptual Model of Historical Trauma: Implications for Public Health Practice and Research." *Journal of Health Disparities Research and Practice* 1, no. 1 (Fall 2006): 93–108.
Southern Africa AIDS Training Programme & the International HIV/AIDS Alliance. *CBO/NGO Support: The Role and Value of NGO Based CBO/NGO Support Providers in the Response to HIV/AIDS in Southern and Eastern Africa:A Case Study of CHEP.* The SHARE Series. Harare: SAT/International HIV/AIDS Alliance, 2004.
Stark, Rodney, and Roger Finke. *Acts of Faith: Explaining the Human Side of Religion.* Berkeley, CA: University of California Press, 2000.
Szreter, Simon, and Michael Woolcock. "Health by Association? Social Capital, Social Theory, and the Political Economy of Public Health." *International Journal of Epidemiology* 33 (2004): 650–67.
———. "Rejoinder: Crafting Rigorous and Relevant Social Theory for Public Health Policy." *International Journal of Epidemiology* 33 (2004): 700–04.
Sztompka, Piotr. *Trust: A Sociological Theory.* Cambridge, UK: Cambridge University Press, 1999.
Thatcher, Margaret. "Interview (Douglas Keay)." *Women's Own,* October 31, 1987.
Thomas, Caroline, and Peter Wilkin. *Globalization, Human Security, and the African Experience.* Critical Security Studies. Boulder, CO: Lynne Rienner Publishers, 1998.
Thomas, Liz, Barbara Schmid, James R Cochrane, Malibongwe Gwele, and Rosamond Ngcubo. "'Let Us Embrace': Role and Significance of an Integrated Faith-Based Initiative for HIV and Aids: Masangane Case Study." Cape Town: African Religious Health Assets Programme, University of Cape Town, 2006.
Thomas, Richard K. *Society and Health: Sociology for Health Professionals.* New York: Kluwer Academic/Plenum Publishers, 2003.
Thumma, Scott, and Warren Bird. "Not Who You Think They Are: The Real Story of People Who Attend America's Megachurches." 1–34. Hartford, CN: Hartford Institute for Religion Research & The Leadership Network, 2009.

Turner, Nicol E., and Randal D. Pinkett. "An Asset-Based Approach to Community Building and Community Technology." Paper presented at the Shaping the Network Society: The Future of the Public Sphere in Cyberspace, Directions and Implications of Advanced Computing, Seattle, WA, May 20–23, 2000.

Turnock, B. J. *Public Health: What It Is and How It Works.* 2nd ed. Gaithersburg, MD: Aspen Publications, 2001.

UCLA. "Whitehead." University of California Los Angeles, School of Public Health. Accessed October 1, 2009. http://www.ph.ucla.edu/epi/Snow/whitehead.html.

United Nations Development Programme. "Human Development Report: International Cooperation at a Crossroads—Aid, Trade and Security in an Unequal World." New York: United Nations, 2005.

Unschuld, Paul U. "Traditional Chinese Medicine: Some Historical and Epistemological Reflections." *Social Science & Medicine* 24 (1987): 1023–29.

van Minnen, Peter. "Medical Care in Late Antiquity." In *Ancient Medicine in Its Socio-Cultural Context, Volume 1*, edited by Ph. J. van der Eijk, H. F. J. Horstmanshoff, and P. H. Schrijvers. The Wellcome Institute Series in the History of Medicine, 153–69. Amsterdam; Atlanta, GA: Rodopi, 1995.

Vásquez, Manuel A., and Marie F. Marquardt. *Globalizing the Sacred: Religion across the Americas.* New Brunswick, NJ: Rutgers University Press, 2003.

Verter, Bradford. "Spiritual Capital: Theorizing Religion with Bourdieu against Bourdieu." *Sociological Theory* 21, no. 2 (June 2003): 150–74.

Vygotsky, Lev. *Mind in Society.* Translated by M. Cole. Cambridge, MA: Harvard University Press, 1978.

Wailoo, Kenneth. *Dying in the City of the Blues: Sickle Cell Anemia and the Politics of Race.* Chapel Hill, NC: University of North Carolina Press, 2001.

Walshe, Peter. *Church Versus State in South Africa: The Case of the Christian Institute.* London; Maryknoll, NY: C. Hurst; Orbis, 1983.

Wesley-Esquimaux, Cynthia C., and Magdalena Smolewski. "Historic Trauma and Aboriginal Healing." 110. Ottawa, ON: Report for The Aboriginal Healing Foundation, 2004.

Whitehead, Henry. "Report on the Cholera Outbreak in the Parish of St. James, Westminster, During the Autumn of 1854." Accessed October 8, 2009. http://john-snow.matrix.msu.edu/work.

Wickkiser, Bronwen L. *Asklepios, Medicine, and the Politics of Healing in Fifth-Century Greece: Between Craft and Cult.* Baltimore, MD: Johns Hopkins University Press, 2008.

Wilkinson, Richard, and Kate Pickett. *The Spirit Level: Why Greater Equality Makes Societies Stronger.* London; New York: Penguin & Bloomsbury Press, 2009.

Wind, James P. "One Congregation's Experience." *Second Opinion,* (March 13, 1990): 77–88.

Wind, James P., and James W. Lewis. *American Congregations Volume 1: Portraits of Twelve Religious Communities.* Chicago: University of Chicago Press, 1998.

———. *American Congregations Volume 2: New Perspectives in the Study of Congregations.* Chicago: The University of Chicago Press, 1998.

Wolf, Stewart, and John S. Bruhn. *The Power of Clan: The Influence of Human Relationships to Reduce Heart Disease.* New Brunswick, NJ: Transaction, 1993.

Woodberry, Robert D. "Researching Spiritual Capital: Promises and Pitfalls." Cambridge, MA. Spiritual Capital Planning Meeting. Accessed February 10, 2010. http://www.spiritualcapitalresearchprogram.com/pdf/woodberry.pdf.

Woodward, Billy, Joel Shurkin, and Debra Gordon. *Scientists Greater Than Einstein: The Biggest Lifesavers of the Twentieth Century.* Fresno, CA: Linden Publishing, 2009.

World Bank. *World Development Report 1993: Investing in Health.* New York: Oxford University Press, 1993.

World Health Organization. *Building from Common Foundations: The World Health Organization and Faith-Based Organizations in Primary Healthcare.* Geneva: World Health Organization, 2008.

———. "A Cross-Cultural Study of Spirituality, Religion, and Personal Beliefs as Components of Quality of Life." *Social Science and Medicine* 62 (2006): 1486–97.

———. "Declaration of Alma-Ata." From the *International Conference on Primary Health Care.* Alma-Ata, USSR: World Health Organization, 1978.

———. *Health by the People.* Geneva: World Health Organization, 1975.

———. *The World Health Report 2008: Primary Health Care—Now More Than Ever.* Geneva: World Health Organization, 2008.

Wright, Kate, Louis Rowitz, Adelaide Merkle, W. Michael Reid, Gary Robinson, Bill Herzog, Diane Weber, *et al.* "Competency Development in Public Health Leadership." *American Journal of Public Health* 90, no. 8 (Aug. 2000): 1202–07.

Yount, Kathryn M., and Joel Gittelsohn. "Comparing Reports of Health-Seeking Behavior from the Integrated Illness History and a Standard Child Morbidity Survey." *Journal of Mixed Methods Research* 2, no. 1 (2008): 23–62.

Zhang, Daqing, and Paul U. Unschuld. "China's Barefoot Doctor: Past, Present, and Future." *The Lancet* 372, no. 9653 (2008): 1865–67.

INDEX